Stage B, a Pre-cursor of Heart Failure, Part I

Guest Editors

JAY N. COHN, MD
GARY S. FRANCIS, MD

HEART FAILURE CLINICS

www.heartfailure.theclinics.com

Consulting Editors
RAGAVENDRA R. BALIGA, MD, MBA
JAMES B. YOUNG, MD

Founding Editor
JAGAT NARULA, MD, PhD

January 2012 • Volume 8 • Number 1

SAUNDERS an imprint of ELSEVIER, Inc.

W.B. SAUNDERS COMPANY
A Division of Elsevier Inc.

1600 John F. Kennedy Boulevard • Suite 1800 • Philadelphia, Pennsylvania 19103-2899

http://www.theclinics.com

HEART FAILURE CLINICS Volume 8, Number 1
January 2012 ISSN 1551-7136, ISBN-13: 978-1-4557-3871-7

Editor: Barbara Cohen-Kligerman
Developmental Editor: Teia Stone

Heart Failure Clinics (ISSN 1551-7136) is published quarterly by Elsevier Inc., 360 Park Avenue South, New York, NY 10010-1710. Months of publication are January, April, July, and October. Business and editorial offices: 1600 John F. Kennedy Boulevard, Suite 1800, Philadelphia, PA 19103-2899. Periodicals postage paid at New York, NY, and additional mailing offices. Subscription prices are USD 224.00 per year for US individuals, USD 347.00 per year for US institutions, USD 76.00 per year for US students and residents, USD 268.00 per year for Canadian individuals, USD 398.00 per year for Canadian institutions, USD 285.00 per year for international individuals, USD 398.00 per year for international institutions, and USD 96.00 per year for Canadian and foreign students/residents. To receive student and resident rate, orders must be accompanied by name of affiliated institution, date of term, and the *signature* of program/residency coordinator on institution letterhead. Orders will be billed at individual rate until proof of status is received. Foreign air speed delivery is included in all *Clinics* subscription prices. All prices are subject to change without notice. **POSTMASTER:** Send address changes to *Heart Failure Clinics*, Elsevier Health Sciences Division, Subscription Customer Service, 3251 Riverport Lane, Maryland Heights, MO 63043. **Customer Service: 1-800-654-2452 (US and Canada). From outside of the US and Canada, call 314-447-8871. Fax: 314-447-8029. For print support, e-mail: JournalsCustomerService-usa@elsevier.com. For online support, e-mail: JournalsOnlineSupport-usa@elsevier.com.**

Reprints. For copies of 100 or more of articles in this publication, please contact the Commercial Reprints Department, Elsevier Inc., 360 Park Avenue South, New York, NY 10010-1710. Tel.: 212-633-3812; Fax: 212-462-1935; E-mail: reprints@elsevier.com.

Heart Failure Clinics is covered in *MEDLINE/PubMed (Index Medicus)*.

Printed and bound by CPI Group (UK) Ltd, Croydon, CR0 4YY

Cover artwork courtesy of Umberto M. Jezek.

Transferred to Digital Printing, 2012

Contributors

CONSULTING EDITORS

RAGAVENDRA R. BALIGA, MD, MBA
Vice Chief and Assistant Division Director,
Professor of Medicine, Division of
Cardiovascular Medicine, The Ohio State
University Medical Center, Columbus, Ohio

JAMES B. YOUNG, MD
Professor of Medicine and Executive Dean,
Cleveland Clinic Lerner College of Medicine,
George and Linda Kaufman Chair, Chairman,
Endocrinology and Metabolism Institute,
Cleveland Clinic, Cleveland, Ohio

GUEST EDITORS

JAY N. COHN, MD, FACC
Professor of Medicine, Cardiovascular
Division, University of Minnesota, Minneapolis,
Minnesota

GARY S. FRANCIS, MD
Professor of Medicine, Cardiovascular
Division; Associate Director, Lilehei Cardiac
Clinical Trials Center, University of Minnesota,
Minneapolis, Minnesota

AUTHORS

ANTONIO ABBATE, MD, PhD, FESC
VCU Pauley Heart Center, Virginia
Commonwealth University, Richmond, Virginia

ARVIND BHIMARAJ, MD, MPH
Staff Cardiologist, Methodist DeBakey
Cardiology Associates, Houston, Texas

JAVED BUTLER, MD, MPH
Professor of Medicine, Emory Clinical
Cardiovascular Research Institute, Atlanta,
Georgia

BLASE A. CARABELLO, MD
W.A. "Tex" and Deborah Moncrief Jr,
Professor of Medicine, Vice Chair, Department
of Medicine, Baylor College of Medicine;
Medical Care Line Executive, Michael E.
DeBakey VA Medical Center, Houston, Texas

RAVI DHINGRA, MD, MPH
Instructor of Medicine, Section of Cardiology,
Heart and Vascular Center, Dartmouth
Hitchcock Medical Center, Lebanon,
New Hampshire

DANIEL A. DUPREZ, MD, PhD
Professor of Medicine, Cardiovascular
Division, University of Minnesota, Minneapolis,
Minnesota

SHAINA R. ECKHOUSE, MD
Research Fellow, Division of Cardiothoracic
Surgery, Department of Surgery, Medical
University of South Carolina, Charleston,
South Carolina

EDWARD D. FROHLICH, MD
Alton Ochsner Distinguished Scientist,
Director, Hypertension Research Laboratory,
Ochsner Clinic Foundation, New Orleans,
Louisiana

VASILIKI V. GEORGIOPOULOU, MD
Assistant Professor of Medicine, Emory Clinical
Cardiovascular Research Institute, Atlanta,
Georgia

A. MARTIN GERDES, PhD
Professor and Chair, Department of
Biomedical Sciences, New York College of
Osteopathic Medicine at New York Institute
of Technology, Old Westbury, New York

BODH I. JUGDUTT, MD, DM
Division of Cardiology, Department of
Medicine, University of Alberta and Hospital,
Edmonton, Alberta, Canada

ANDREAS P. KALOGEROPOULOS, MD
Assistant Professor of Medicine, Emory Clinical
Cardiovascular Research Institute, Atlanta,
Georgia

EDWARD G. LAKATTA, MD
Chief, Laboratory of Cardiovascular Science,
Intramural Research Program, Gerontology
Research Center, National Institute on Aging,
National Institutes of Health, Baltimore,
Maryland

BERNHARD MAISCH, MD, FACC, FESC
Professor of Internal Medicine, Director,
Division of Cardiology, Department
of Internal Medicine, Faculty of Medicine,
Philipps-University, UKGM GmbH,
Marburg, Germany

**JAGAT NARULA, MD, PhD, FACC, FAHA,
FRCP(Edin)**
Philip J. and Harriet L. Goodhart Chair in
Cardiology; Professor of Medicine; Associate
Dean for Global Health, Director,
Cardiovascular Imaging Program, Zena and
Michael A. Wiener Cardiovascular Institute,
Marie-Josée and Henry R. Kravis Center for
Cardiovascular Health, Mount Sinai School
of Medicine, New York, New York

MICHEL NOUTSIAS, MD
Assistant Professor, Division of Cardiology,
Department of Internal Medicine, UKGM
GmbH, Marburg, Germany

SABINE PANKUWEIT, PhD
Assistant Professor, Division of Cardiology,
Department of Internal Medicine, UKGM
GmbH, Marburg, Germany

KAUSHIK P. PATEL, PhD
Professor, Department of Cellular and
Integrative Physiology, University of Nebraska
Medical Center, Omaha, Nebraska

ANETTE RICHTER, MD
Division of Cardiology, Department of Internal
Medicine, UKGM GmbH, Marburg, Germany

VOLKER RUPPERT, PhD
Division of Cardiology, Department of Internal
Medicine, UKGM GmbH, Marburg, Germany

OLGA V. SAVINOVA, PhD
Post-Doctoral Fellow, Cardiovascular Health
Research Center, Sanford Research,
University of South Dakota, Sioux Falls,
South Dakota

HAROLD D. SCHULTZ, PhD
Professor, Department of Cellular and
Integrative Physiology, University of Nebraska
Medical Center, Omaha, Nebraska

FRANCIS G. SPINALE, MD, PhD
Professor of Personalized Medicine,
Department of Cell Biology and Anatomy,
University of South Carolina School of
Medicine, Columbia; Professor, Department
of Surgery, Medical University of South
Carolina, Charleston, South Carolina

JAMES B. STRAIT, MD, PhD
Head, Human Cardiovascular Studies,
Laboratory of Cardiovascular Science,
Intramural Research Program; Staff Clinician,
Clinical Research Branch, National Institute
on Aging, National Institutes of Health,
Harbor Hospital, Baltimore, Maryland

DINKO SUSIC, MD, PhD
Staff Scientist, Hypertension Research
Laboratory, Division of Research, Ochsner
Clinic Foundation, New Orleans, Louisiana

W.H. WILSON TANG, MD
Research Director, Section of Heart Failure and
Cardiac Transplantation Medicine, Heart and
Vascular Institute; Associate Professor,
Cleveland Clinic Lerner College of Medicine
at Case Western Reserve University,
Cleveland Clinic, Cleveland, Ohio

**RAMACHANDRAN S. VASAN, MD, DM,
FACC, FAHA**
Chief, Section of Preventive Medicine and
Epidemiology, Department of Medicine, The
Framingham Heart Study, Boston University
School of Medicine, Framingham,
Massachusetts

IRVING H. ZUCKER, PhD
Department of Cellular and Integrative
Physiology, University of Nebraska Medical
Center, Omaha, Nebraska

Contents

> Structural remodeling is a major feature of heart failure and typically precedes the development of symptomatic disease. Structural remodeling of the heart reflects changes in myocyte morphology. Disproportional myocyte growth is observed in pathologic concentric hypertrophy (myocyte thickening) and in eccentric dilated hypertrophy (myocyte lengthening). Alterations in myocyte shape lead to changes in chamber geometry and wall stress. Human and animal studies indicate that changes in myocyte morphology are reversible. Normalization or reversal of maladaptive cardiomyocyte remodeling should be a therapeutic aim that can prevent deterioration or improve cardiac function in heart failure.

> The myocardial interstitium is highly organized and orchestrated, whereby small disruptions in composition, spatial relationships, or content lead to altered myocardial systolic and/or diastolic performance. These changes in extracellular matrix structure and function are important in the progression to heart failure in pressure overload hypertrophy, dilated cardiomyopathy, and ischemic heart disease. The myocardial interstitium is not a passive entity, but rather a complex and dynamic microenvironment that represents an important structural and signaling system within the myocardium.

> This review discusses cardiac consequences of pressure overload. In response to elevated pressure, the ventricular hypertrophy compensates for the increased wall stress. However, the ventricular hypertrophy involves numerous structural adaptations that may lead to ventricular dysfunction and, eventually, heart failure. Particular emphasis is placed on molecular mechanisms that govern the development of hypertrophy and that may lead to maladaptive structural changes resulting in adverse cardiac events.

> Structural cardiac volume overload comprises a group of heterogeneous diseases, each creating a nearly unique set of loading conditions on the left ventricle and/or

right ventricle. In turn, the heart responds to each with unique patterns of remodeling, leading to both adaptive and maladaptive consequences. An understanding of these different patterns of hypertrophy and/or remodeling should be useful in developing strategies for the timing and correction of cardiac volume overload.

Myocardial infarction (MI) accounts for most incidences of heart failure (HF) and low ejection fraction. Evidence suggests that acute MI leads to early cardiac remodeling, with changes in ventricular geometry and structure that in turn lead to a vicious cycle of ventricular dilation, increased wall stress, hypertrophy and more ventricular dilation and dysfunction, and worsening of HF. The early geometric and structural changes contribute to early mechanical complications and subsequent progressive ventricular remodeling and the development of chronic HF. A clear understanding of the underlying mechanisms is helpful in developing optimal preventive and therapeutic strategies for HF.

This article comments on the recent classifications of cardiomyopathies by the American Heart Association and the European Society of Cardiology with respect to their clinical applicability. Taking them and the statement on the role of endomyocardial biopsies in different clinical scenarios together, the clinician is now able to identify genetic, autoimmune, and viral causative factors by using a thorough and logical approach to reach a diagnosis in patients with familial and nonfamilial forms of the underlying structural heart muscle diseases. In this overview, a special emphasis is also placed on the management of inflammatory and viral cardiomyopathies.

Apoptosis is a key feature in the progression of heart disease. Stage B heart failure is characterized by a structurally abnormal heart in which the remodeled myocardium is prone to apoptosis. Elimination of the proapoptotic stimuli or inhibition of the apoptotic cascade could presumably rescue the myocardium and halt the progression of adverse remodeling and heart failure. In this article, the authors review the role of apoptosis (or programmed cell death) in determining the evolution of symptomatic heart failure and particularly the adverse remodeling in the aftermath of acute myocardial infarction.

The temporal relationship between the development of heart failure and activation of the neurohumoral systems involved in chronic heart failure (CHF) has not been precisely defined. When a compensatory mechanism switches to a deleterious contributing factor in the progression of the disease is unclear. This article addresses these issues through evaluating the contribution of various cardiovascular reflexes and cellular mechanisms to the sympathoexcitation in CHF. It also sheds light on some of the important central mechanisms that contribute to the increase in sympathetic nerve activity in CHF.

Oxidative stress represents a persistent imbalance between the production and the compensation of reactive oxygen species. Though predominantly found in advanced heart failure, the most frequent "at-risk" condition has been associated with underlying oxidative stress. It is therefore conceivable that timely detection and early intervention to reduce oxidative stress processes provide an opportunity to prevent disease progression to overt heart failure. This article reviews the current understanding of the current evidence of oxidative stress involvement in the pathophysiology of human heart failure and its potential therapeutic interventions in patients with Stage A and B heart failure.

Elevated levels of circulating proinflammatory cytokines and adipokines have been repeatedly associated with increased risk for clinically manifest (Stage C) heart failure in large cohort studies. However, the role of low-grade, subclinical inflammatory activity in the transition from risk factors (Stage A heart failure) to structural heart disease (Stage B heart failure) is less well understood. Recent evidence suggests that chronic low-grade inflammatory activity is involved in most mechanisms underlying progression of structural heart disease, including ventricular remodeling after ischemic injury, response to pressure and volume overload, and myocardial fibrosis. Inflammation also contributes to progression of peripheral vascular changes.

Prevalence of diabetes and heart failure are increasing exponentially worldwide. Diabetes is well-known to increase the risk of heart failure independent of other traditional risk factors and ischemia. Current evidence indicates the presence of several biochemical and molecular changes associated with diabetes that lead to diastolic dysfunction or American Heart Association stage B heart failure. Some, if not all, changes may also predate the development of frank diabetes. In this review, the authors present some of the epidemiologic evidence and a brief description of major mechanistic pathways that favor the development of heart failure in prediabetic and diabetic states.

Arterial stiffness/elasticity plays a major role in the pathogenesis of heart failure beyond arterial blood pressure. Arterial wave reflections are generated from the periphery of the vascular system, especially at the level of the small arteries. The pattern change of the arterial wave reflections can alter the ventricular-vascular coupling in a pathologic manner, leading to heart failure. Several noninvasive techniques are used to estimate arterial stiffness/elasticity. Small artery elasticity has important predictive value for the diagnosis of heart failure. The beneficial effect of

Heart Failure Clinics

ACCESS THE CLINICS ONLINE!

Available at:
http://www.theclinics.com

Editorial

Reducing the Burden of Stage B Heart Failure Will Require Connecting the Dots Between "Knowns" and "Known Unknowns"

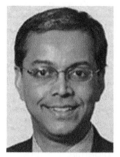 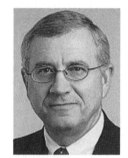

Ragavendra R. Baliga, MD, MBA   James B. Young, MD
Consulting Editors

There are known knowns; there are things we know we know.

We also know there are known unknowns; that is to say we know there are some things we do not know.

But there are also unknown unknowns—the ones we don't know we don't know.

—*Former United States Secretary of Defense Donald Rumsfeld*[1]

The American College of Cardiology/American Heart Association heart failure guidelines define Stage B heart failure as patients with structural heart disease but no current or prior symptoms of heart failure[2] and include patients with prior myocardial infarction, left ventricular hypertrophy, valvular heart disease, regional wall-motion abnormality, left ventricular enlargement, and systolic and diastolic dysfunction.[3] Despite their lack of symptoms, these patients with systolic dysfunction have a nearly five-fold risk of developing heart failure[4] (**Fig. 1**). The common causes of stage B heart failure include ischemic heart disease and hypertension[5–7] (**Box 1**). It is estimated that the prevalence of stage B heart failure is four times as great as that of stages C and D heart failure patients put together. One recent population-based study estimates that 34% of individuals >45 years

of age have stage B heart failure.[8] This burden is projected to increase as the prevalence of tobacco use, obesity,[9,10] hypertension,[11] hyperglycemia,[12] dyslipidemia,[13] and consequently ischemic heart disease continues to increase worldwide.[14] Efforts to reduce this burden will require reducing risk at an individual level[3,15,16] and a population-based approach[17] (**Fig. 2**)—an integrated approach that has successfully achieved near global eradication of communicable diseases such as poliomyelitis.

It is estimated that about 5%-10% of the population are at very high risk of developing cardiovascular events (**Fig. 2**), whereas a much larger proportion of the population is at moderate risk.[17–20] Individuals at the tail end of the distribution are more prone to fatal and nonfatal cardiovascular events, whereas more individuals with moderate risk will develop cardiovascular events because the whole burden of moderate risk individuals is much larger.[9,11–13] Therefore, it is vital that population-based strategies be pursued to shift the risk distribution of the population as a whole to the left, using both lifestyle changes and pharmacotherapy.[17,21] These include reduction of salt intake[22] and trans-fatty acids[23,24] at a population level through, arguably, legislation[25] and with a focus on health education,[26,27] using

Heart Failure Clin 8 (2012) xi–xv
doi:10.1016/j.hfc.2011.10.001
1551-7136/12/$ – see front matter © 2012 Elsevier Inc. All rights reserved.

heartfailure.theclinics.com

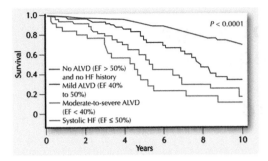

Fig. 1. Kaplan–Meier curves for survival. Referent group consists of subjects with normal left ventricular systolic function (EF >50%) and no history of congestive heart failure. Mild ALVD indicates mild asymptomatic left ventricular systolic dysfunction (EF 40% to 50%); mod/sev ALVD, moderate-to-severe asymptomatic left ventricular systolic dysfunction (EF <40%); systolic CHF, congestive heart failure with EF ≤50%. (*From* Wang TJ, Evans JC, Benjamin EJ, et al. Natural history of asymptomatic left ventricular systolic dysfunction in the community. Circulation 2003;108(8):977–82; with permission.)

mass media with attention paid to blood pressure, cholesterol, and obesity[28,29] control, which are known to be cost effective.[18–20] The benefits of preventive guidelines and continuing medical education are increasingly becoming apparent,

> **Box 1**
> **Causes of stage B heart failure**
>
> - Ischemic etiology
> - Nonischemic cause
>   - Hypertension
>   - Valvular heart disease
>   - Cardiotoxin exposure particularly chemotherapy[52]
>   - Post-viral infection/myocarditis
>   - Familial idiopathic dilated cardiomyopathy

as evidenced by recent declines in heart failure mortality and hospitalizations.[30,31]

Reducing risk at an individual level will clearly require lifestyle changes, adherence to pharmacotherapy,[32–34] and possibly mechanical cardiac resynchronization.[35–37] The lack of physical activity, increased caloric intake, and use of tobacco result in hypertension,[5,11] dyslipidemia,[13,38] and hyperglycemia,[12] which in turn have been attributed to 75% of the cardiovascular event risk factors. Other established risk factors for cardiovascular disease include age, gender, obesity, past history of cardiovascular disease, family history of cardiovascular disease, and socioeconomic position.[39]

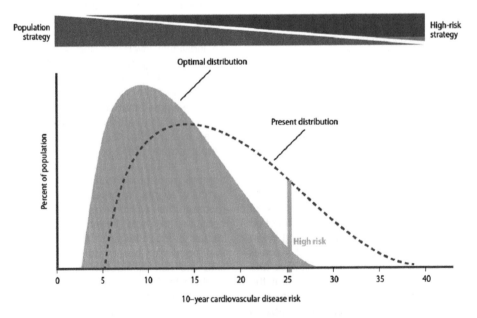

Fig. 2. At any given time, about 5%–10% of the population are at very high risk of developing cardiovascular events. A much larger segment of the population is at moderate risk. If no preventive action is taken, individuals at the tail end of the distribution will develop fatal and nonfatal cardiovascular events. Many more events will occur in the segment of the population with modest elevation of risk, as the number of individuals in this segment is larger. (*From* Mendis S. Cardiovascular risk assessment and management in developing countries. Vasc Health Risk Manag 2005;1(1):15–8.)

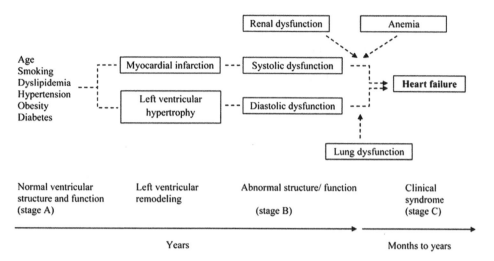

Fig. 3. Interaction of cardiac and noncardiac dysfunctions and progression to heart failure. (*From* Klein L. Omnes Viae Romam Ducunt: asymptomatic cardiac and noncardiac organ system dysfunction leads to heart failure. Circulation 2011;124:4–6; with permission.)

These, for obvious reasons, are much harder to address with a goal of improvising outcomes. Also, a recent study reported that dysfunction of non-cardiac organs—particularly the renal, pulmonary, and hematopoietic systems—was associated with a 30% increase in overall risk of heart failure and the risk increased proportionally if more than one organ was involved.[40,41] In this study, the average age of the participants was 76 years and most were women with a history of hypertension; not many had diabetes or coronary artery disease. These investigators found that dysfunction of the non-cardiac organs was relatively "mild" as reflected by serum creatinine >1.05 mg/dL, hemoglobin <13 g/dL, or FEV1/FVC ratio <91% predicted. These findings support earlier data regarding the additive effects of cardio-renal-anemia syndrome[42] and the effect of impaired lung function on both systolic and diastolic cardiac performance.[43,44] Therefore, it has been argued that reducing risk at the individual level will require attention to both traditional risk factors and non-cardiac organ dysfunction (**Fig. 3**).

Although there are established strategies to reduce individual risk[18–20] and population-based risk, there is no definitive method to identify patients with stage B heart failure (**Box 2**).[45] Identification of the individual with stage B heart failure involves screening of populations and promising strategies include using biomarkers.[46–51] To discuss such challenges pertaining to the management of stage B heart failure, Drs Jay Cohn and Gary Francis have assembled an international panel of experts. These expert opinions

Box 2
Summary of proposed research designs[45]

1. Determine the incidence of asymptomatic LVSD in community-based cohorts.

2. Characterize the natural history of asymptomatic LVSD in the community:

   a. Natural history in individuals with different degrees of LVSD

   b. Natural history in individuals with LVSD without previous MI

3. Examine the natural history of subclinical left ventricular diastolic dysfunction.

4. Examine the cost-effectiveness of various screening strategies for identifying left ventricular dysfunction and develop better screening tools.

5. Address the role of medications other than ACE inhibitors in managing patients with asymptomatic LVSD.

6. Increase representation of the following types of patients in clinical trials: patients with mild LVSD, those with LVSD and no history of MI, and those with isolated left ventricular diastolic dysfunction

ACE, angiotensin-converting enzyme; LVSD, left ventricular systolic dysfunction; MI, myocardial infarction.
From Wang TJ, Levy D, Benjamin EJ, et al. The epidemiology of "asymptomatic" left ventricular systolic dysfunction: implications for screening. Ann Intern Med 2003;138(11):907–16; with permission.

provide ample food for thought on developing an effective strategy to manage stage B pre-heart failure. We hope that these insightful articles will allow "connecting the dots" between what we know and the "known unknowns" of stage B pre-heart failure.

Ragavendra R. Baliga, MD, MBA
Division of Cardiovascular Medicine
Ohio State University Medical Center
Columbus, OH, USA

James B. Young, MD
Lerner College of Medicine
Endocrinology and Metabolism Institute
Cleveland Clinic
Cleveland, OH, USA

E-mail addresses:
Ragavendra.baliga@osumc.edu (R.R. Baliga)
youngj@ccf.org (J.B. Young)

REFERENCES

1. Rumsfeld D. "There are known unknowns. That is to say, there are things we now know we don't know. But there are also unknown unknowns. These are the things we do not know we don't know". NATO HQ, Brussels, Press Conference by U.S. Secretary of Defense Donald Rumsfeld; June 6, 2002.
2. Hunt SA, Abraham WT, Chin MH, et al. 2009 Focused Update Incorporated into the ACC/AHA 2005 Guidelines for the Diagnosis and Management of Heart Failure in Adults: A Report of the American College of Cardiology Foundation/American Heart Association Task Force on Practice Guidelines Developed in Collaboration with the International Society for Heart and Lung Transplantation. J Am Coll Cardiol 2009;53(15):e1–90.
3. Greenberg B. Pre-clinical diastolic dysfunction in diabetic patients: where do we go from here? J Am Coll Cardiol 2010;55(4):306–8.
4. Wang TJ, Evans JC, Benjamin EJ, et al. Natural history of asymptomatic left ventricular systolic dysfunction in the community. Circulation 2003;108(8):977–82.
5. Bakris GL, Baliga RR. Hypertension. Oxford: Oxford University Press; 2012.
6. Krishnamoorthy A, Brown T, Ayers CR, et al. Progression from normal to reduced left ventricular ejection fraction in patients with concentric left ventricular hypertrophy after long-term follow-up. Am J Cardiol 2011;108(7):997–1001.
7. Milani RV, Drazner MH, Lavie CJ, et al. Progression from concentric left ventricular hypertrophy and normal ejection fraction to left ventricular dysfunction. Am J Cardiol 2011;108(7):992–6.
8. Ammar KA, Jacobsen SJ, Mahoney DW, et al. Prevalence and prognostic significance of heart failure stages. Circulation 2007;115(12):1563–70.
9. Finucane MM, Stevens GA, Cowan MJ, et al. National, regional, and global trends in body-mass index since 1980: systematic analysis of health examination surveys and epidemiological studies with 960 country-years and 9.1 million participants. Lancet 2011;377(9765):557–67.
10. Anand SS, Yusuf S. Stemming the global tsunami of cardiovascular disease. Lancet 2011;377(9765):529–32.
11. Danaei G, Finucane MM, Lin JK, et al. National, regional, and global trends in systolic blood pressure since 1980: systematic analysis of health examination surveys and epidemiological studies with 786 country-years and 5.4 million participants. Lancet 2011;377(9765):568–77.
12. Danaei G, Finucane MM, Lu Y, et al. National, regional, and global trends in fasting plasma glucose and diabetes prevalence since 1980: systematic analysis of health examination surveys and epidemiological studies with 370 country-years and 2.7 million participants. Lancet 2011;378(9785):31–40.
13. Farzadfar F, Finucane MM, Danaei G, et al. National, regional, and global trends in serum total cholesterol since 1980: systematic analysis of health examination surveys and epidemiological studies with 321 country-years and 3.0 million participants. Lancet 2011;377(9765):578–86.
14. Mackay J, Mensah GA, Mendis S, et al. World Health Organization. The atlas of heart disease and stroke. Geneva: World Health Organization; 2004.
15. Goldberg LR, Jessup M. Stage B heart failure: management of asymptomatic left ventricular systolic dysfunction. Circulation 2006;113(24):2851–60.
16. Frieden TR, Berwick DM. The "Million Hearts" initiative–preventing heart attacks and strokes. N Engl J Med 2011;365(13):e27.
17. Mendis S. Cardiovascular risk assessment and management in developing countries. Vasc Health Risk Manag 2005;1(1):15–8.
18. Daniels SR, Pratt CA, Hayman LL. Reduction of risk for cardiovascular disease in children and adolescents. Circulation 2011;124(15):1673–86.
19. Weintraub WS, Daniels SR, Burke LE, et al. Value of primordial and primary prevention for cardiovascular disease: a policy statement from the American Heart Association. Circulation 2011;124(8):967–90.
20. Balagopal PB, de Ferranti SD, Cook S, et al. Nontraditional risk factors and biomarkers for cardiovascular disease: mechanistic, research, and clinical considerations for youth: a scientific statement from the American Heart Association. Circulation 2011;123(23):2749–69.
21. Heagerty AM. Secondary prevention of heart disease and stroke: work to do. Lancet 2011;378(9798):1200–2.

22. Baliga RR, Narula J. Salt never calls itself sweet. Indian J Med Res 2009;129(5):472–7.
23. Angell SY, Silver LD, Goldstein GP, et al. Cholesterol control beyond the clinic: New York City's trans fat restriction. Ann Intern Med 2009;151(2):129–34.
24. Mello MM. New York City's war on fat. N Engl J Med 2009;360(19):2015–20.
25. Dumanovsky T, Huang CY, Nonas CA, et al. Changes in energy content of lunchtime purchases from fast food restaurants after introduction of calorie labelling: cross sectional customer surveys. BMJ 2011;343:d4464.
26. Farewell Brown J. Food pyramid. CDS Rev 2011; 104(4):22–3.
27. Garg A, Guez G. Food pyramid replaced by plate. Dent Implantol Update 2011;22(7):52–4.
28. Benac N. First lady aims to trim American waist sizes. CMAJ 2010;182(9):E385–6.
29. Tanne JH. Michelle Obama launches programme to combat US childhood obesity. BMJ 2010;340:c948.
30. Chen J, Normand SL, Wang Y, et al. National and regional trends in heart failure hospitalization and mortality rates for Medicare beneficiaries, 1998-2008. JAMA 2011;306(15):1669–78.
31. Gheorghiade M, Braunwald E. Hospitalizations for heart failure in the United States—a sign of hope. JAMA 2011;306(15):1705–6.
32. Frigerio M, Oliva F, Turazza FM, et al. Prevention and management of chronic heart failure in management of asymptomatic patients. Am J Cardiol 2003;91(9A): 4F–9F.
33. Yusuf S, Islam S, Chow CK, et al. Use of secondary prevention drugs for cardiovascular disease in the community in high-income, middle-income, and low-income countries (the PURE Study): a prospective epidemiological survey. Lancet 2011;378(9798): 1231–43.
34. Klapholz M. Beta-blocker use for the stages of heart failure. Mayo Clin Proc 2009;84(8):718–29.
35. Linde C, Abraham WT, Gold MR, et al. Cardiac resynchronization therapy in asymptomatic or mildly symptomatic heart failure patients in relation to etiology: results from the REVERSE (REsynchronization reVErses Remodeling in Systolic Left vEntricular Dysfunction) study. J Am Coll Cardiol 2008;56(22): 1826–31.
36. St John Sutton M, Ghio S, Plappert T, et al. Cardiac resynchronization induces major structural and functional reverse remodeling in patients with New York Heart Association class I/II heart failure. Circulation 2009;120(19):1858–65.
37. Moss AJ, Hall WJ, Cannom DS, et al. Cardiac-resynchronization therapy for the prevention of heart-failure events. N Engl J Med 2009;361(14):1329–38.
38. Baliga RR, Cannon CP. Dyslipidemia. Oxford: Oxford University Press; 2011.
39. Baliga RR. Cardiology. New York: McGraw-Hill Medical; 2011.
40. Lam CSP, Lyass A, Kraigher-Krainer E, et al. Cardiac dysfunction and noncardiac dysfunction as precursors of heart failure with reduced and preserved ejection fraction in the community / clinical perspective. Circulation 2011;124(1):24–30.
41. Klein L. Omnes Viae Romam Ducunt. Circulation 2011;124(1):4–6.
42. Baliga RR, Young JB, Fonarow GC, et al. Staying in the pink of health for patients with cardiorenal anemia requires a multidisciplinary approach. Heart Fail Clin 2010;6(3):xi–xvi.
43. Barr RG, Bluemke DA, Ahmed FS, et al. Percent emphysema, airflow obstruction, and impaired left ventricular filling. N Engl J Med 2010;362(3):217–27.
44. Guazzi M. Alveolar gas diffusion abnormalities in heart failure. J Card Fail 2008;14(8):695–702.
45. Wang TJ, Levy D, Benjamin EJ, et al. The epidemiology of "asymptomatic" left ventricular systolic dysfunction: implications for screening. Ann Intern Med 2003;138(11):907–16.
46. Daniels LB, Clopton P, Jiang K, et al. Prognosis of stage A or B heart failure patients with elevated B-type natriuretic peptide levels. J Card Fail 2010; 16(2):93–8.
47. Heidenreich PA, Gubens MA, Fonarow GC, et al. Cost-effectiveness of screening with B-type natriuretic peptide to identify patients with reduced left ventricular ejection fraction. J Am Coll Cardiol 2004;43(6):1019–26.
48. Macheret F, Boerrigter G, McKie P, et al. Pro-B-type natriuretic peptide1-108 circulates in the general community: plasma determinants and detection of left ventricular dysfunction. J Am Coll Cardiol 2011; 57(12):1386–95.
49. Velagaleti RS, Gona P, Levy D, et al. Relations of biomarkers representing distinct biological pathways to left ventricular geometry. Circulation 2008; 118(22):2252–8.
50. Gupta S, Rohatgi A, Ayers CR, et al. Risk scores versus natriuretic peptides for identifying prevalent stage B heart failure. Am Heart J 2011;161(5): 923–30, e922.
51. Poppe KK, Whalley GA, Richards AM, et al. Prediction of ACC/AHA Stage B heart failure by clinical and neurohormonal profiling among patients in the community. J Card Fail 2011;16(12):957–63.
52. Baliga RR, Young JB. Early detection and monitoring of vulnerable myocardium in patients receiving chemotherapy: is it time to change tracks? Heart Fail Clin 2011;7(3):xiii–xix.

Preface

Stage B, a Pre-cursor of Heart Failure

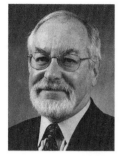 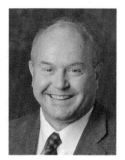

Jay N. Cohn, MD   Gary S. Francis, MD
Guest Editors

The concept that structural changes in the left ventricle antedate the clinical syndrome of heart failure was emphasized by the American College of Cardiology/American Heart Association committee that prepared their guideline document in 2005 and its revision in 2009. By designating this structural alteration "Stage B" and identifying this patient population as "at risk for heart failure," a they supported the view that the clinical syndrome occurs as the culmination of a progressive process that can be identified long before the patient becomes symptomatic and enters a management phase with high morbidity and mortality. We have therefore elected to label the condition as "Stage B, a pre-cursor of heart failure."

The structural basis of this Stage B phase, the mechanisms that may contribute to its development and progression, the clinical tools that may be used to detect and monitor it, and the therapeutic approaches that may favorably influence its course have not been comprehensively explored. Therefore, the purpose of having two issues of *Heart Failure Clinics*, this one and a second one to be published in April 2012, is to provide an in-depth discussion of all aspects of the description, mechanisms, detection, and potential management of Stage B. Furthermore,

we explore the rationale for screening to detect structural abnormalities likely to progress.

Since heart failure occurs as a consequence of a wide variety of cardiac disorders, the structural abnormalities that precede the symptomatic phase can be similarly diverse. In this first issue the structural changes in the myocyte and interstitium are reviewed. Changes in size and shape of myocytes and changes in content of the interstitium are fundamental to structural remodeling. Understanding the factors that induce, contribute to, and orchestrate this remodeling process is key to developing strategies to restrain and reverse it.

The hemodynamic stresses and disease processes that induce remodeling may account in part for differences in the structural response. We therefore explore the structural changes in pressure and volume overload, ischemia, and various cardiomyopathies. The molecular and cellular contributors to these processes will continue to be the focus of fundamental research.

Factors that may contribute to the progression of remodeling are critical to the development of effective therapies. The second section of this issue therefore explores apoptosis, neurohormonal stimulation, oxidative stress, and inflammation as well as the contributions of diabetes,

Heart Failure Clin 8 (2012) xvii–xviii
doi:10.1016/j.hfc.2011.08.015

arterial stiffness, and aging. The interaction of these factors is probably critical to understanding progression of the structural process in individual patients.

The second issue of this series discusses clinical aspects of the structural process. Monitoring tools, therapeutic approaches, and the rationale for screening are reviewed in depth.

For this text, we, as authors, have sought individuals who have made major contributions to our understanding of heart failure. Their willingness to participate and the quality of their articles lend remarkable credibility to the endeavor. We are grateful for their participation and for their skill in providing such insightful reviews of the data.

Accomplishing the formidable task of collecting and editing these articles would not have been possible without the dedication and skill of Cheryl (Kitty) Tincher at the University of Minnesota and Barbara Cohen-Kligerman at Elsevier. We are indebted to them for their assistance.

Jay N. Cohn, MD
Gary S. Francis, MD

University of Minnesota Medical School
Minneapolis, MN 55455, USA

E-mail addresses:
cohnx001@umn.edu (J.N. Cohn)
franc354@umn.edu (G.S. Francis)

Myocyte Changes in Heart Failure

Olga V. Savinova, PhD[a], A. Martin Gerdes, PhD[b],*

KEYWORDS

- Cardiomyocyte • Structural remodeling • Heart failure
- Cardiac hypertrophy

Heart failure (HF) is often described as an inability of the heart to meet hemodynamic needs of the body. HF is a syndrome that can represent the end stage of different forms of heart disease. In the Western world, the prevalence and incidence of HF are increasing.[1] Survival after the onset of overt HF is grim, with a 5-year survival rate as low as 25% in men and 38% in women according to a Framingham study.[2]

The American College of Cardiology and American Heart Association developed a new approach to the classification of HF by introducing a staging system that emphasizes both the development and progression of the disease.[3,4] Stage A and B patients are defined as those with risk factors that predispose toward the development of HF. For example, stage A patients might present with coronary artery disease, hypertension, or diabetes mellitus but not demonstrate clear left ventricular (LV) structural disease or functional impairment, whereas patients who demonstrate LV hypertrophy or impaired LV function but remain asymptomatic for HF would be designated as stage B. Stage C denotes patients with current or past symptoms of HF associated with underlying structural heart disease, and stage D designates patients with truly refractory HF.

This classification recognizes that therapeutic interventions introduced even before the appearance of LV dysfunction or symptoms can reduce the population morbidity and mortality of HF because such therapeutic interventions will address established risk factors and structural pathologies early in the course of the disease. The identification of the mechanisms responsible for the cardiac structural abnormalities is important because some conditions that lead to LV dysfunction are potentially reversible. At present, stage B patients will typically remain untreated for structural heart disease because of the absence of HF symptoms. The exception is patients recovering from myocardial infarction (MI).[3]

STRUCTURAL REMODELING OF THE HEART REFLECTS CHANGES IN MYOCYTE MORPHOLOGY

It has been known for many years that structural remodeling is a major feature of HF. The failing heart is characterized by a dilated, relatively thin-walled ventricle. It is important to include the term relative because actual wall thickness may or may not be increased, depending on the patient history related to hypertension. Because of the spatial arrangement of myocytes within the ventricular wall, cell length contributes to chamber circumference (diameter), whereas cell diameter is primarily responsible for changes in wall thickness. Consequently, changes in myocyte dimensions should largely provide the cellular analogue of chamber diameter/wall thickness alterations affecting wall stress. An understanding of how myocyte shape is altered in the progression to failure should, therefore, provide considerable insight into pathologic cardiac remodeling.

The authors have nothing to disclose.

[a] Cardiovascular Health Research Center, Sanford Research, University of South Dakota, 2301 East 60th Street North, Sioux Falls, SD 57104, USA

[b] Department of Biomedical Sciences, New York College of Osteopathic Medicine at New York Institute of Technology, Northern Boulevard, PO Box 8000, Old Westbury, NY 11568-8000, USA

* Corresponding author.

E-mail address: agerdes@nyit.edu

Heart Failure Clin 8 (2012) 1–6

doi:10.1016/j.hfc.2011.08.004

Historically, it has been thought that the contribution of cardiomyocytes to cardiac remodeling is primarily caused by hypertrophy rather than hyperplasia (ie, that cardiomyocytes are able to grow in size but not in number). A useful and consistent measure to characterize cardiomyocyte morphology is their length-to-width ratio, which is approximately 7:1 in the healthy myocardium of all mammalian species studied to date.[5] Indeed, this constant is the cellular analogue to the similar and consistent LV chamber diameter/ wall thickness ratio found in mammals regardless of size. Myocyte number, rather than size, accounts for the difference in heart mass of mammals from small to large. The normal mammalian heart contains approximately 25 million myocytes per gram of LV tissue.[6] Myocyte length-to-width ratio increases with dilated HF but may be reduced with compensated hypertension, reflecting gross anatomic features of the LV.

PATHOLOGIC CHANGES IN MYOCYTE SHAPE

Cardiomyocyte morphology exhibits distinct variation in various pathologic conditions.[7] Chronic ischemic heart disease may lead to ventricular dilation and congestive HF. The authors compared cells from patients with normal coronary arteries with myocytes from explanted hearts from patients with chronic ischemic heart disease.[8] Chronic ischemic heart disease manifested in a 40% increase in myocyte length (141 ± 9 vs 197 ± 8 μm, P<.01). Cell width was not significantly different, and cell length-to-width ratio was 49% greater in the ischemic hearts. The extent of myocyte lengthening was comparable to the increase in end-diastolic diameter. These data suggest that increased myocyte length is largely responsible for the chamber dilation in ischemic heart disease. Furthermore, maladaptive remodeling of myocyte shape may contribute to the elevated wall stress (eg, increased chamber radius/wall thickness). Zaferiedes and colleagues[9] later confirmed these changes in myocyte shape in failing human hearts.

Another study in dogs showed that cardiac pacing induced dilated HF, which was accompanied (among other pathologic changes) by a 23% increase in the cardiomyocyte length-to-width ratio.[10]

After MI, LV remodeling is characterized by cavity dilatation, eccentric hypertrophy, and regional mechanical dysfunction. A study conducted in a sheep model of MI correlated cellular hypertrophy with the function of noninfarcted myocardium assessed by magnetic resonance imaging.[11] Intramyocardial circumferential shortening was reduced after MI in the region adjacent to the infarct, whereas function in the remote region did not change. Adjacent intramyocardial circumferential shortening correlated inversely with adjacent myocyte volume (r = −0.72, P<.009) and cell length (r = −0.70, P<.02). Thus, this model indicated that disproportionate cellular hypertrophy occurs (predominantly caused by an increase in cell length) in mechanically dysfunctional noninfarcted regions adjacent to a chronic transmural MI.

A study of spontaneously hypertensive HF (SHHF) rats demonstrated that during progression to HF, cardiomyocytes length correlated well with LV chamber diameter (**Fig. 1**). Importantly, during this transition to dilated failure, there was no change in the myocyte cross-sectional area. Indeed, the authors' data have consistently shown that increased myocyte length without a change in myocyte diameter seems to be a common feature of progression from stable hypertrophy to dilated failure of all causes.

MYOCYTE SHAPE AND VENTRICULAR WALL STRESS

Calculation of relative wall thickness (RWT) by the formula RWT = 2 × PWTd/LVIDd (where *PWTd* and *LVIDd* denote posterior wall thickness and LV internal diameter at diastole) permits categorization of an increase in LV mass as either concentric (RWT >0.42) or eccentric (RWT <0.42) hypertrophy and allows identification of concentric remodeling (normal LV mass with increased RWT).[12] It is worth noting that the term eccentric

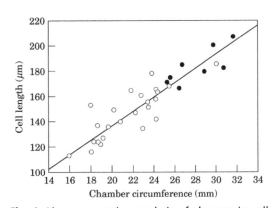

Fig. 1. Linear regression analysis of changes in cell length and chamber circumference in aging SHHF rats. Open circles, pre-HF; closed circles, in HF; r = 0.93. (*From* Tamura T, Onodera T, Said S, et al. Correlation of myocyte lengthening to chamber dilation in the spontaneously hypertensive heart failure (SHHF) rat. J Mol Cell Cardiol 1998;30:2175; with permission.)

hypertrophy was originally used to describe a volume-overloaded heart that was eccentric or displaced to the left of midline. In recent years, eccentric hypertrophy has often been used to describe a dilated, failing heart. Perhaps it might be better to describe compensated volume overloading as compensated, eccentric hypertrophy and dilated failure as decompensated, eccentric hypertrophy.

Many years ago, it was hypothesized by Grossman[13] that myocyte shape alterations during cardiac hypertrophy parallel changes in ventricular anatomy. After first developing and validating a precise and comprehensive method to assess cell size[6] and applying this method to many animal models of heart disease, cumulative data collected by the authors laboratory over many years have confirmed Grossman's theory (reviewed in Gerdes[5]). It is worth noting that the comprehensive cell-sizing approach used allows direct comparison of all published data because the values closely approach absolute values.

Cardiac and skeletal muscles are both comprised of longitudinal arrays of thick and thin filaments in a repeating unit called the sarcomere. Sarcomeric proteins undergo constant molecular turnover. Thus, a direction of vectors for assembly and disassembly of sarcomeres as a unit could determine the shape of cardiomyocytes.[5,14,15] Recent computational modeling of eccentric and concentric cardiac growth through sarcomerogenesis indeed shows that both models (strain-driven eccentric growth and stress-driven concentric growth) closely recapitulate changes in chamber geometry.[16] It is plausible that cardiomyocyte remodeling that occurs at the cellular level is the underlying reason for pathologic LV hypertrophy.

One particular change in cardiomyocyte morphologic dynamics is arrested or impaired cross-sectional growth in the presence of longitudinal growth. This growth could lead to the increase in LV chamber diameter characteristic of dilated cardiomyopathy. Increase in LV chamber diameter in the absence of wall thickening is directly related to increased diastolic wall stress: $\sigma = P*r/h$; where P is the end-diastolic pressure, r is the end-diastolic radius, and h is wall thickness.[13] According to this equation, normalization of cross-sectional growth of cardiomyocytes in the dilated heart could increase wall thickness and reduce LV wall stress.

Because coronary blood flow predominantly occurs during relaxation of the heart muscle, normalization of diastolic wall stress could also lead to better oxygenation and improved pump function. Coronary flow reserve was studied in patients with dilated cardiomyopathy.[17] The investigators found that coronary flow reserve (the ratio of maximal to resting coronary flow) negatively correlated with LV end-diastolic pressure ($r = -0.69$; $P<.05$), LV end-diastolic volume index ($r = -0.7$; $P<.05$), and LV end-diastolic wall stress ($r = -0.84$; $P<.001$).

HUMAN GENETICS

Identification of causative mutations in familial cardiomyopathies provides insights into the general mechanisms of structural remodeling of cardiac myocytes preceding symptoms of HF. Hypertrophic cardiomyopathy seems to be a disease of the sarcomere because most of the disease-causing mutations have been identified in genes encoding many of the sarcomeric proteins.[18] These genes include beta-myosin heavy chain,[19] α-tropomyosin and troponin T,[20] cardiac myosin binding protein-C,[21,22] the myosin regulatory light chain and myosin essential light chain,[23] troponin I,[24] and actin.[25] Dilated cardiomyopathy, on the other hand, is primarily caused by mutations in a set of genes coding for cytoskeletal proteins: dystrophin,[26,27] desmin,[28] metavinculin,[29] and actin (mutated close to a dystrophin-binding site).[30]

MOLECULAR MECHANISMS OF CARDIOMYOCYTE GROWTH REGULATION

Kehat and Molkentin[31] recently reviewed molecular pathways underlying pathologic cardiac hypertrophy. In addition, the reader is referred to the discussion of mechanical stress-induced sarcomere assembly during cardiac muscle growth by Russell and colleagues.[32] Here the authors would like to focus on a few studies that address the bidirectional effects of several molecular players on cardiomyocyte growth.

The protein melusin was found to interact with and relay signals from the cytoplasmic domain of integrin b1 in LV hypertrophy induced by pressure overload. After the surgical induction of pressure overload, melusin-deficient mice displayed increased dilation accompanied by LV dysfunction and reduced survival.[33] Moreover, when compared with wild-type (WT) mice, melusin-deficient mice developed a similar degree of LV hypertrophy in response to the chronic administration of the classical prohypertrophic agonists angiotensin II or phenylephrine. In contrast, cardiac-specific overexpression of melusin resulted in concentric LV hypertrophy after pressure overload compared with WT animals that displayed eccentric LV hypertrophy culminating in HF.[34] These findings suggest that melusin might be a mechanical sensor that regulates cardiomyocyte cross-sectional growth.

Effects of renin and PPAR-γ were studied in cultured adult rat ventricular cardiomyocytes. Renin directly caused an unexpected lengthening of cardiomyocytes in culture. Cardiomyocytes isolated from TGR(mRen2)27 rats, overexpressing renin, were longer than those of nontransgenic littermates. Cell length was reduced by feeding these rats pioglitazone, a PPAR-γ agonist. Pioglitazone affected cell length independent of blood pressure.[35] This study showed that increased cardiac afterload can directly lead to eccentric hypertrophy (cell lengthening) but the effect of renin on blood pressure and cardiomyocyte length can be decoupled by activation of PPAR-γ.

An increase in cardiac afterload typically produces concentric hypertrophy characterized by an increase in cardiomyocyte width, whereas volume overload or exercise results in eccentric growth characterized by cellular elongation from addition of sarcomeres in series and proportional growth of myocyte diameter. The signaling pathways that control eccentric versus concentric heart growth were studied using mice lacking 2 ERK proteins (ERK1/2) in the heart and in mice expressing activated form of mitogen-activated protein kinase 1 (Mek1) in the heart, which induces ERK1/2 signaling.[36] Cardiomyocytes from hearts of ERK1/2-deficient mice showed preferential eccentric growth (lengthening) in response to pressure overload, whereas myocytes from Mek1 transgenic hearts showed concentric growth (width increase). Isolated adult myocytes, in which ERK1/2 signaling was acutely inhibited by adenoviral transfer of dominant negative form of Mek1 and dual specificity phosphatase 6, showed spontaneous lengthening. In contrast, infection of isolated myocytes with an adenovirus encoding activated Mek1 promoted constitutive ERK1/2 signaling and increased myocyte width. This study demonstrated that the ERK1/2 signaling pathway regulates the balance between eccentric and concentric growth of the heart.

REVERSE REMODELING IN HUMAN AND ANIMAL STUDIES

Reverse remodeling describes the regression of pathologic myocardial hypertrophy, chamber shape distortions, and dysfunction that may occur spontaneously or in response to therapeutic interventions (recently reviewed by Hellawell and Margulies[37]). There is now extensive evidence supporting considerable potential for reverse remodeling among patients with chronic HF and significant distortions of normal myocardial geometry. This body of evidence includes large-scale clinical trials and case series documenting responses to pharmacologic, device-based, and surgical interventions.

Restrictive mitral annuloplasty (RMA) often leads to reverse LV remodeling in patients with advanced cardiomyopathy and functional mitral regurgitation. Multidetector computed tomography (MDCT) was used to assess stress-shortening relations before and after RMA.[38] The study suggests that the decrease in afterload after the reduction in volume overload was responsible for postoperative reverse LV remodeling after RMA.

Another study illustrates that early correction of the underlying cause of pathologic remodeling can lead to the reversal of remodeling presumably because of the inherent plasticity of cardiomyocytes. Performing mitral valve repair before the development of significant secondary tricuspid valve regurgitation and the reduction in ejection fraction is associated with a greater likelihood of significant regression of LV mass, possibly predicting improved recovery of normal LV function after surgical intervention.[39]

Echocardiographic changes in patients enrolled in the Multicenter Automatic Defibrillator Implantation Trial-Cardiac Resynchronization Therapy (CRT) trial showed that improvement in outcomes (reduction of the risk of death or HF event) with CRT was associated with favorable alterations in cardiac size and function.[40]

Patients with chronic advanced HF unloaded by LV assist devices can show improvement in their myocardial function and some can show reverse remodeling to the extent that their myocardial function improves sufficiently for the device to be removed (reviewed by Birks[41]). Data also suggest that combining mechanical support with adjuvant drug therapy targeting remodeling can increase the rate of recovery.[42]

After the insertion of an LV assist device, the Margulies group[9] was first to show that series removal of sarcomeres can occur in the dilated, failing human heart. The authors' group showed series removal of sarcomeres in SHHF rats near failure after treatment with an ACE inhibitor or angiotensin type 1 receptor blocker.[43] Thus, cardiac myocytes from failing hearts clearly possess the ability to reverse remodel to a more normal phenotype after either mechanically or pharmacologically induced unloading. The authors also studied reversal of eccentric hypertrophy after the relief of surgical volume overload.[44] To determine whether the series addition of sarcomeres observed during eccentric hypertrophic growth is reversible on removal of the initiating stimulus, an aortocaval fistula was created and myocyte geometry was evaluated at 2 and 12 weeks after shunt occlusion. A 76% cardiac enlargement was produced in rats with an aorto-caval fistula. As is typical of compensated hyper-trophy from volume overloading, increases in myocyte length and width contributed approxi-mately equally to the increase in myocyte volume. The extent of LV hypertrophy was reduced to 22% and 18% at 2 and 12 weeks of fistula reversal, respectively. Significant reduction in myocyte length from series sarcomere removal was noted in 2 of the 3 regions examined. This study was the first to show that myocytes possess the neces-sary machinery to remove series sarcomeres, returning altered pump function, and dilated ventricular chamber geometry toward control values.

SUMMARY

Cardiomyocyte remodeling is a universal change in structural heart disease characteristic of stage B HF. Because of the plasticity of cardiomyocyte architecture, the process of remodeling can be reversed. The detailed description of the mecha-nisms responsible for cardiomyocyte growth regulation will aid in development of preventive therapeutics to attenuate or prevent the progres-sion of HF from asymptomatic stage B to full-blown debilitating disease.

REFERENCES

1. Kannel WB. Incidence and epidemiology of heart failure. Heart Fail Rev 2000;5(2):167–73.
2. Kannel WB, Ho K, Thom T. Changing epidemiolog-ical features of cardiac failure. Br Heart J 1994; 72(Suppl 2):S3–9.
3. Hunt SA, Abraham WT, Chin MH, et al. 2009 focused update incorporated into the ACC/AHA 2005 guide-lines for the diagnosis and management of heart failure in adults: a report of the American College of Cardiology Foundation/American Heart Associa-tion Task Force on Practice Guidelines: developed in collaboration with the International Society for Heart and Lung Transplantation. Circulation 2009; 119(14):e391–479.
4. Hunt SA. ACC/AHA 2005 guideline update for the diagnosis and management of chronic heart failure in the adult: a report of the American College of Cardiology/American Heart Association Task Force on Practice Guidelines (writing committee to update the 2001 guidelines for the evaluation and manage-ment of heart failure). J Am Coll Cardiol 2005;46(6): e1–82.
5. Gerdes AM. Cardiac myocyte remodeling in hyper-trophy and progression to failure. J Card Fail 2002; 8(Suppl 6):S264–8.
6. Gerdes AM, Moore JA, Hines JM, et al. Regional differences in myocyte size in normal rat heart. Anat Rec 1986;215(4):420–6.
7. Gerdes AM, Capasso JM. Structural remodeling and mechanical dysfunction of cardiac myocytes in heart failure. J Mol Cell Cardiol 1995;27(3):849–56.
8. Gerdes AM, Kellerman SE, Moore JA, et al. Struc-tural remodeling of cardiac myocytes in patients with ischemic cardiomyopathy. Circulation 1992; 86(2):426–30.
9. Zafeiridis A, Jeevanandam V, Houser SR, et al. Regression of cellular hypertrophy after left ventricular assist device support. Circulation 1998;98(7):656–62.
10. Kajstura J, Zhang X, Liu Y, et al. The cellular basis of pacing-induced dilated cardiomyopathy. Myocyte cell loss and myocyte cellular reactive hypertrophy. Circulation 1995;92(8):2306–17.
11. Kramer CM, Rogers WJ, Park CS, et al. Regional myocyte hypertrophy parallels regional myocardial dysfunction during post-infarct remodeling. J Mol Cell Cardiol 1998;30(9):1773–8.
12. Lang RM, Bierig M, Devereux RB, et al. Recommen-dations for chamber quantification. Eur J Echocar-diogr 2006;7(2):79–108.
13. Grossman W, Jones D, McLaurin LP. Wall stress and patterns of hypertrophy in the human left ventricle. J Clin Invest 1975;56(1):56–64.
14. Thomas TA, Kuzman JA, Anderson BE, et al. Thyroid hormones induce unique and potentially beneficial changes in cardiac myocyte shape in hypertensive rats near heart failure. Am J Physiol Heart Circ Phys-iol 2005;288(5):H2118–22.
15. Russell B, Motlagh D, Ashley WW. Form follows function: how muscle shape is regulated by work. J Appl Physiol 2000;88(3):1127–32.
16. Goktepe S, Abilez OJ, Parker KK, et al. A multiscale model for eccentric and concentric cardiac growth through sarcomerogenesis. J Theor Biol 2010; 265(3):433–42.
17. Inoue T, Sakai Y, Morooka S, et al. Coronary flow reserve in patients with dilated cardiomyopathy. Am Heart J 1993;125(1):93–8.
18. Bowles NE, Bowles KR, Towbin JA. The "final common pathway" hypothesis and inherited cardio-vascular disease. The role of cytoskeletal proteins in dilated cardiomyopathy. Herz 2000;25(3):168–75.
19. Geisterfer-Lowrance AA, Kass S, Tanigawa G, et al. A molecular basis for familial hypertrophic cardio-myopathy: a beta cardiac myosin heavy chain gene missense mutation. Cell 1990;62(5):999–1006.
20. Thierfelder L, Watkins H, MacRae C, et al. Alpha-tropomyosin and cardiac troponin T mutations cause familial hypertrophic cardiomyopathy: a disease of the sarcomere. Cell 1994;77(5):701–12.

21. Bonne G, Carrier L, Bercovici J, et al. Cardiac myosin binding protein-C gene splice acceptor site mutation is associated with familial hypertrophic cardiomyopathy. Nat Genet 1995;11(4):438–40.

22. Watkins H, Conner D, Thierfelder L, et al. Mutations in the cardiac myosin binding protein-C gene on chromosome 11 cause familial hypertrophic cardiomyopathy. Nat Genet 1995;11(4):434–7.

23. Poetter K, Jiang H, Hassanzadeh S, et al. Mutations in either the essential or regulatory light chains of myosin are associated with a rare myopathy in human heart and skeletal muscle. Nat Genet 1996; 13(1):63–9.

24. Kimura A, Harada H, Park JE, et al. Mutations in the cardiac troponin I gene associated with hypertrophic cardiomyopathy. Nat Genet 1997;16(4):379–82.

25. Mogensen J, Klausen IC, Pedersen AK, et al. Alpha-cardiac actin is a novel disease gene in familial hypertrophic cardiomyopathy. J Clin Invest 1999; 103(10):R39–43.

26. Towbin JA, Hejtmancik JF, Brink P, et al. X-linked dilated cardiomyopathy. Molecular genetic evidence of linkage to the Duchenne muscular dystrophy (dystrophin) gene at the Xp21 locus. Circulation 1993;87(6):1854–65.

27. Ortiz-Lopez R, Li H, Su J, et al. Evidence for a dystrophin missense mutation as a cause of X-linked dilated cardiomyopathy. Circulation 1997;95(10): 2434–40.

28. Li D, Tapscoft T, Gonzalez O, et al. Desmin mutation responsible for idiopathic dilated cardiomyopathy. Circulation 1999;100(5):461–4.

29. Maeda M, Holder E, Lowes B, et al. Dilated cardiomyopathy associated with deficiency of the cytoskeletal protein metavinculin. Circulation 1997; 95(1):17–20.

30. Olson TM, Michels VV, Thibodeau SN, et al. Actin mutations in dilated cardiomyopathy, a heritable form of heart failure. Science 1998;280(5364):750–2.

31. Kehat I, Molkentin JD. Molecular pathways underlying cardiac remodeling during pathophysiological stimulation. Circulation 2010;122(25):2727–35.

32. Russell B, Curtis MW, Koshman YE, et al. Mechanical stress-induced sarcomere assembly for cardiac muscle growth in length and width. J Mol Cell Cardiol 2010;48(5):817–23.

33. Brancaccio M, Fratta L, Notte A, et al. Melusin, a muscle-specific integrin beta1-interacting protein,

is required to prevent cardiac failure in response to chronic pressure overload. Nat Med 2003;9(1): 68–75.

34. Sbroggio M, Ferretti R, Percivalle E, et al. The mammalian CHORD-containing protein melusin is a stress response protein interacting with Hsp90 and Sgt1. FEBS Lett 2008;582(13):1788–94.

35. Hinrichs S, Heger J, Schreckenberg R, et al. Controlling cardiomyocyte length: the role of renin and PPAR-{gamma}. Cardiovasc Res 2011;89(2): 344–52.

36. Kehat I, Davis J, Tiburcy M, et al. Extracellular signal-regulated kinases 1 and 2 regulate the balance between eccentric and concentric cardiac growth. Circ Res 2011;108(2):176–83.

37. Hellawell JL, Margulies KB. Myocardial reverse remodeling. Cardiovasc Ther 2010. [Epub ahead of print].

38. Takeda K, Taniguchi K, Shudo Y, et al. Mechanism of beneficial effects of restrictive mitral annuloplasty in patients with dilated cardiomyopathy and functional mitral regurgitation. Circulation 2010;122(Suppl 11): S3–9.

39. Stulak JM, Suri RM, Dearani JA, et al. Does early surgical intervention improve left ventricular mass regression after mitral valve repair for leaflet prolapse? J Thorac Cardiovasc Surg 2011;141(1): 122–9.

40. Solomon SD, Foster E, Bourgoun M, et al. Effect of cardiac resynchronization therapy on reverse remodeling and relation to outcome: multicenter automatic defibrillator implantation trial: cardiac resynchronization therapy. Circulation 2010; 122(10):985–92.

41. Birks EJ. Myocardial recovery in patients with chronic heart failure: is it real? J Card Surg 2010; 25(4):472–7.

42. Birks EJ, Tansley PD, Hardy J, et al. Left ventricular assist device and drug therapy for the reversal of heart failure. N Engl J Med 2006;355(18):1873–84.

43. Tamura T, Said S, Harris J, et al. Reverse remodeling of cardiac myocyte hypertrophy in hypertension and failure by targeting of the renin-angiotensin system. Circulation 2000;102(2):253–9.

44. Gerdes AM, Clark LC, Capasso JM. Regression of cardiac hypertrophy after closing an aortocaval fistula in rats. Am J Physiol 1995;268(6 Pt 2): H2345–51.

Changes in the Myocardial Interstitium and Contribution to the Progression of Heart Failure

Shaina R. Eckhouse, MD[a], Francis G. Spinale, MD, PhD[b,c],*

KEYWORDS

- Interstitium • Extracellular matrix • Heart failure
- Pressure overload hypertrophy • Dilated cardiomyopathy
- Myocardial infarction

With a prolonged cardiovascular stress or pathophysiologic stimuli, a cascade of structural events occurs, defined as myocardial remodeling, as a continuum of changes in the structure and function of the myocardium. Adverse left ventricular (LV) myocardial events have been shown to affect cellular signaling and extracellular signaling processes. Changes occurring in the cellular constituents of the myocardium that accompany remodeling are discussed in an article elsewhere in this issue; therefore, the significant alterations in the structure and composition of the myocardial interstitium will be the focus of this article. Historically, the myocardial interstitium was considered a static entity with a passive and nonresponsive structure composed of a fibrillar collagen network; however, it has now been shown to be a dynamic structure that plays a fundamental role in myocardial adaptation to a pathologic stress facilitating the remodeling process. Therefore, the purpose of this article is threefold. First, present an up-to-date overview of myocardial extracellular matrix structure and function. Second, briefly show how the myocardial interstitium is altered in important disease states that can progress to chronic heart failure: pressure overload hypertrophy (POH) in context of hypertension and aortic stenosis, ischemic heart disease in the context myocardial infarction (MI), and dilated cardiomyopathy (DCM). Third, identify potential diagnostic and therapeutic strategies relevant to myocardial matrix remodeling in the context of these cardiac disease states.

MYOCARDIAL INTERSTITIUM STRUCTURE AND FUNCTION

Traditionally, the myocardial interstitium was thought to be composed mainly of fibrillar collagen; however, a wide array of molecules

This research was supported by NIH grants HL57952, HL59165, HL95608, and HL78825 and a Merit Award from the Veterans' Affairs Health Administration. Dr Eckhouse's research was supported by NIH grant T32 HL007260. Dr Spinale is a consultant for Boston Scientific Corporation.

[a] Division of Cardiothoracic Surgery, Department of Surgery, Medical University of South Carolina, 114 Doughty Street, Suite 326, Charleston, SC 29425, USA
[b] Department of Cell Biology and Anatomy, University of South Carolina School of Medicine, CVCTRC, Columbia, SC 29208, USA
[c] Department of Surgery, Medical University of South Carolina, Charleston, SC, USA
* Corresponding author. Department of Cell Biology and Anatomy, University of South Carolina School of Medicine, CVCTRC, Columbia, SC 29208.
E-mail address: cvctrc@uscmed.sc.edu

Heart Failure Clin 8 (2012) 7–20
doi:10.1016/j.hfc.2011.08.012
1551-7136/12/$ – see front matter Published by Elsevier Inc.

besides collagen are now known to constitute greater than 95% of the extracellular matrix.[1,2] Specifically, it contains noncollagen matrix proteins, proteoglycans, glycosaminoglycans, and a large reservoir of bioactive signaling molecules.[3–16] The interstitium is highly organized and orchestrated, whereby small disruptions in composition, spatial relationships, or content lead to altered myocardial systolic and/or diastolic performance. For example, the fibrillar collagens ensure structural integrity of adjoining myocytes, provide the means through which myocyte shortening is translated into overall left ventricular pump function, and are essential for maintaining alignment of myofibrils within the myocyte through a collagen-integrin-cytoskeletal-myofibril relation.[17–23] Using a papillary muscle preparation, Baicu and colleagues[24] showed that proteolytic digestion of the myocardial interstitium reduces the extent and velocity of cardiomyocyte shortening. In contrast, isolated cardiomyocyte shortening was preserved. These findings are summarized in **Fig. 1** and underscore the importance of the interstitium to transduce myocyte shortening into overall myocardial ejection. This section reviews the different molecules that compose and contribute

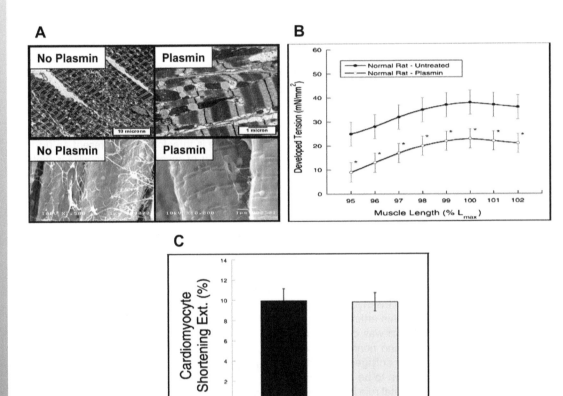

Fig. 1. Transmission and scanning electron microscopy (EM) were performed on papillary muscle samples that had been fixed at a maximum length preload. The images are of normal myocardium and normal myocardium treated with plasmin, a serine protease that activates matrix metalloproteinases to cleave interstitial proteins, including fibrillar collagen. (A) The top left transmission EM depicts intact sarcolemma with individual myofibrils. The bottom left scanning EM of normal myocardium depicts a fine fibrillar collagen weave within the interstitium. The bottom right scanning EM image depicts the myocardium after treatment with plasmin, showing a significant loss of fibrillar collagen. The top right transmission EM shows no gross changes in sarcolemma architecture or evidence of myocyte injury. (B) The normal myocardium treated with plasmin develops less force at a specific muscle length compared with untreated myocardium. Overall, plasmin treatment moved the developed force versus muscle length relationship downward. Muscle length is graphed as the percent of the maximal papillary muscle length that resulted in peak active tension (%Lmax). (C) The graph shows that no change in cardiomyocyte shortening extent occurred with plasmin treatment of normal (NML) cardiomyocytes, further supporting the concept that extracellular matrix degradation does not affect the function of the isolated cardiomyocyte. (*From* Baicu CF, Stroud JD, Livesay VA, et al. Changes in extracellular collagen matrix alter myocardial systolic performance. Am J Physiol Heart Circ Physiol 2003;284(1):H122–32; with permission.)

to the structure and function of the myocardial extracellular matrix. Although this article is not meant to provide an exhaustive overview, it provides the prototypical examples to illustrate the diversity of constituents that exist within the myocardial interstitium.

Structural Matrix Proteins

Structural matrix proteins are collagen and noncollagen proteins that constitute the organization of the myocardial interstitium. The noncollagen matrix proteins compose the basement membrane, which forms anchoring points for the fibrillar collagen matrix and contact points for other proteoglycans within the extracellular matrix.

Fibrillar collagen

Initially, the fibrillar collagen matrix, composed mainly of collagen I and III, was considered to be a static complex, but these structural proteins are now well understood to have the ability to undergo rapid degradation and turnover.[1,17–23,25] Early in its modification, collagen fibril formation entails posttranslational changes during which the amino terminal and carboxy terminal ends of the procollagen fibril are cleaved through proteolytic reactions. These collagen-derived peptides (procollagen type III amino terminal propeptide [PIIIP] and procollagen type I carboxy terminal propeptide [PIP], respectively) can be detected in the plasma and used as biomarkers of matrix synthesis, which is discussed later. The result of these modifications causes a necessary conformational change for collagen fibril cross-linking and triple helix formation.[26] Although the newly formed, un–cross-linked collagen fibrils are vulnerable to degradation, the triple-helical collagen fiber is resistant to nonspecific proteolysis, and further degradation requires specific enzymatic cleavage, as is discussed in a subsequent paragraph.

The importance of collagen cross-linking with respect to overall left ventricular geometry and function has been shown in several animal models and clinical studies.[17,27–30] For instance, inhibition of lysyl hydroxylase, a critical enzyme in collagen cross-linking, with β-aminopropionitrile results in a collagen disease in humans known as lathyrism.[31] Treatment with β-aminopropionitrile in a porcine model causes a decrease in collagen cross-linking and content, resulting in a decrease in myocardial stiffness.[29] In patients with severe left ventricular dilation (DCM), reduced collagen cross-linking of fibrils has been reported. Therefore, not only is total collagen content relevant but also the degree of collagen cross-linking holds functional and clinical importance in the context of heart failure.[17,29,30]

Integrins

The integrins are a family of transmembrane proteins that aid in multiple functions affecting myocardial structure and function.[20,21,25] The binding interface with proteins constituting the basement membrane consists of integrins, which directly influence myocyte growth and geometry through ligand binding. More specifically, integrins affect cell migration and survival during normal cardiac development and myocardial remodeling. Although numerous integrin ligands exist, they most commonly act as receptors for collagen I and III, laminin, fibronectin, and thrombospondin in the basement membrane.[2,32] Although genetic polymorphisms have been shown to affect the concentration of integrins within the basement membrane in platelets, this relationship remains to be studied in the myocardial interstitium, where it may play an important role in the setting of cardiac disease.[32]

Laminin and fibronectin

Laminin and fibronectin are heavily glycosylated glycoproteins in the basement membrane of cardiac myocytes that associate with many myocardial interstitium factors, including fibrillar collagen and cell membrane receptors. For example, the change in content and distribution of these glycoproteins will affect hydration within the extracellular space and subsequent myocardial compliance.[33–36] These highly charged molecules within the myocardial interstitium result in the formation of a hydrated gel, which serves as a reservoir for signaling molecules and bioactive peptides. Furthermore, fibronectin binds to integrins, which activate a profibrotic pathway that leads to extracellular matrix deposition.[37] Although laminin and fibronectin play a role in determining receptor-to-ligand interaction within the myocardial interstitium, these glycoproteins have been overlooked in the context of heart failure.

Matrix Signaling and Associative Proteins

It is becoming recognized that the myocardial interstitium is composed of a vast array of nonstructural proteins. Specifically, these proteins influence collagen fibril assembly and morphology and regulate signaling between cells and the extracellular matrix. Some illustrative examples of the wide portfolio of matrix proteins are provided.

Secreted protein and rich in cysteine

Secreted protein and rich in cysteine (SPARC, also known as *osteonectin*) is a matricellular protein that serves as an accessory protein composed of three modular domains that regulate matrix assembly into mature fibrils, specifically collagen types I and III.[38,39] In a transgenic mouse model, SPARC gene deletion is associated with impaired collagen production and collagen fibril disorganization. Overall, an inefficiency of incorporation of collagen into fibrils occurs in the absence of SPARC, which results in premature myocardial rupture.[40] With overexpression of SPARC, enhanced collagen deposition is noted with increased formation of mature fibers, which leads to ventricular hypertrophy.[39,41]

Thrombospondin

Thrombospondin is a family of glycoproteins that participate in the communication between the cardiomyocyte and the myocardial interstitium in both embyogenesis and cardiac disease states, such as POH and DCM.[42–44] Specifically, thrombospondin seems to modulate cell-to-matrix interactions through the coalescence of membrane proteins and signaling molecules at specific contact points on the cell surface.[42,45,46] One of the most important functions of thrombospondin is its downstream induction of fibrillar collagen expression and synthesis.[44,46] In a murine model with gene deletion of thrombospondin, multiple processes were affected in the interstitium, including decreased collagen cross-linking and increased matrix protease activity.[47] Ultimately, the lack of thrombospondin caused a decrease in collagen content and, combined with the decrease in collagen cross-linking, LV dilation occurred with increasing rates of myocardial rupture.[43]

Galectin-3

The ß-galactoside–binding protein galectin-3 has been identified as an interstitial chaperone protein that regulates extracellular matrix growth, structure, and function in cardiac disease, such as POH.[48,49] Expression and activation of galectin-3 is stimulated by cardiac inflammation, specifically the macrophages and neutrophils. Galectin-3 binds to several interstitial ligands that include fibrillar collagens, basement membranes, and integrins, and this in turn affects collagen synthesis and degradation.[49]

Transforming growth factor

As a family of three regulatory cytokines (ß1, ß2, and ß3), transforming growth factor (TGF) plays an important role in stimulating production of extracellular matrix in the myocardium.[50–53] In this article, TGF is referred to in general terms. TGF is released in an inactive form in the interstitial space, where it is activated by proteolytic cleavage and has been shown to influence a wide array of processes, including inflammation, apoptosis, cardiac development, and myocardial remodeling.[50–53] Active TGF binds to TGF type I and II receptors and results in downstream activation of a variety of events, which prototypically include fibrillar collagen expression.[50,51] In a transgenic model of TGF overexpression, increased deposition of collagen types I and III occurred, whereas in a mouse MI model, inhibition of TGF decreased collagen deposition and increased LV dilation.[54,55] Thus, TGF seems to be a critical signaling molecule in maintaining normal extracellular matrix homeostasis and regulating increased collagen expression in myocardial remodeling during cardiac disease.

Matrix metalloproteinases

The matrix metalloproteinases (MMPs) are a family of zinc-dependent myocardial interstitium proteases that play several roles in myocardial remodeling.[56–61] More than 25 distinct human MMPs have been identified and characterized; expression of MMPs has been shown to be ubiquitous in tissue remodeling processes.[58–61] **Table 1** lists the identifications of specific MMPs in cardiac disease states. Historically, MMPs were thought to be only involved in proteolysis of the myocardial interstitium; however, MMPs are now well understood to possess a large portfolio of biologic functions pertaining to myocardial remodeling.[60–62] Initially, MMPs are synthesized as inactive zymogens that are secreted as proenzymes into the myocardial interstitium. The proenzyme form then binds specific myocardial interstitium proteins and remains ezymatically quiescent until the propeptide domain is cleaved. Although the MMPs were initially thought to be secreted only in a soluble proenzyme form, a unique subfamily of MMPs, the membrane-type MMPs, are fully active enzymes inserted into the cell membrane after secretion.[56] Because the membrane-type MMPs are inserted into the cell membrane already activated, a localized, pericellular site of myocardial interstitium proteolytic activity is established. Multiple clinical studies of cardiac disease have shown a clear cause-and-effect relationship between MMPs and myocardial interstitial remodeling and ventricular dysfunction, which is discussed later.

Tissue inhibitors of MMPs

A critical control point of MMP activity is through the inhibition of the activated enzyme by the actions of a group of specific MMP inhibitors termed *tissue inhibitors of MMPs* (TIMPs).[63–65] In general, TIMPs are low-molecular-weight proteins that bind to the catalytic domain of active MMPs and thereby prevent access to substrates. Historically, the predominant role of TIMPs was thought to be the inhibition of active MMPs; however,

Table 1
Studies evaluating MMPs and TIMPs in different cardiac diseases

Classification	MMP/TIMP	POH	MI	DCM
Collagenase	MMP-1	79	—	63, 64, 85
—	MMP-8	107	95, 102	—
Gelatinase	MMP-2	103, 107	95, 98, 99	63, 64, 87
—	MMP-9	103	95, 98, 99, 101, 105	63–65, 87
Stromelysins	MMP-3	—	95	63, 64
Membrane type	MMP-14	103	—	64, 87
Tissue inhibitors	TIMP-1	79, 80, 81, 103	105, 108	63, 65, 85
—	TIMP-2	103	105	63, 65
—	TIMP-3	—	—	65, 85, 87
—	TIMP-4	107	105	65

Abbreviation: TIMP, tissue inhibitors of MMPs.

studies have shown that TIMPs are also be involved in MMP activation along with actions independent of MMPs.[66,67]

EXTRACELLULAR REMODELING IN CARDIAC DISEASE

The causes that give rise to heart failure are diverse, as are the structural and functional changes of prototypical causes. Stylized summations of the structural changes, as seen in POH, DCM, and MI, are depicted in **Fig. 2**.

Myocardial Remodeling with Pressure Overload Hypertrophy

Matrix remodeling and LV function
In addition to myocyte hypertrophy, the hallmark of myocardial structural remodeling with POH is extracellular matrix accumulation.[68–74] Moreover, prolonged POH is associated with significantly increased collagen accumulation between individual myocytes and myocyte fascicles, and the highly organized architecture of the myocardial interstitium is replaced with a thickened, poorly organized structure. Clinical studies of POH showed increased myocardial interstitial matrix accumulation and increased LV stiffness.[71–74] For example, increased collagen accumulation was seen in LV myocardial samples taken from patients with POH secondary to aortic stenosis, and was associated with increased myocardial stiffness.[71] As shown in the histopathologic images of **Fig. 3**A, amplification of matrix accumulation occurs and causes the fundamental pathophysiologic change seen in POH, myocardial stiffness, which gives rise to impairments in diastolic filling, as shown in **Fig. 3**B.[75,76] Therefore,

in POH, the structural abnormalities within the matrix leads to impaired LV filling and increased filling pressures, such as increased LV end diastolic pressures and left atrial pressures.

In summary, changes in the matrix can directly contribute to the progression of heart failure symptoms in patients with POH.

Changes in myocardial interstitium determinants in POH
The preponderance of studies evaluating myocardial biopsies obtained from patients with POH, irrespective of aortic stenosis or hypertensive heart disease, uniformly shows increased accumulation of collagen.[43,70,71,75,77] Furthermore, changes in critical determinants that effect collagen levels are altered in the remodeling process that occurs with POH. Myocardial samples from patients with POH secondary to aortic stenosis show increases in the matrix-signaling molecule thrombospondin; therefore, parallel induction of thrombospondin occurs to increase collagen deposition.[43] Several studies present increases in myocardial expression of TGF in patients with POH secondary to aortic stenosis, and the increase in TGF positively correlates with levels of collagen I and III in patients with POH.[70,77] Moreover, dynamic changes in MMP and TIMP levels have been reported. For example, Fielitz and colleagues[68] identified robustly increased levels of TIMPs, which would in turn favor greater inhibition of MMP-induced matrix degradation. Thus, as shown in **Fig. 2**C, increased induction of profibrotic signaling molecules and inhibition of collagen breakdown promote matrix remodeling through favoring increased collagen accumulation.

A Normal Interstitium

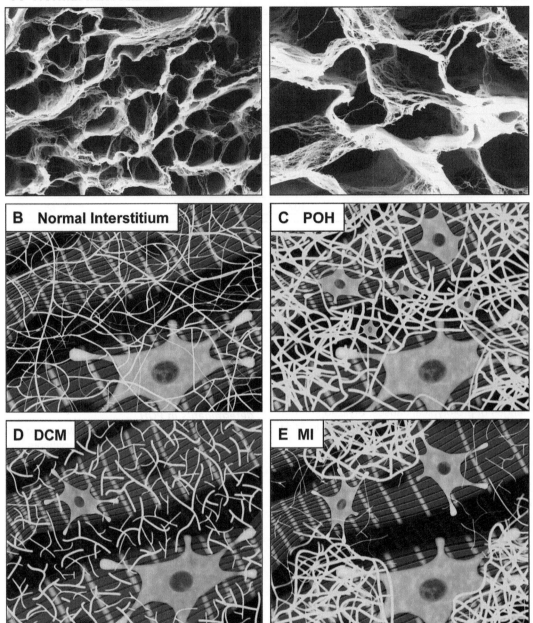

Fig. 2. (*A*) Scanning electron microscopy showing normal myocardial interstitium organization. The schematic illustration depicts the extracellular matrix surrounding the cardiomyocytes in (*B*) normal myocardium, (*C*) POH, (*D*) DCM, and (*E*) MI. (*B*) In the normal myocardium, the interstitium forms a highly organized continuum between cardiomyocytes to provide a structural support system and a functional depot for a wide array of non-collagen matrix proteins, signaling molecules, and other cell types, such as fibroblasts. (*C*) In POH secondary to aortic stenosis or hypertension, the schematic illustrates the diffuse collagen accumulation that occurs along with an increase in fibroblast proliferation that leads to myocardial matrix accumulation and diastolic dysfunction. (*D*) In DCM, the schematic shows the increase in extracellular matrix turnover, with the hallmarks of increased fibrillar collagen and decreased collagen cross-linking. (*E*) In ischemic heart disease secondary to MI, the myocardial remodeling process is region-dependent and not uniform, with both collagen accumulation (*the infarct region*) and degradation occurring (*the border zone*).

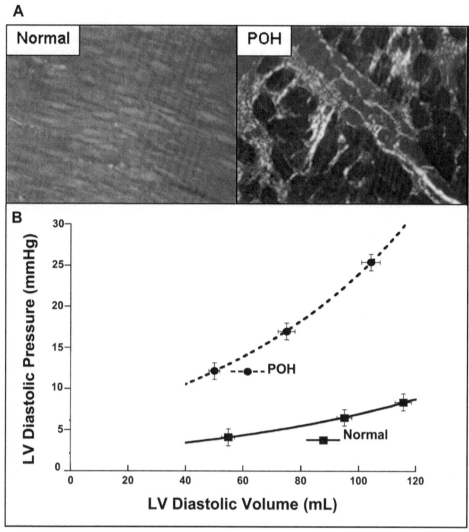

Fig. 3. (A) Histopathologic images of normal myocardium compared with myocardium that has undergone extra-cellular matrix remodeling secondary to pressure overload hypertrophy. Note the significant collagen accumulation in the myocardium affected by POH (*white and blue areas*). (B) The graph illustrates the relationship between pressure and volume of the LV during diastole in both normal patients and patients with POH. With the same diastolic volume during filling, the graph illustrates that patients with POH have increased diastolic pressures compared with controls. This finding indicates a decrease in compliance of the myocardium with long-standing POH. [(A) *Adapted from* Villari B, Campbell SE, Hess OM, et al. Influence of collagen network on left ventricular systolic and diastolic function in aortic valve disease. J Am Coll Cardiol 1993;22(5):1477–84; with permission. (B) *From* Zile MR, Baicu CF, Gaasch WH. Diastolic heart failure–abnormalities in active relaxation and passive stiffness of the left ventricle. N Engl J Med 2004;350(19):1953–9; with permission.]

Changes in matrix determinants detected in the plasma in POH

Collagen-derived peptides, such as PIP and PIIIP, enter the circulation in quantities that likely reflect collagen synthesis and can be measured in the plasma.[78,79] For example, Laviades and colleagues[79] measured increased levels of PIP and PIIIP with no change in levels of the marker for collagen degradation in patients with POH secondary to hypertension. Plasma levels of the signaling molecule galectin-3 were increased in patients with POH.[48] Moreover, plasma levels of TIMP-1 have been widely shown to be increased in POH secondary to hypertension.[80,81] The disproportionate increase in TIMP levels promotes inhibition of MMP-activated interstitial collagen turnover because of a shift in the overall ratio of MMPs to TIMPs.[80,81]

In summary, plasma profiling has shown that determinants of synthesis, signaling proteins, and inhibitors of collagen degradation are all increased and correlate with collagen accumulation in the setting of POH.

Myocardial Remodeling with DCM

Myocardial interstitial remodeling and LV function

In contrast to POH, the underlying pathophysiology of DCM is LV dilation and reduced systolic performance. DCM is a diverse classification of primary myocardial disease states, which uniformly causes an increase in LV chamber radius compared with wall thickness.[58,59] With respect to the myocardial matrix in patients with DCM, changes in normal structure and composition occur, which can result in a loss of appropriate alignment of cardiomyocyte fascicles, which in turn may contribute to LV dilation. In general, a heterogeneous matrix remodeling process occurs in DCM, which results in structural discontinuity and in turn the loss of normal matrix cellular support, such as the matrix-myocyte interfaces. The failure of a cohesive matrix-myocyte interface would in turn defeat normal transduction of myocyte shortening to myocardial ejection. Thus, significant disruptions in the normal matrix architecture can contribute to both LV dilation and decreased systolic performance.

Changes in myocardial interstitium determinants in DCM

In DCM, a dysregulation between matrix synthetic and degradative pathways occur, which results in defective matrix architecture.[63–65,82–86] Multiple studies have shown that collagen expression and collagen content are increased in DCM.[17,84,87] However, defects in collagen cross-linking occur with the development of DCM, which increases susceptibility to proteolysis and matrix instability. In several reports, the matrix signaling molecule thrombospondin was decreased in patients with end-stage DCM.[43,88] The reduction of thrombospondin results in a loss of normal matrix signaling and the synthetic pathways of collagen. TGF expression is simultaneously augmented in DCM, underscoring the differential changes occurring within the myocardial interstitium.[43,88] Increased posttranslational modification and degradation of collagen in DCM is also occurring within the myocardial matrix, as exemplified by the alterations in MMP and TIMP levels. More specifically, increases in MMP-2, MMP-3, MMP-9, MMP-13, and membrane type 1 MMP occur with concurrent decreases in MMP-1, TIMP-2, TIMP-3, and TIMP-4 in DCM. The overall change in ratio of MMPs to

TIMPs shifts, favoring MMP-mediated matrix proteolysis.[56,57,63–65] Therefore, in summary, an increase in matrix profibrotic signaling coupled with an increase in interstitial proteolytic pathways seems to occur, which would create a futile cycle in terms of matrix accumulation and stability in patients with DCM. The resulting architecture of the defective myocardial interstitium is depicted in **Fig. 2**D.

Changes in matrix determinants detected in the plasma in DCM

DCM is the most common indication for cardiac transplantation, and therefore myocardial sampling can be readily performed in these patients. Thus, few studies have focused primarily on plasma profiling for extracellular matrix remodeling. However, in conjunction with myocardial biopsies, Bruggink and colleagues[89] evaluated plasma samples and measured increased levels of PIP and PIIIP in both the myocardium and the plasma before and after implantation of an LV-assist device in patients with end-stage DCM.

Myocardial Remodeling with Ischemic Heart Disease

Myocardial interstitial remodeling and LV function

It is now recognized that several structural events occur within the myocardial interstitium after MI, which involves both the MI and non-MI regions.[56,57,90–93] The LV remodeling process after MI occurs in two phases, the acute phase and the chronic remodeling phase. The acute phase involves myocyte necrosis, an influx of inflammatory cells, and interstitial remodeling primarily within the MI region. In addition, a new region emerges, the border zone region, which consists of viable myocytes, an influx of inflammatory cells, and proliferating fibroblasts, which results in a site of continuous matrix turnover.[90,93,94] In the chronic adaptive phase, the MI region undergoes increased matrix accumulation and scar formation. However, the border zone region continues to undergo both matrix accumulation and proteolysis.[90,93,94] This type of matrix instability is not dissimilar to that described in patients with DCM. The structural changes that occur within the MI and border zone regions can result in dyskinetic contraction patterns. This dyskinesia can cause abnormal stress and strain patterns during the cardiac cycle, and continued matrix turnover, and potentially yield MI expansion and LV dilation.[57,90–94] This post-MI remodeling process is exemplified in **Fig. 4**A, wherein LV dilation occurs in patients as a function of time post-MI. Despite uniform standards of pharmacologic therapy, LV

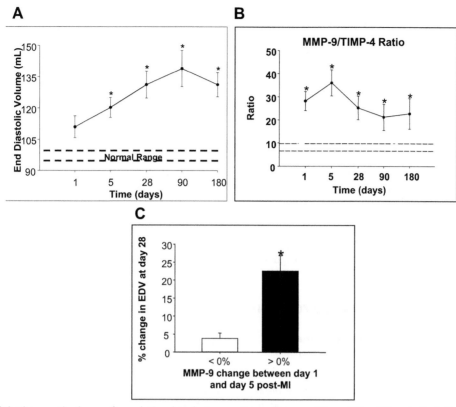

Fig. 4. (*A*) The graph shows the relationship between time after an MI and the LV end diastolic volume. Compared with patients without an MI (normal range), a significant increase is seen in LV end diastolic volume after an MI. (*B*) A significant increase in the ratio of MMP-9 to TIMP-4 levels is seen in patients after an MI compared with patients without an MI (range of ratio illustrated by the *two dashed lines*). (*C*) When the percent change in MMP-9 levels from day 1 to 5 is compared with the percent change in LV end diastolic volume 1 month after an MI, a significant increase is seen in the percent change in LV end diastolic volume, with an increase in MMP-9 from day 1 to 5. (*From* Ahmed SH, Clark LL, Pennington WR, et al. Matrix metalloproteinases/tissue inhibitors of metalloproteinases: relationship between changes in proteolytic determinants of matrix composition and structural, functional, and clinical manifestations of hypertensive heart disease. Circulation 2006;113(17):2089–96; with permission.)

remodeling occurs in most patients post-MI, underscoring the need for matrix-specific therapeutic interventions. The dynamic changes occurring in the different regions of the myocardium promote significant architectural changes that are depicted in a stylized manner in **Fig. 2E**.

Changes in myocardial interstitium determinants in ischemic heart disease

Although clinical studies have documented a relationship between plasma levels of matrix signaling proteins and the progression of ischemic heart disease secondary to MI, few have evaluated the structure and function of the myocardial interstitium directly.[56,57,90–92,95] Using a microdialysis system, dynamic changes in interstitial MMP activity were shown in patients during and after a period of myocardial arrest and subsequent reperfusion.[95]

This study underscores that rapid and time-specific changes within the human myocardial interstitium occur with respect to determinants of matrix remodeling.

Changes in matrix determinants detected in the plasma in ischemic heart disease

A large number of studies have been performed that clearly show time-specific changes in plasma profiles of the synthetic and degradative matrix pathways post-MI.[18,56,57,90–92,96–101] One example showed that PIIIP and the plasma marker for collagen degradation, CITP, were increased in patients at the onset of the MI.[90] The acute elevation in these determinants of collagen composition suggest that a simultaneous increase in collagen synthesis and degradation occurs, which is consistent with the acute phase of post-MI remodeling.

Several studies have provided data to show that increased plasma levels of MMPs were measured post-MI.[96,97,102–105] For example, increased levels of MMP-8 and MMP-9 were shown in the plasma 3 days after MI, whereby MMP-8 levels subsequently decreased and MMP-9 levels remained elevated for 6 months.[94] Concurrently, TIMP-1 plasma levels were increased with no change in levels of TIMP-2 and TIMP-4 for 6 months after MI.[97] Overall, the post-MI ratio of MMP levels to TIMP levels shifted in favor of a heightened matrix proteolytic state. For example, the ratio of MMP-9 levels to TIMP-4 levels increased by more than 200% for 6 months post-MI, as illustrated in **Fig. 4**B.[105] Thus, the plasma signature in patients post-MI suggests a heterogeneity in matrix remodeling, which includes prosynthetic and degradative pathways that can culminate in a heterogeneous matrix, as shown in **Fig. 2**E.

CLINICAL APPLICATION OF THE MYOCARDIAL INTERSTITIUM
The Myocardial Interstitium and the Diagnostic and Prognostic Potential in Heart Failure

One potential clinical application in the context of developing heart failure is to monitor myocardial interstitial remodeling through plasma profiling determinants of matrix synthesis and degradation. For example, one study showed that plasma levels of PIP and PIIIP can be used in determining prognosis in patients with heart failure.[106] Higher plasma levels of these collagen synthesis markers were associated with increased hospitalization and mortality. In patients presenting with acute dyspnea, levels of the matrix signaling molecule galectin-3 were increased in those with an underlying myocardial cause, which may hold diagnostic relevance.[48,49] In addition, increased plasma galectin-3 was associated with increased hospitalizations and mortality in patients with heart failure.[48] Plasma levels of TIMP-1 have also been evaluated as a diagnostic tool in determining the transition to heart failure in POH secondary to hypertension.[103,107] For example, a specific cassette of matrix determinants, which included TIMP-1, can be predictive for the development of heart failure in patients with POH.[107] Plasma levels of MMPs and TIMPs have shown potential prognostic value with respect to cardiovascular events and mortality.[108] For example, the degree of LV dilation post-MI, which is a predictor of outcomes, has been associated with the magnitude of change in plasma MMP-9 (see **Fig. 4**C).[105] In another example, patients from the Framingham Heart Study showed a relationship between increased

plasma TIMP-1 levels and morbidity and mortality in heart failure.[108] Thus, plasma profiling of matrix signaling molecules and matrix proteases may have a role in monitoring the progression and predicting outcomes of patients in heart failure.

With respect to therapeutic interventions in heart failure, plasma profiling of myocardial matrix structural proteins and proteases may reflect the efficacy of therapy. In a substudy of the Eplerenone Post-Acute MI Heart Failure Efficacy and Survival Study (EPHESUS), selective aldosterone receptor antagonists resulted in clear changes in markers of collagen synthesis and degradation, which were associated with a decrease in all-cause mortality and the composite end point of cardiovascular death or heart failure hospitalization in patients post-MI.[109] In patients with POH secondary to hypertension, angiotensin-converting enzyme inhibitors have been shown to decrease plasma levels of TIMP-1.[79] In patients with end-stage heart failure secondary to DCM, LV assist device placement resulted in a time-dependent increase in plasma levels of PIP and PIIIP and decreased levels of MMP-9.[85,89] These findings suggest that a shift in matrix synthesis and degradation occurs, wherein LV assist devices promote a stabilization of the collagen matrix.

The myocardial interstitium is not a passive entity, but rather a complex and dynamic microenvironment that represents an important structural and signaling system within the myocardium. Future clinical research focusing on the molecular and cellular mechanisms that regulate the extracellular matrix structure and function will likely contribute to an improved understanding of the LV remodeling process in heart failure and yield novel diagnostic, prognostic, and therapeutic targets.

REFERENCES

1. Brower GL, Gardner JD, Forman MF, et al. The relationship between myocardial extracellular matrix remodeling and ventricular function. Eur J Cardiothorac Surg 2006;30(4):604–10.
2. Bowers SL, Banerjee I, Baudino TA. The extracellular matrix: at the center of it all. J Mol Cell Cardiol 2010;48(3):474–82.
3. Baumgarten G, Knuefermann P, Kalra D, et al. Load-dependent and -independent regulation of proinflammatory cytokine and cytokine receptor gene expression in the adult mammalian heart. Circulation 2002;105(18):2192–7.
4. Booz GW, Baker KM. Molecular signalling mechanisms controlling growth and function of cardiac fibroblasts. Cardiovasc Res 1995;30(4):537–43.
5. Briest W, Homagk L, Rassler B, et al. Norepinephrine-induced changes in cardiac transforming

growth factor-beta isoform expression pattern of female and male rats. Hypertension 2004;44(4):410–8.

6. Chen K, Mehta JL, Li D, et al. Transforming growth factor beta receptor endoglin is expressed in cardiac fibroblasts and modulates profibrogenic actions of angiotensin II. Circ Res 2004;95(12):1167–73.

7. Dell'Italia LJ, Meng QC, Balcells E, et al. Compartmentalization of angiotensin II generation in the dog heart. Evidence for independent mechanisms in intravascular and interstitial spaces. J Clin Invest 1997;100(2):253–8.

8. Diwan A, Dibbs Z, Nemoto S, et al. Targeted overexpression of noncleavable and secreted forms of tumor necrosis factor provokes disparate cardiac phenotypes. Circulation 2004;109(2):262–8.

9. Ergul A, Walker CA, Goldberg A, et al. ET-1 in the myocardial interstitium: relation to myocyte ECE activity and expression. Am J Physiol Heart Circ Physiol 2000;278(6):H2050–6.

10. Filion RJ, Popel AS. Intracoronary administration of FGF-2: a computational model of myocardial deposition and retention. Am J Physiol Heart Circ Physiol 2005;288(1):H263–79.

11. Frangogiannis NG, Ren G, Dewald O, et al. Critical role of endogenous thrombospondin-1 in preventing expansion of healing myocardial infarcts. Circulation 2005;111(22):2935–42.

12. Fuchs S, Skwara A, Bloch M, et al. Differential induction and regulation of matrix metalloproteinases in osteoarthritic tissue and fluid synovial fibroblasts. Osteoarthr Cartil 2004;12(5):409–18.

13. Multani MM, Ikonomidis JS, Kim PY, et al. Dynamic and differential changes in myocardial and plasma endothelin in patients undergoing cardiopulmonary bypass. J Thorac Cardiovasc Surg 2005;129(3):584–90.

14. Rodriguez-Vita J, Ruiz-Ortega M, Ruperez M, et al. Endothelin-1, via ETA receptor and independently of transforming growth factor-beta, increases the connective tissue growth factor in vascular smooth muscle cells. Circ Res 2005;97(2):125–34.

15. Romero JR, Rivera A, Lanca V, et al. Na+/Ca2+ exchanger activity modulates connective tissue growth factor mRNA expression in transforming growth factor beta1- and Des-Arg10-kallidin-stimulated myofibroblasts. J Biol Chem 2005;280(15):14378–84.

16. Wei CC, Meng QC, Palmer R, et al. Evidence for angiotensin-converting enzyme- and chymase-mediated angiotensin II formation in the interstitial fluid space of the dog heart in vivo. Circulation 1999;99(19):2583–9.

17. Gunja-Smith Z, Morales AR, Romanelli R, et al. Remodeling of human myocardial collagen in idiopathic dilated cardiomyopathy. Role of metalloproteinases and pyridinoline cross-links. Am J Pathol 1996;148(5):1639–48.

18. Burlew BS, Weber KT. Connective tissue and the heart. Functional significance and regulatory mechanisms. Cardiol Clin 2000;18(3):435–42.

19. Cleutjens JP, Verluyten MJ, Smiths JF, et al. Collagen remodeling after myocardial infarction in the rat heart. Am J Pathol 1995;147(2):325–38.

20. Keller RS, Shai SY, Babbitt CJ, et al. Disruption of integrin function in the murine myocardium leads to perinatal lethality, fibrosis, and abnormal cardiac performance. Am J Pathol 2001;158(3):1079–90.

21. Hornberger LK, Singhroy S, Cavalle-Garrido T, et al. Synthesis of extracellular matrix and adhesion through beta(1) integrins are critical for fetal ventricular myocyte proliferation. Circ Res 2000;87(6):508–15.

22. Spinale FG, Tomita M, Zellner JL, et al. Collagen remodeling and changes in LV function during development and recovery from supraventricular tachycardia. Am J Physiol 1991;261(2 Pt 2):H308–18.

23. Stroud JD, Baicu CF, Barnes MA, et al. Viscoelastic properties of pressure overload hypertrophied myocardium: effect of serine protease treatment. Am J Physiol Heart Circ Physiol 2002;282(6):H2324–35.

24. Baicu CF, Stroud JD, Livesay VA, et al. Changes in extracellular collagen matrix alter myocardial systolic performance. Am J Physiol Heart Circ Physiol 2003;284(1):H122–32.

25. Ross RS, Borg TK. Integrins and the myocardium. Circ Res 2001;88(11):1112–9.

26. Nimni ME. Fibrillar collagens: their biosynthesis, molecular structure, and mode of assembly. In: Zern MA, Reid LM, editors. Extracellular matrix. New York: Marcel Dekker, Inc; 1993. p. 121–48.

27. Borg TK, Klevay LM, Gay RE, et al. Alteration of the connective tissue network of striated muscle in copper deficient rats. J Mol Cell Cardiol 1985;17(12):1173–83.

28. Fomovsky GM, Thomopoulos S, Holmes JW. Contribution of extracellular matrix to the mechanical properties of the heart. J Mol Cell Cardiol 2010;48(3):490–6.

29. Kato S, Spinale FG, Tanaka R, et al. Inhibition of collagen cross-linking: effects on fibrillar collagen and ventricular diastolic function. Am J Physiol 1995;269(3 Pt 2):H863–8.

30. Asif M, Egan J, Vasan S, et al. An advanced glycation endproduct cross-link breaker can reverse age-related increases in myocardial stiffness. Proc Natl Acad Sci U S A 2000;97(6):2809–13.

31. Levene CI. Diseases of the collagen molecule. J Clin Pathol Suppl (R Coll Pathol) 1978;12:82–94.

32. Kunicki TJ. The role of platelet collagen receptor (glycoprotein Ia/IIa; integrin alpha2 beta1) polymorphisms in thrombotic disease. Curr Opin Hematol 2001;8(5):277–85.

33. Kuettner KE, Kimura JH. Proteoglycans: an overview. J Cell Biochem 1985;27(4):327–36.

34. Sivasubramanian N, Coker ML, Kurrelmeyer KM, et al. Left ventricular remodeling in transgenic mice with cardiac restricted overexpression of tumor necrosis factor. Circulation 2001;104(7):826–31.

35. Bradham WS, Bozkurt B, Gunasinghe H, et al. Tumor necrosis factor-alpha and myocardial remodeling in progression of heart failure: a current perspective. Cardiovasc Res 2002;53(4):822–30.

36. Fowlkes JL, Winkler MK. Exploring the interface between metallo-proteinase activity and growth factor and cytokine bioavailability. Cytokine Growth Factor Rev 2002;13(3):277–87.

37. Ogawa E, Saito Y, Harada M, et al. Outside-in signalling of fibronectin stimulates cardiomyocyte hypertrophy in cultured neonatal rat ventricular myocytes. J Mol Cell Cardiol 2000;32(5):765–76.

38. Bradshaw AD, Sage EH. SPARC, a matricellular protein that functions in cellular differentiation and tissue response to injury. J Clin Invest 2001; 107(9):1049–54.

39. McCurdy S, Baicu CF, Heymans S, et al. Cardiac extracellular matrix remodeling: fibrillar collagens and Secreted Protein Acidic and Rich in Cysteine (SPARC). J Mol Cell Cardiol 2010;48(3):544–9.

40. Schellings MW, Vanhoutte D, Swinnen M, et al. Absence of SPARC results in increased cardiac rupture and dysfunction after acute myocardial infarction. J Exp Med 2009;206(1):113–23.

41. Bradshaw AD, Baicu CF, Rentz TJ, et al. Pressure overload-induced alterations in fibrillar collagen content and myocardial diastolic function: role of secreted protein acidic and rich in cysteine (SPARC) in post-synthetic procollagen processing. Circulation 2009;119(2):269–80.

42. Bornstein P. Thrombospondins as matricellular modulators of cell function. J Clin Invest 2001; 107(8):929–34.

43. Schroen B, Heymans S, Sharma U, et al. Thrombospondin-2 is essential for myocardial matrix integrity: increased expression identifies failure-prone cardiac hypertrophy. Circ Res 2004;95(5):515–22.

44. Schellings MW, Pinto YM, Heymans S. Matricellular proteins in the heart: possible role during stress and remodeling. Cardiovasc Res 2004;64(1):24–31.

45. Murphy-Ullrich JE, Gurusiddappa S, Frazier WA, et al. Heparin-binding peptides from thrombospondins 1 and 2 contain focal adhesion-labilizing activity. J Biol Chem 1993;268(35):26784–9.

46. Spinale FG. Cell-matrix signaling and thrombospondin: another link to myocardial matrix remodeling. Circ Res 2004;95(5):446–8.

47. Swinnen M, Vanhoutte D, Van Almen GC, et al. Absence of thrombospondin-2 causes age-related dilated cardiomyopathy. Circulation 2009; 120(16):1585–97.

48. Shah RV, Chen-Tournoux AA, Picard MH, et al. Galectin-3, cardiac structure and function, and long-term mortality in patients with acutely decompensated heart failure. Eur J Heart Fail 2010;12(8): 826–32.

49. Zile MR, DeSantis SM, Baicu CF, et al. Plasma galectin-3 levels and relation to left ventricular function and the determinants of matrix composition in hypertensive heart disease. Circulation 2010;122(Suppl 21):A12433.

50. Border WA, Noble NA. Transforming growth factor beta in tissue fibrosis. N Engl J Med 1994; 331(19):1286–92.

51. Leask A. TGFbeta, cardiac fibroblasts, and the fibrotic response. Cardiovasc Res 2007;74(2): 207–12.

52. Lijnen PJ, Petrov VV, Fagard RH. Induction of cardiac fibrosis by transforming growth factor-beta(1). Mol Genet Metab 2000;71(1–2):418–35.

53. Hausenloy DJ, Yellon DM. Cardioprotective growth factors. Cardiovasc Res 2009;83(2):179–94.

54. Seeland U, Haeuseler C, Hinrichs R, et al. Myocardial fibrosis in transforming growth factor-beta(1) (TGF-beta(1)) transgenic mice is associated with inhibition of interstitial collagenase. Eur J Clin Invest 2002;32(5):295–303.

55. Frantz S, Hu K, Adamek A, et al. Transforming growth factor beta inhibition increases mortality and left ventricular dilatation after myocardial infarction. Basic Res Cardiol 2008;103(5):485–92.

56. Spinale FG. Myocardial matrix remodeling and the matrix metalloproteinases: influence on cardiac form and function. Physiol Rev 2007;87(4):1285–342.

57. Chapman RE, Spinale FG. Extracellular protease activation and unraveling of the myocardial interstitium: critical steps toward clinical applications. Am J Physiol Heart Circ Physiol 2004;286(1):H1–10.

58. Poole-Wilson PA. Relation of pathophysiologic mechanisms to outcome in heart failure. J Am Coll Cardiol 1993;22(4 Suppl A):22A–9A.

59. Douglas PS, Morrow R, Ioli A, et al. Left ventricular shape, afterload and survival in idiopathic dilated cardiomyopathy. J Am Coll Cardiol 1989;13(2): 311–5.

60. Nagase H, Visse R, Murphy G. Structure and function of matrix metalloproteinases and TIMPs. Cardiovasc Res 2006;69(3):562–73.

61. Malemud CJ. Matrix metalloproteinases (MMPs) in health and disease: an overview. Front Biosci 2006; 11:1696–701.

62. Hwang IK, Park SM, Kim SY, et al. A proteomic approach to identify substrates of matrix metalloproteinase-14 in human plasma. Biochim Biophys Acta 2004;1702(1):79–87.

63. Thomas CV, Coker ML, Zellner JL, et al. Increased matrix metalloproteinase activity and selective upregulation in LV myocardium from patients with

end-stage dilated cardiomyopathy. Circulation 1998;97(17):1708–15.

64. Spinale FG, Coker ML, Heung LJ, et al. A matrix metalloproteinase induction/activation system exists in the human left ventricular myocardium and is upregulated in heart failure. Circulation 2000;102(16):1944–9.

65. Li YY, Feldman AM, Sun Y, et al. Differential expression of tissue inhibitors of metalloproteinases in the failing human heart. Circulation 1998;98(17):1728–34.

66. Lovelock JD, Baker AH, Gao F, et al. Heterogeneous effects of tissue inhibitors of matrix metalloproteinases on cardiac fibroblasts. Am J Physiol Heart Circ Physiol 2005;288(2):H461–8.

67. Guedez L, Stetler-Stevenson WG, Wolff L, et al. In vitro suppression of programmed cell death of B cells by tissue inhibitor of metalloproteinases-1. J Clin Invest 1998;102(11):2002–10.

68. Fielitz J, Leuschner M, Zurbrugg HR, et al. Regulation of matrix metalloproteinases and their inhibitors in the left ventricular myocardium of patients with aortic stenosis. J Mol Med 2004;82(12):809–20.

69. Polyakova V, Hein S, Kostin S, et al. Matrix metalloproteinases and their tissue inhibitors in pressure-overloaded human myocardium during heart failure progression. J Am Coll Cardiol 2004;44(8):1609–18.

70. Heymans S, Schroen B, Vermeersch P, et al. Increased cardiac expression of tissue inhibitor of metalloproteinase-1 and tissue inhibitor of metalloproteinase-2 is related to cardiac fibrosis and dysfunction in the chronic pressure-overloaded human heart. Circulation 2005;112(8):1136–44.

71. Hess OM, Ritter M, Schneider J, et al. Diastolic stiffness and myocardial structure in aortic valve disease before and after valve replacement. Circulation 1984;69(5):855–65.

72. Monrad ES, Hess OM, Murakami T, et al. Time course of regression of left ventricular hypertrophy after aortic valve replacement. Circulation 1988; 77(6):1345–55.

73. Villari B, Vassalli G, Monrad ES, et al. Normalization of diastolic dysfunction in aortic stenosis late after valve replacement. Circulation 1995;91(9):2353–8.

74. Krayenbuehl HP, Hess OM, Monrad ES, et al. Left ventricular myocardial structure in aortic valve disease before, intermediate, and late after aortic valve replacement. Circulation 1989;79(4):744–55.

75. Villari B, Campbell SE, Hess OM, et al. Influence of collagen network on left ventricular systolic and diastolic function in aortic valve disease. J Am Coll Cardiol 1993;22(5):1477–84.

76. Zile MR, Baicu CF, Gaasch WH. Diastolic heart failure–abnormalities in active relaxation and passive stiffness of the left ventricle. N Engl J Med 2004;350(19):1953–9.

77. Villar AV, Llano M, Cobo M, et al. Gender differences of echocardiographic and gene expression patterns in human pressure overload left ventricular hypertrophy. J Mol Cell Cardiol 2009;46(4):526–35.

78. Lopez B, Gonzalez A, Querejeta R, et al. The use of collagen-derived serum peptides for the clinical assessment of hypertensive heart disease. J Hypertens 2005;23(8):1445–51.

79. Laviades C, Varo N, Fernandez J, et al. Abnormalities of the extracellular degradation of collagen type I in essential hypertension. Circulation 1998; 98(6):535–40.

80. Timms PM, Wright A, Maxwell P, et al. Plasma tissue inhibitor of metalloproteinase-1 levels are elevated in essential hypertension and related to left ventricular hypertrophy. Am J Hypertens 2002;15(3):269–72.

81. Tayebjee MH, Nadar SK, MacFadyen RJ, et al. Tissue inhibitor of metalloproteinase-1 and matrix metalloproteinase-9 levels in patients with hypertension Relationship to tissue Doppler indices of diastolic relaxation. Am J Hypertens 2004;17(9): 770–4.

82. Barton PJ, Birks EJ, Felkin LE, et al. Increased expression of extracellular matrix regulators TIMP1 and MMP1 in deteriorating heart failure. J Heart Lung Transplant 2003;22(7):738–44.

83. Herpel E, Singer S, Flechtenmacher C, et al. Extracellular matrix proteins and matrix metalloproteinases differ between various right and left ventricular sites in end-stage cardiomyopathies. Virchows Arch 2005;446(4):369–78.

84. Klotz S, Foronjy RF, Dickstein ML, et al. Mechanical unloading during left ventricular assist device support increases left ventricular collagen cross-linking and myocardial stiffness. Circulation 2005; 112(3):364–74.

85. Li YY, Feng Y, McTiernan CF, et al. Downregulation of matrix metalloproteinases and reduction in collagen damage in the failing human heart after support with left ventricular assist devices. Circulation 2001;104(10):1147–52.

86. Mukherjee R, Herron AR, Lowry AS, et al. Selective induction of matrix metalloproteinases and tissue inhibitor of metalloproteinases in atrial and ventricular myocardium in patients with atrial fibrillation. Am J Cardiol 2006;97(4):532–7.

87. Felkin LE, Lara-Pezzi E, George R, et al. Expression of extracellular matrix genes during myocardial recovery from heart failure after left ventricular assist device support. J Heart Lung Transplant 2009;28(2):117–22.

88. Batlle M, Perez-Villa F, Lazaro A, et al. Decreased expression of thrombospondin-1 in failing hearts may favor ventricular remodeling. Transplant Proc 2009;41(6):2231–3.

89. Bruggink AH, van Oosterhout MF, de Jonge N, et al. Reverse remodeling of the myocardial extracellular matrix after prolonged left ventricular assist

device support follows a biphasic pattern. J Heart Lung Transplant 2006;25(9):1091–8.

90. Erlebacher JA, Weiss JL, Weisfeldt ML, et al. Early dilation of the infarcted segment in acute transmural myocardial infarction: role of infarct expansion in acute left ventricular enlargement. J Am Coll Cardiol 1984;4(2):201–8.

91. Pfeffer MA, Braunwald E. Ventricular remodeling after myocardial infarction. Experimental observations and clinical implications. Circulation 1990; 81(4):1161–72.

92. Sutton MG, Sharpe N. Left ventricular remodeling after myocardial infarction: pathophysiology and therapy. Circulation 2000;101(25):2981–8.

93. St John Sutton M, Pfeffer MA, Plappert T, et al. Quantitative two-dimensional echocardiographic measurements are major predictors of adverse cardiovascular events after acute myocardial infarction. The protective effects of captopril. Circulation 1994;89(1):68–75.

94. Doughty RN, Whalley GA, Gamble G, et al. Left ventricular remodeling with carvedilol in patients with congestive heart failure due to ischemic heart disease. Australia-New Zealand Heart Failure Research Collaborative Group. J Am Coll Cardiol 1997;29(5):1060–6.

95. Spinale FG, Koval CN, Deschamps AM, et al. Dynamic changes in matrix metalloproteinase activity within the human myocardial interstitium during myocardial arrest and reperfusion. Circulation 2008;118(Suppl 14):S16–23.

96. Dinh W, Futh R, Scheffold T, et al. Increased serum levels of tissue inhibitor of metalloproteinase-1 in patients with acute myocardial infarction. Int Heart J 2009;50(4):421–31.

97. McGavigan AD, Maxwell PR, Dunn FG. Serological evidence of altered collagen homeostasis reflects early ventricular remodeling following acute myocardial infarction. Int J Cardiol 2006;111(2):267–74.

98. Hlatky MA, Ashley E, Quertermous T, et al. Matrix metalloproteinase circulating levels, genetic polymorphisms, and susceptibility to acute myocardial infarction among patients with coronary artery disease. Am Heart J 2007;154(6):1043–51.

99. Kai H, Ikeda H, Yasukawa H, et al. Peripheral blood levels of matrix metalloproteases-2 and -9 are elevated in patients with acute coronary syndromes. J Am Coll Cardiol 1998;32(2):368–72.

100. Squire IB, Evans J, Ng LL, et al. Plasma MMP-9 and MMP-2 following acute myocardial infarction in man: correlation with echocardiographic and neurohumoral parameters of left ventricular dysfunction. J Card Fail 2004;10(4):328–33.

101. Wagner DR, Delagardelle C, Ernens I, et al. Matrix metalloproteinase-9 is a marker of heart failure after acute myocardial infarction. J Card Fail 2006;12(1): 66–72.

102. van den Borne SW, Cleutjens JP, Hanemaaijer R, et al. Increased matrix metalloproteinase-8 and -9 activity in patients with infarct rupture after myocardial infarction. Cardiovasc Pathol 2009;18(1): 37–43.

103. Ahmed SH, Clark LL, Pennington WR, et al. Matrix metalloproteinases/tissue inhibitors of metalloproteinases: relationship between changes in proteolytic determinants of matrix composition and structural, functional, and clinical manifestations of hypertensive heart disease. Circulation 2006; 113(17):2089–96.

104. Kelly D, Cockerill G, Ng LL, et al. Plasma matrix metalloproteinase-9 and left ventricular remodelling after acute myocardial infarction in man: a prospective cohort study. Eur Heart J 2007;28(6):711–8.

105. Webb CS, Bonnema DD, Ahmed SH, et al. Specific temporal profile of matrix metalloproteinase release occurs in patients after myocardial infarction: relation to left ventricular remodeling. Circulation 2006; 114(10):1020–7.

106. Zannad F, Alla F, Dousset B, et al. Limitation of excessive extracellular matrix turnover may contribute to survival benefit of spironolactone therapy in patients with congestive heart failure: insights from the randomized aldactone evaluation study (RALES). Rales Investigators. Circulation 2000;102(22):2700–6.

107. Zile MR, DeSantis SM, Baicu CF, et al. Plasma biomarkers that reflect determinants of matrix composition identify the presence of left ventricular hypertrophy and diastolic heart failure. Circ Heart Fail 2011;4(3):246–56.

108. Sundstrom J, Evans JC, Benjamin EJ, et al. Relations of plasma total TIMP-1 levels to cardiovascular risk factors and echocardiographic measures: the Framingham heart study. Eur Heart J 2004;25(17): 1509–16.

109. Iraqi W, Rossignol P, Angioi M, et al. Extracellular cardiac matrix biomarkers in patients with acute myocardial infarction complicated by left ventricular dysfunction and heart failure: insights from the Eplerenone Post-Acute Myocardial Infarction Heart Failure Efficacy and Survival Study (EPHESUS) study. Circulation 2009;119(18):2471–9.

Pressure Overload

Edward D. Frohlich, MD[a],*, Dinko Susic, MD, PhD[b]

KEYWORDS

- Ventricular hypertrophy • Ventricular dysfunction
- Molecular mechanisms of myocardial hypertrophy
- Heart failure

Pressure overload imposes hemodynamic burden on the left ventricle (LV), which, in turn, initiates a series of events leading to ventricular remodeling, hypertrophy, and eventually heart failure (HF). According to classical concept, pressure overload leads to left (LVH) through the growth of cardiomyocytes and nonmyocytic components of the myocardium. Apparently, the pattern of ventricular remodeling depends on the form of cardiac stress. Thus, concentric hypertrophy develops in response to pressure load and eccentric hypertrophy develops in response to volume overload, whereas in response to the loss of myocardial tissue (after infarction), stretch and dilation of infarcted tissue increases ventricular volume, which is accompanied by hypertrophy of the noninfarcted myocardial tissue. Further, this process is regarded as an adaptive and, at least initially, beneficial event that serves to normalize wall stress and, therefore, to mechanically compensate the heart. Thereafter, this apparently compensated hypertrophy transitions to HF. The question is at what point in the natural history of ventricular hypertrophy does this adaptive, beneficial event become maladaptive resulting in a failing heart? The classical descriptions by Meerson and Grossman[1–3] clearly distinguished a compensated phase from a decompensated phase. However, novel studies indicate that ventricular remodeling in response to stress includes both adaptive and maladaptive myocardial reactions and that any degree of hypertrophy is detrimental for function and eventually survival.[4]

This article reviews the effects of pressure overload (hypertension, aortic stenosis, coarctation of the aorta) on the ventricles, including structural, functional, cellular, and molecular aspects. Most of the data relate to the LV but similar principles may presumably be applied to the right.

PRESSURE OVERLOAD: DEFINITION

Pressure overload is one of the numerous forms of cardiac stress that may induce ventricular remodeling, involving changes in the chamber architecture, cardiomyocytes, and in nonmyocytic elements. The term remodeling was originally used to describe ventricular changes that occur after myocardial infarction but now it is widely used to describe myocardial responses to various stressors, including pressure and volume overloads, loss of tissue caused by infarction, neurohumoral activation, and so forth.[5,6] The most common disease entities that exert pressure overload are essential hypertension, aortic stenosis, subvalvular aortic stenosis (also known as subaortic stenosis), and coarctation of the aorta (**Box 1**). It is generally accepted that the mechanical stress (ie, an increase in pressure) initiates a series of events that eventually result in the ventricular remodeling. However, an isolated increase in pressure (ie, pure mechanical stress) without simultaneous neurohumoral activation of varying degrees seldom, if ever, occurs in a living organism. Thus, in addition to pure mechanical stress, pressure overload also implies neural and

The authors have nothing to disclose.
[a] Hypertension Research Laboratory, Ochsner Clinic Foundation, 1514 Jefferson Highway, New Orleans, LA 70121, USA
[b] Hypertension Research Laboratory, Division of Research, Ochsner Clinic Foundation, 1514 Jefferson Highway, New Orleans, LA 70121, USA
* Corresponding author.
E-mail address: efrohlich@ochsner.org

Heart Failure Clin 8 (2012) 21–32
doi:10.1016/j.hfc.2011.08.005

humoral influences that may modify, exacerbate, or inhibit ventricular responses. It is worth noting that the possible involvement of neural and humoral factors in ventricular response to mechanical stress feeds long-lasting controversies over the role of nonpressure factors in the development of ventricular hypertrophy and on whether some antihypertensive agents are better than others in preventing or reversing hypertrophy.

Cautionary Factors

When discussing pressure-overload hypertrophy, several disease entities, such as essential hypertension, aortic stenosis, subvalvular aortic stenosis, and coarctation of the aorta, are usually considered. Each of these disorders has one common denominator: increased LV pressure. On the other hand, there are also numerous differences between them. Several earlier studies were related to aortic and subvalvular aortic stenosis and the results were extrapolated to patients with essential hypertension. However, there is an enormous difference between them in systemic hemodynamics. Arterial pressure and total peripheral resistance are normal in patients with aortic stenosis. On the other hand, in essential hypertension, there is an increase in systolic and diastolic pressure and an increase in peripheral resistance with arteriolar changes throughout the body that may result in neurohumoral disturbances and local changes, including myocardial ischemia. Therefore, although LV pressure may be the same, the myocardium may be exposed to different influences in different disorders. Furthermore, aortic stenosis and subvalvular aortic stenosis are often accompanied by varying degrees of valvular insufficiency and, consequently, in addition to pressure volume factors, may also be operative. Similarly, the myocardial consequences of secondary hypertension, such as renovascular hypertension or hyperaldosteronism, may differ from those in essential hypertension. Thus, it is of importance to be cautious when extrapolating results obtained from different diseases, although they may have common abnormalities and consequences.

Confounding Factors

In addition to neurohumoral activation, several other pathologic confounding factors may modify the myocardial response to mechanical load. These factors include concomitant obesity; concomitant diseases, such as diabetes; coronary arterial disease; the aging process; genetic and racial factors; and sodium intake. Some of these confounders (obesity, sodium intake) may be associated with an additional increased volume load on the ventricle and the others may directly affect myocardium through ischemia, inflammation, or protein deposition. It is also worth noting that sodium intake should be considered an important confounding factor in pressure-overload hypertrophy, although it is often disregarded. Because a clear correlation was found between sodium intake and arterial pressure in clinical and experimental studies, it is usually assumed that sodium exerts adverse cardiovascular effect indirectly through the increase in arterial pressure.[7,8] However, a great deal of experimental studies conclusively demonstrated that excessive sodium intake exerted adverse cardiovascular and renal effects independent of arterial pressure. Thus, in normotensive rats, although sodium excess need not increase arterial pressure, it significantly increases LV mass and myocardial collagen deposition and decreases ventricular function.[8–10] Furthermore, in salt-loaded, spontaneously hypertensive rats, therapy with agents that inhibit the renin-angiotensin system prevented the development of ventricular hypertrophy but did not prevent the increase in arterial pressure.[11,12] There are no clinical studies that specifically addressed this subject, but the results of a recent long-term observational study demonstrated a significant (25%) reduction in cardiovascular end points in patients with lower salt intake even after accounting for confounding factors.[13]

CARDIAC CONSEQUENCES OF PRESSURE OVERLOAD
Structural Remodeling of the Myocardium

In response to prolonged pressure overload the ventricle hypertrophies. This is an adaptive, compensatory phenomenon as is expressed in Laplace law,

$$T = (P \times R) / M$$

tension in the wall (T) is proportional to the pressure difference between the ventricle and surrounding environment (P) and to ventricular radius (*R*), whereas it is inversely proportional to wall thickness (*M*). Thus, in response to increased pressure and the consequent increase in ventricular wall tension and stress, wall thickness and mass increase, in the presence of unchanged volume, result in the normalization of wall stress.[2] This type of hypertrophy is called concentric.[2] The consequent hypertrophy then reduces the wall stress, which together with the switch to slower contraction and anaerobic metabolism (as discussed later) ultimately results in better-adapted muscle.[14]

Adult cardiomyocytes were considered terminally differentiated cells unable to divide, and, therefore, ventricular hypertrophy was thought to result from the growth (hypertrophy) of individual myocytes and hypertrophy and hyperplasia of nonmyocytic cells.[15,16] However, recent experimental studies conclusively demonstrated the hyperplastic growth of myocardial cells, at least under certain specific conditions.[17–19] Some earlier morphometric clinical studies of human hearts also demonstrated that myocytic proliferation may occur in severely hypertrophic hearts.[20,21] Furthermore, more recent studies unequivocally demonstrated that myocyte regeneration occurs in humans and animals after myocardial infarction, after prolonged pressure overload, and in the senescent decompensated heart.[22–25] The origin of the replicating cardiomyocytes is not clear. They may be derived from resident cardiac stem cells or from circulating stem cells that have homed to the heart.[26] All of these observations have challenged the view of the heart as a postmitotic organ and have proposed a new paradigm in which parenchymal and nonparenchymal cells are continuously replaced by newly formed, younger populations of myocytes as well as by vascular smooth muscle and endothelial cells.[26,27] Thus, it seems that the increased cardiac mass in LVH may result from a combination of hypertrophy and hyperplasia of both myocytes and nonmyocytic cells, although there may still be opposing views.[28]

At the cellular level, concentric LVH is characterized by an increase in the cardiomyocytes width, mostly caused by the parallel addition of new sarcomeres.[29] In contrast, in eccentric VH, resulting from volume overload, there is an increase in cardiomyocyte length, which is caused by the addition of new sarcomeres in series. The intricate mechanism for this difference in cellular response to pressure versus volume overload still remains unknown. The hypertrophied ventricle is also associated with hyperplasia of fibroblasts, increased synthesis of extracellular matrix proteins, and fibrosis.[30–33] Excessive fibroblast

proliferation accompanied by the accumulation of collagen and fibrosis induces myocardial stiffening, which is an important pathophysiologic facet of cardiac dysfunction.[34,35] In LVH, there is also a change in the amount and composition of various cell proteins, enzymes, and structures.[36] Actually, the first report of protein modifications in cardiac overload was a change in myosin isoforms.[37] In small animals, with a faster heart rate, pressure overload induces a switch from *alpha* to *beta* myosin isoform that results in decreased myosin ATPase activity and shortening velocity.[38] In larger animals, including man, with slower heart rates, cardiac myocytes contain almost exclusively *beta* myosin isoform, and this switch does not occur. However, the small amount of *alpha* myosin that is expressed in human hearts switches to *beta* isoform in HF and this may contribute to contractile dysfunction.[39] There are also changes in some cytoskeletal proteins, such as titin in LVH, which may be involved in the development of hypertrophy.[40,41]

Cardiac Function in LVH

LVH has been long recognized as an independent risk factor for cardiovascular morbidity and mortality, including sudden cardiac death and dysrhythmia, heart failure, ventricular ischemia, and coronary heart disease.[3,32,33,42–44] Thus, it is obvious that structural and functional changes in the myocardium that occur with LVH constitute the basis for that increased risk, although, at least in the early stages, hypertrophy may seem to be a beneficial, adaptive phenomenon. Both clinical and experimental studies demonstrate that the progression of functional changes in LVH progresses in parallel with structural changes from normal ventricle and myocyte function to hypertrophied ventricle and normal myocyte function to hypertrophied ventricle with myocyte dysfunction. These changes involve electrical and mechanical properties of the myocardium as well as coronary circulation.

Electrical properties of the myocardium in LVH

The existence of LVH is a strong predictor for the development of cardiac arrhythmias, including atrial fibrillation, ventricular ectopy, and sudden cardiac death.[45] A finding that antihypertensive therapy significantly reduced VH and improved functional capacity and electrical stability of the ventricle further confirms the causal relationship between LVH and cardiac dysrhythmias.[46] However, pathophysiological mechanisms involved in this increased arrhythmogenic propensity of hypertrophied myocardium are still not completely understood.

Apparently, an interaction of several factors contributes to the development of atrial fibrillation. Increased left atrial pressure with consequent distension, stretching, and increased atrial size may alter atrial electrophysiological properties, including the shortening of the effective refractory period and the increased dispersion of refractoriness with subsequent increase in arrhythmogenicity.[47–49] Atrial fibrosis is another factor in the development of fibrillation.[50] Neurohumoral activation, particularly activation of the renin-angiotensin-aldosterone system, through its proinflammatory properties (increase in reactive oxygen species, inflammatory cytokines, and adhesion molecules), is also considered as one of the mechanisms in the development of fibrillation.[51,52]

Similarly, several factors are responsible for ventricular arrhythmogenicity in LVH including myocardial fibrosis and ischemia as well as neurohumoral activation.[45] The excessive accumulation of fibrillar collagen is a characteristic feature of hypertensive heart disease. The increased myocardial fibrosis may lead to the distortion of the tissue structure and increased stiffness of the myocardium to promote diastolic dysfunction.[53,54] These structural changes in the myocardium related to fibrosis can lead to the nonhomogeneous propagation of electrical impulses and give rise to ventricular arrhythmias caused by reentry.[45] Furthermore, microvascular dysfunction with myocardial ischemia has been reported in patients with hypertension and LVH, and the presence of myocardial ischemia may trigger the onset of ventricular arrhythmia and sudden death in those patients.[55] Neuroendocrine activation is also thought to play a role in the development of ventricular arrhythmias in LVH. Thus, sympathetic activation has been shown to exert a direct proarrhythmic effect that may lead to ventricular arrhythmia and sudden cardiac death.[56] Although no direct link has been demonstrated between angiotensin II and ventricular arrhythmias, angiotensin II leads to LVH via direct trophic actions on the heart that subsequently increase vulnerability to ventricular arrhythmias.[57] Electrophysiologically, it has been well established that prolongation and dispersion of ventricular repolarization as it occurs in LVH are associated with an increased risk of ventricular tachyarrhythmias.[58] Further, prolongation of the QT interval similar to a pharmacologically induced proarrhythmic effect has also been observed in LVH.[59] At a cellular level, structural remodeling induced by hypertension is associated with impaired cell-cell communication at the gap junction and increased susceptibility to ventricular arrhythmia.[60] It should be noted that vulnerability to ventricular dysrhythmias is not necessarily related to abnormal calcium channel handling.[61]

Finally, although the direct causal relationship between LVH and sudden cardiac death has not been established, the results of the Framingham Heart Study demonstrate that an incremental increase in left ventricular (LV) mass for 50 g/m^2 conferred a 45% higher risk of sudden death in patients aged more than 40 years.[62]

Mechanical properties of the myocardium in LVH

Hypertrophy is a response to the increased LV afterload (elevated vascular resistance and arterial pressure) as well as an adaptive and protective process up to a certain point. Beyond that, a variety of dysfunctions occur, including alterations in ventricular wall mechanics and function. Even before LVH develops in patients with hypertension, it is possible to detect changes in ventricular function. Thus, the earliest functional changes are in LV diastolic function, with a lower E/A ratio and prolonged isovolumic relaxation time.[63,64] With the progression of hypertension and increasing hemodynamic load, either systolic or diastolic dysfunction becomes apparent and then progresses to HF.[65]

Mechanical function of the hypertrophied heart has been studied at different levels, from those of isolated myocytes to intact circulation. The results of these studies have demonstrated numerous alterations in myocardial contraction and relaxation as well as in the cardiac properties at rest.[66–68] A characteristic of pressure overload LVH is the existence of so-called isolated diastolic dysfunction or diastolic dysfunction with normal ejection fraction.[66,67,69] Pathophysiological mechanisms leading to alterations in cardiac performance in LVH include changes in cardiomyocytes, extracellular matrix, myocardial perfusion, and neurohumoral factors.[66–68,70,71] Alterations in myocytes include changes in the expression of contractile proteins, enzymes (lactic dehydrogenase, creatine kinase, nitric oxide synthase, Ca^{2+}-ATPase of sarcoplasmic reticulum), humoral factors (atrial natriuretic factors, components of the renin-angiotensin system), and cytoskeletal proteins.[42,70,71] Calcium homeostasis is disturbed because of the changes in sarcolemmal Ca^{2+} channels responsible for the short- and long-term extrusion of calcium from the cytosol; decreased sarcoplasmic reticulum calcium Ca^{2+} reuptake caused by a decrease in Ca^{2+} ATPase; and the altered phosphorylation of calcium-handling proteins, such as phospholamban, calmodulin, and calsequestrin.[42,70,72] These changes may promote abnormalities in excitation-contraction coupling as well as active relaxation and passive stiffness of cardiomyocytes.[42,70,73] Energy metabolism in the cardiomyocytes may also be altered, which may also affect the relaxation process.[42,70] Furthermore, changes in cytoskeletal proteins (titin, desmin) have been shown to alter diastolic function.[41,42]

Pressure-overload LVH is invariably accompanied by the accumulation of fibrillar collagen in the extracellular matrix.[74] Collagens (mostly types I and III in myocardium) are synthetized by fibroblast and their function is to support myocytes and maintain their alignment. Their tensile strength and resilience resist the deformation, maintain the shape and thickness, prevent the rupture, and contribute to the passive and active stiffness of the myocardium. In the hypertrophic process that accompanies a pressure overload, increased collagen synthesis, fibroblast proliferation, and a structural and biochemical remodeling of the matrix are seen. This myocardial fibrosis alters myocardial stiffness and consequently affects myocardial function.[33,34,74] There is general agreement that extracellular matrix remodeling may exert a profound effect on diastolic function.[74,75] On the other hand, a definite cause-and-effect relationship between excessive collagen accumulation and systolic function has not been established.[75] Furthermore, there is evidence that indicates that the reduction in myocardial collagen matrix could exacerbate the severity of HF.[75] Abnormalities in the collagen scaffold facilitate alterations in physiologic orientation of the muscular fibers resulting in the impairment of the transmission of contractile force through the myocardial wall.[76] It has been suggested that the architecture of the scaffold plays a significant role in determining ventricular function.[76] Myocardial ischemia may also participate in the deterioration of myocardial function in LVH.[42,68]

Neurohumoral activation may participate in determining cardiac function, which includes the production of local, cardiac components of the renin-angiotensin system, cytokines, and growth factors.[42,77] Aside from the circulating renin-angiotensin systems, its components are synthesized locally by cardiomyocytes and fibroblasts and, by acting in the autocrine or paracrine manner, may affect ventricular remodeling and function.[77–79] Although there are still many unresolved issues, recent evidence suggests that under normal loading conditions, cardiac angiotensin II does not affect cardiac size or function. However, in hypertension, cardiac angiotensin, acting via angiotensin II, type 1, receptors, enhances inflammation, oxidative stress, and cell death.[77–79] In this manner, it contributes to alterations in hypertrophic remodeling, progression of fibrosis, and cardiac function. The expression of numerous growth factors and cytokines is increased in VH, which may also contribute to the development and progression of hypertrophy.[70,71]

Coronary circulation in LVH

Both myocardial oxygen demand and perfusion through coronary circulation are altered in VH. Oxygen demand of hypertrophic ventricle is increased because of the increased work load and myocardial mass.[80] Morphologic studies of hypertrophied hearts from experimental animals and patients with pressure-overload hypertrophy show that the ratio of capillaries to myocytes is not different from normal hearts.[81] However, because of the myocytic hypertrophic growth, relative capillary density (number of capillaries per unit of mass) is decreased.[3,82] Therefore, even in the absence of large vessel occlusion caused by atherosclerotic coronary artery disease, there is a mismatch between oxygen demand and supply. This mismatch translates into the reduced capacity of hypertrophied myocardium to adequately increase flow in response to increased demand. It may not be apparent at rest but ischemia of varying degrees may become apparent when demand is increased, with exercise for instance. Pathophysiologically, it is manifested as increased minimal coronary vascular resistance and decreased coronary flow reserve (the difference between basal and maximal coronary blood flow) during maximal vasodilation.[3,82] The main mechanisms controlling coronary artery tone are metabolic, myogenic, neurohormonal, and endothelial. Apparently, large coronary arteries have a greater dependency on endothelium-dependent mechanisms for the maintenance of proper tone, whereas smaller arterioles depend more on metabolic and myogenic mechanisms.[83] Nitric oxide produced by vascular endothelium is the primary dilator of large epicardial coronary arteries, and several studies have suggested that altered nitric oxide bioavailability contributes to the altered vasomotion seen in hypertension.[83] Therapy with a nitric oxide precursor has been reported to improve altered coronary circulation.[84]

Box 2 summarizes cardiac consequences of pressure overload.

CLINICAL CORRELATES

Clinically, long-standing pressure overload results in ventricular hypertrophy; in essential

> **Box 2**
> **Cardiac consequences of pressure overload**
>
> 1. Structural remodeling of the myocardium
>
>   Cardiomyocytes
>
>   Nonmyocytic cells
>
>   Extracellular matrix
>
> 2. Alterations in cardiac function
>
>   Electrical properties of the myocardium
>
>   Mechanical properties of the myocardium
>
>   Coronary circulation

hypertension it is LVH. Electrocardiography and echocardiography are the two most common methods for the assessment of LVH, with electrocardiography having a high specificity but low sensitivity. In patients with hypertension, the prevalence of LVH increases with the severity of hypertension, age, and obesity. It ranges from 20% in patients with mild hypertension to almost 100% in those with severe or complicated hypertension, as determined by echocardiography.[85] LVH is also an independent risk factor for cardiovascular morbidity and mortality.[43,86] Furthermore, several studies demonstrated that the geometric pattern of hypertrophy translates into different levels of risk, with concentric hypertrophy having the greatest risk.[87,88] The underlying factors for the association between LVH and the risk of cardiovascular disease may include a combination of electrophysiological alterations, myocardial structural changes, and increased sympathetic and renin-angiotensin system activity.[89,90] Finally, the results of several studies demonstrated conclusively that the regression of hypertrophy is associated with the reduction of cardiovascular risk, a finding that supports the notion of a causal relationship between LVH and cardiovascular risk.[91,92]

Hypertrophy of the ventricle normalizes wall stress and, at least at the beginning of ventricular function, seems to be normal. However, with the progression of time, signs and symptoms of heart dysfunction slowly develop.[43,66,86,93] As already mentioned, the earliest functional changes involve LV diastolic function and the may develop even before LVH becomes apparent.[94] Diastolic dysfunction is characteristic of concentric, pressure-overloaded hypertrophy and it involves abnormalities in ventricular filling, including decreased distensibility and impaired relaxation.[66,93] Of course, systolic dysfunction may also develop, particularly in cases whereby

myocardial mass is reduced because of ischemia and apoptosis or when calcium handling by myocytes is affected.[68] With time, ventricular dysfunction slowly progresses to HF, with either preserved or reduced ejection fraction.[95] In patients who have hypertension with pressure-overload hypertrophy, the proportion of patients that have HF with preserved ejection fraction (diastolic failure) is relatively high.[66,95] It also increases with age, from 46% in patients aged younger than 45 years to 59% in patients aged older than 85 years.[95] In terms of function and symptoms, systolic and diastolic dysfunction are practically identical. However, structural and echocardiographic features differ significantly.[42,66,68] For instance, interstitial collagen is increased in diastolic HF but normal or decreased in systolic HF. There are numerous therapeutic options in the treatment of HF in VH.[42,96,97] However, despite the development of novel drugs and new generations of old drugs, the prognosis of HF still remained grim.[98] As in many other disorders, cardiac delivery of transgenes and stem cell therapy are now regarded as possible new and potent therapeutic tools.[28,99] To date, bone marrow stem cells, endogenous populations of cardiac stem cells, embryonic stem cells, and induced pluripotent stem cells have been investigated for their ability to regenerate myocardium.[99,100] Strategies for regenerating the heart are being realized because both animal and clinical trials suggest that these new approaches provide a short-term improvement of cardiac function.[25,101] However, a more complete understanding of the underlying mechanisms and applications is necessary to sustain longer-term therapeutic success.

MOLECULAR MECHANISMS OF VH

There is general agreement on the basic principles involved in the cardiac response to pressure overload. Several extensive and excellent reviews that cover this topic have been published in the last decade and the authors provide only an outline herein.[4,6,70,71,80] There are 3 basic steps:

1. The remodeling of the heart in VH is activated by biomechanical stress resulting from the causal disorder, increased pressure in essential hypertension for instance. This biomechanical stress combines diverse degrees of diastolic stretching and systolic overload and varying degrees of neurohumoral activation, either local myocardial or systemic. Mechanical stress is most likely sensed by membrane and sarcomere coupled stretch receptors, whereas neurohumoral stress is sensed by various

membrane receptors, including G-protein coupled receptors.[4,80]

2. These mechanical and neurohumoral factors activate numerous intracellular signaling pathways, integrated into a complex web, which transmits the signal to the nucleus. The 2 key enzymes that activate transcription factors are calcium dependent.[4] These enzymes are CaM-KII, a serine/threonine kinase that phosphorylates several key proteins, and Calcineurin, a Ca/calmodulin-dependent phosphatase.[4,80] On the other hand, G-protein coupled receptors signal through G proteins, such as Gαq, Gαs, and Rho family members.[4,80] Modulation of phospholipase C and adenylyl and guanylyl cyclases directly control downstream effectors such as kinases and phosphatases.[80]

3. Through these signaling pathways, transcriptional factors are activated with the resulting expression of various genes in the cardiac myocytes and nonmyocytic cells and consequent phenotype changes. An interesting approach has been used to detect transcription factors involved in gene activation in myocardial hypertrophy. Thus, Hannenhalli and colleagues[102] searched for enriched transcription factor binding sites in the promoters of genes that were differentially expressed in hypertrophy. They found that the most overrepresented transcription binding sites included nuclear factor of activated T cells, myocyte enhancer factor, globin transcription factor, interferon regulatory factor, and so forth.[4] All of these foregoing events culminate in an altered transcription that includes the re-induction of the fetal gene program and new cellular growth.[70,80]

Oversimplifying the hypertrophy process, it seems that the activation of some of the pathways leads to beneficial, adaptive remodeling, whereas the activation of others has maladaptive, harmful results.[80,102] The predominance of maladaptive over beneficial signaling would then result in the progression of disease toward HF. Thus, the classic paradigm conceptualized LVH as a process required for the normalization of wall stress, as required by the law of Laplace.[2] With the progression of a disease that caused hypertrophy, LVH would then in some cases progress to maladaptive form, characterized by increased fibrosis and progression to HF. As already discussed, because LVH is by itself a significant risk factor for cardiovascular morbidity and mortality, this concept has been challenged.[103,104] Furthermore, the results of recent experimental studies showed that the blockade of some signaling pathways (calcineurin for instance) may prevent or ameliorate the development of hypertrophy.[103,104] However, as pointed out by Samuel and Swynghedauw,[105] before changing the paradigm it would be necessary to clearly demonstrate that prevention of LVH by the blockade of signaling pathways would not alter myocardial function.[105] Nevertheless, regardless of paradigms, newly discovered signaling pathways in LVH represent potential targets for the new generation of cardiovascular drugs.[104]

TRANSITION FROM COMPENSATED HYPERTROPHY TO HF

According to the classic hypothesis, pressure overload causes myocytes to grow in width to increase wall thickness and in this way normalizes pressure-related wall stress. Then, the following question arises: why or how could an essentially beneficial, adaptive process eventually lead to HF? Evidence shows that in addition to adaptive processes, initial stimulus may also evoke a maladaptive response within myocardium.[6,33,34,106] These maladaptive changes involve cardiomyocytes, nonmyocytic cells, extracellular matrix, and the intramyocardial vasculature with the resulting development of ventricular dysfunction and HF.[6,33,34,106]

There are several potentially detrimental changes at the cardiomyocyte level in LVH. First, there is a change in energy metabolism toward a greater use of glucose and a diminished use of fatty acids, with the resulting decrease in ATP production and energy starvation.[70,107] In addition, the decreased use of fatty acids may lead to the accumulation of lipids within myocytes and, consequently, to contractile dysfunction.[108] Furthermore, apoptosis of cardiomyocytes is greatly enhanced in hypertensive heart disease, which may lead to the reduction in contractile mass and affect contractility.[109] Autophagy, a lysosomal-mediated process of intracellular protein and organelle recycling, is also stimulated in cardiomyocytes in response to pressure overload.[110] Unrestrained autophagy has been shown to induce cell death and consequently could lead to the reduction in the number of myocytes and contractile dysfunction.[110]

In the pressure-overloaded ventricle, there is an exaggerated deposition of collagen fibers (type I and III) in the extracellular matrix, in both the interstitium and perivascularly.[111] This increase in myocardial collagen content is a result of several alterations in collagen metabolism, including increased procollagen synthesis by fibroblasts and myofibroblasts, increased conversion of procollagen into collage, increased collagen cross-linking, and unchanged or decreased collagen degradation by matrix metalloproteinases.[111] Depending on its location and magnitude, collagen fiber cross-linking and the relative abundance of type I and III collagens, fibrosis can adversely increase myocardial stiffness, leading to diastolic dysfunction and HF.[74,75] Perivascular accumulation of collagen may, on the other hand, reduce wall distensibility of intramural coronary vessels and, thus, contribute to myocardial ischemia.[42] Furthermore, extracellular accumulation of collage fibers also induces electrical heterogeneity of the myocardium, which predisposes to ventricular dysrhytmias.[112]

Finally, changes in myocardial vasculature, independent of any atherosclerotic alterations, may reduce the coronary flow reserve and cause myocardial ischemia when oxygen demand increases, such as during exercise.[113] These changes include structural alterations, such as an increase in the wall-to-lumen ratio of small arteries and arterioles caused by the hypertrophy of vascular smooth muscle.[113] There is also rarefaction of myocardial capillary network. Finally, perivascular fibrosis in hypertrophied ventricles may affect the distensibility of coronary vessels and decrease coronary flow reserve. Thus, a positive correlation and linear regression between myocardial collagen concentration and minimal vascular resistance were found for both ventricles of spontaneously hypertensive rats and normotensive Wistar rats.[114] The importance of periarteriolar collagen for the coronary flow reserve was further confirmed by findings that the normalization of blood pressure after the debanding of the rat aorta induced regression of media hypertrophy, but the normalization of the coronary flow reserve was achieved only after the additional reversal of collagen accumulation by pharmacologic means.[115] The consequences of these structural changes are further aggravated by vascular functional alterations resulting from endothelial dysfunction and reduction in nitric oxide availability.[116]

SUMMARY

Pressure-overload–induced ventricular hypertrophy is one of the major risk factors for cardiovascular-related morbidity and mortality. The risk inherent in ventricular hypertrophy resides in hypertrophied cardiomyocytes and the remodeling of myocardium: fibrosis, ischemia, and loss of myocardial mass. Recent discoveries of molecular mechanisms involved in the development of myocardial hypertrophy opened new avenues in the therapeutic approach to the problem. It is now clear that ventricular hypertrophy, although possibly beneficial in some aspects, is essentially a maladaptive process that should be either prevented (preferably) or reversed.

REFERENCES

1. Meerson FZ. Compensatory hyperfunction of the heart and cardiac insufficiency. Circ Res 1962;10: 250–8.
2. Grossman W, Jones D, McLaurin I. Wall stress and patterns of hypertrophy in the human left ventricle. J Clin Invest 1975;56:50–8.
3. Frohlich ED, Apstein C, Chobanian A, et al. The heart in hypertension. N Engl J Med 1992;327: 998–1008.
4. Barry SP, Townsend PA. What causes a broken heart – molecular insights into heart failure. Int Rev Cell Mol Biol 2010;284:113–79.
5. Pfeffer JM, Pfeffer MA, Braunwald E. Influence of chronic captopril therapy on the infracted left ventricle of the rat. Circ Res 1985;57:84–95.
6. Opie LH, Commerford PJ, Gersh BJ, et al. Controversies in ventricular remodeling. Lancet 2006;367: 356–67.
7. Intersalt Cooperative Research Group. Intersalt: an international study of electrolyte excretion and blood pressure: results of 24-hour urinary sodium and potassium excretion. BMJ 1988;297:319–28.
8. Yu HC, Burrell LM, Black MJ, et al. Salt induces myocardial and renal fibrosis in normotensive and hypertensive rats. Circulation 1999;98:2621–8.
9. Yuan BX, Leenen FH. Dietary sodium intake and left ventricular hypertrophy in normotensive rats. Am J Physiol 1991;261:H1397–401.
10. Varagic J, Frohlich ED, Díez J, et al. Myocardial fibrosis, impaired coronary hemodynamics, and biventricular dysfunction in salt- loaded SHR. Am J Physiol Heart Circ Physiol 2006;290:H1503–9.
11. Varagic J, Frohlich ED, Susic D, et al. AT1 receptor antagonism attenuates target organ effect of salt excess in SHRs without affecting pressure. Am J Physiol Heart Circ Physiol 2008;294:H853–8.
12. Susic D, Varagic J, Frohlich ED. Cardiovascular effects of inhibition of renin- angiotensin-aldosterone system components in hypertensive rats given salt excess. Am J Physiol Heart Circ Physiol 2010;298: H1177–81.
13. Cook NR, Cutler JA, Obarzanek E, et al. Long term effects of dietary sodium reduction on cardiovascular disease outcomes: observational follow-up of the trials of hypertension prevention (TOHP). BMJ 2007;334:885–8.
14. Alpert NR, Mulieri LA. Increased myothermal economy of isometric force generation in compensated cardiac hypertrophy induced by

pulmonary artery constriction in the rabbit. Circ Res 1982;50:491–500.

15. Grove D, Zak R, Nair KG, et al. Biochemical correlates of cardiac hypertrophy. IV. Observations on the cellular organization of growth during myocardial hypertrophy in the rat. Circ Res 1969;25:473–85.

16. Nair KG, Cutilletta F, Zak R, et al. Biochemical correlates of cardiac hypertrophy. I. Experimental model, changes in heart weight, RNA content and nuclear RNA polymerase activity. Circ Res 1968; 23:451–62.

17. Bruel A, Christofersen TE, Nyengaard JR. Growth hormone increases the proliferation of the existing cardiac myocytes and the total number of cardiac myocytes in the rat heart. Circ Res 2007;76:400–8.

18. Leeuwenburgh BP, Helbing WA, Wenink AC, et al. Chronic right ventricular pressure overload results in hyperplastic rather than hypertrophic response. J Anat 2008;212:286–94.

19. Du Y, Plante E, Janicki JS, et al. Temporal evaluation of cardiac myocyte hypertrophy and hyperplasia in male rats secondary to chronic volume overload. Am J Pathol 2010;177:1155–63.

20. Astorri E, Bolognesi R, Colla B, et al. Left ventricular hypertrophy: a cytometric study on 42 human hearts. J Mol Cell Cardiol 1977;9:763–75.

21. Linzbach AJ. Heart failure from the point of view of quantitative anatomy. Am J Cardiol 1960;5:370–81.

22. Kajstura J, Leri A, Finato N, et al. Myocardial proliferation in end-stage cardiac failure in humans. Proc Natl Acad Sci U S A 1998;95:8801–5.

23. Beltrami CA, Urbanek K, Kajstura J, et al. Evidence that human cardiac myocytes divide after infarction. N Engl J Med 2001;344:1750–7.

24. Urbanek K, Quaini F, Tasca G, et al. Intense myocyte formation from cardiac stem cells in human cardiac hypertrophy. Proc Natl Acad Sci U S A 2003;100:10440–5.

25. Linke A, Muller P, Nurzynska D, et al. Cardiac stem cells in the dog regenerate infarcted myocardium improving cardiac performance. Proc Natl Acad Sci U S A 2005;102:8966–71.

26. Anversa P, Nadal-Ginard B. Myocyte renewal and ventricular remodeling. Nature 2002;415:240–3.

27. Anversa P, Leri A, Kajstura J. Cardiac regeneration. J Am Coll Cardiol 2006;47:1769–76.

28. Chien KR. Stem cells: lost in translation. Nature 2004;428:607–8.

29. Anversa P, Ricci R, Olivetti G. Quantitative structural analysis of the myocardium during physiologic growth and induced cardiac hypertrophy: a review. J Am Coll Cardiol 1986;7:1140–9.

30. Jalil JE, Doering CW, Janicki JS, et al. Fibrillar collagen and myocardial stiffness in the intact hypertrophied rat left ventricle. Circ Res 1989;64: 1041–50.

31. Camelitti P, Borg TK, Kohl P. Structural and functional characterization of cardiac fibroblasts. Cardiovasc Res 2005;65:40–51.

32. Diez J, Frohlich ED. A translational approach to hypertensive heart disease. Hypertension 2010; 55:1–8.

33. Frohlich ED, Gonzales A, Diez J. Hypertensive left ventricular hypertrophy risk: beyond adaptive cardiomyocyte hypertrophy. J Hypertens 2011;29: 17–26.

34. Weber KT, Janicki JS, Shroff SG, et al. Collagen remodeling of the pressure overloaded, hypertrophied nonhuman primate myocardium. Circ Res 1988;62:756–65.

35. Weber KT, Brilla CG. Pathological hypertrophy and cardiac interstitium. Fibrosis and the renin-angiotensin-aldosterone system. Circulation 1991; 83:1849–65.

36. Swynghedauw B. Phenotypic plasticity of adult myocardium: molecular mechanisms. J Exp Biol 2006;209:2320–7.

37. Lompre AM, Schwartz K, D'Albis A, et al. Myosin isozymes redistribution in chronic heart loading. Nature 1979;282:105–7.

38. Swynghedauw B. Developmental and functional adaptation of contractile proteins in cardiac and skeletal muscle. Physiol Rev 1986;66:710–71.

39. Miyata S, Minobe W, Bristow MR, et al. Myosin heavy chain isoform expression in the failing and nonfailing human heart. Circ Res 2000;86: 386–90.

40. Linke WA. Sense and stretchability: the role of titin and titin-associated proteins in myocardial stress-sensing and mechanical dysfunction. Cardiovasc Res 2008;77:637.

41. Zile MR, Brutsaert DL. New concepts in diastolic function and diastolic heart failure: part II: causal mechanisms and treatment. Circulation 2002;105: 1503–8.

42. Frohlich ED. Fibrosis and ischemia: the real risk in hypertensive heart disease. Am J Hypertens 2001;14:194s–9s.

43. Kannel WB, Castelli WP, McNamara PM, et al. Role of blood pressure in the development of congestive heart failure: the Framingham study. N Engl J Med 1972;287:781–7.

44. Dunn FG, Pringle SD. Left ventricular hypertrophy and myocardial ischemia in systemic hypertension. Am J Cardiol 1987;60:191–221.

45. Yiu KH, Tse HF. Hypertension and cardiac arrhythmias: a review of epidemiology, pathophysiology and clinical implications. J Hum Hypertens 2008; 22:380–8.

46. Manolis AJ, Beldekos D, Handanis S, et al. Comparison of spirapril, isradipine or combination in hypertensive patients with left ventricular

hypertrophy: effects on LVH regression and arrhythmogenic propensity. J Hypertens 2002;11: 1445–50.

47. Tarazi RC, Miller A, Frohlich ED, et al. Electrocardiographic changes reflecting left atrial abnormality in hypertension. Circulation 1966;34:818–22.

48. Dunn FG, Pfeffer MA, Frohlich ED. ECG alterations with progressive left ventricular hypertrophy in spontaneous hypertension. Clin Exp Hypertens 1978;1:67–86.

49. Ravelli F, Allessie M. Effects of atrial dilatation on refractory period and vulnerability to atrial fibrillation in the isolated Langendorff-perfused rabbit heart. Circulation 1997;90:1686–95.

50. Tanaka K, Zlochiver S, Vikstrom KL, et al. The spatial distribution of fibrosis governs fibrillation wave dynamics in the posterior left atrium during heart failure. Circ Res 2007;101:839–47.

51. Goette A, Staack T, Rocken C, et al. Increased expression of extracellular signal regulated kinase and angiotensin-converting enzyme in human atria during atrial fibrillation. J Am Coll Cardiol 2000;35: 1669–77.

52. Brasier AR, Recinos A III, Eledrisi MS. Vascular inflammation and the renin– angiotensin system. Arterioscler Thromb Vasc Biol 2002;22:1257–66.

53. Frohlich ED, Tarazi RC, Dustan HP. Clinical-physiological correlations in the development of hypertensive heart disease. Circulation 1971;44:446–55.

54. Muller-Brunotte R, Kahan T, Lopez B, et al. Myocardial fibrosis and diastolic dysfunction in patients with hypertension: results from the Swedish Irbesartan Left Ventricular Hypertrophy Investigation versus Atenolol (SILVHIA). J Hypertens 2007;25: 1958–66.

55. Erdogan D, Yildirim I, Ciftci O, et al. Effects of normal blood pressure, prehypertension, and hypertension on coronary microvascular function. Circulation 2007;115:593–9.

56. Barron HV, Lesh MD. Autonomic nervous system and sudden cardiac death. J Am Coll Cardiol 1996;27:1053–60.

57. Harrap SB, Mitchell GA, Casley DJ, et al. Angiotensin II, sodium, and cardiovascular hypertrophy in spontaneously hypertensive rats. Hypertension 1993;21:50–5.

58. Hart G. Cellular electrophysiology in cardiac hypertrophy and failure. Cardiovasc Res 1994;28:933–46.

59. Savelieva I, Yap YG, Yi G, et al. Relation of ventricular repolarization to cardiac cycle length in normal subjects, hypertrophic cardiomyopathy, and patients with myocardial infarction. Clin Cardiol 1999;22:649–54.

60. Tribulova N, Okruhlicova L, Novakova S, et al. Hypertension-related intermyocyte junction remodeling is associated with a higher incidence of low-K(+)-induced lethal arrhythmias in isolated rat heart. Exp Physiol 2002;87:195–205.

61. Zaugg CE, Wu ST, Lee RJ, et al. Intracellular Ca2+ handling and vulnerability to ventricular fibrillation in spontaneously hypertensive rats. Hypertension 1997;30:461–7.

62. Haider AW, Larson MG, Benjamin EJ, et al. Increased left ventricular mass and hypertrophy are associated with increased risk for sudden death. J Am Coll Cardiol 1998;32:1454–9.

63. Dunn FG, Chandraratna P, de Carvalho JGR, et al. Pathophysiologic assessment of hypertensive heart disease with echocardiography. Am J Cardiol 1977;39:789–95.

64. Dreslinski GR, Frohlich ED, Dunn FG, et al. Echocardiographic diastolic ventricular abnormality in hypertensive heart disease: atrial emptying index. Am J Cardiol 1981;47:1087–90.

65. Aeschbacher BC, Hutter D, Fuhrer J, et al. Diastolic dysfunction precedes myocardial hypertrophy in the development of hypertension. Am J Hypertens 2001;14:106–13.

66. Shepherd RF, Zachariah PK, Shub C. Hypertension and left ventricular diastolic function. Mayo Clin Proc 1989;64:1521–32.

67. Zile MR, Brutsaert DL. New concepts in diastolic dysfunction and diastolic heart failure: part I: diagnosis, prognosis and measurements of diastolic function. Circulation 2002;105:1503–8.

68. Brutsaert DL. Cardiac dysfunction in heart failure: the cardiologist's love affair with time. Prog Cardiovasc Dis 2006;49:157–81.

69. Yip GW, Fung JW, Tan YT, et al. Hypertension and heart failure: a dysfunction of systole, diastole or both. J Hum Hypertens 2009;23:295–306.

70. Fouad FM, Slominski JM, Tarazi RC. Left ventricular diastolic function in hypertension: relation to left ventricular mass and systolic function. J Am Coll Cardiol 1984;53:1387–93.

71. Swynghedauw B. Molecular mechanisms of myocardial remodeling. Physiol Rev 1999;79:216–62.

72. Swinghedauw B. Molecular mechanisms in evolutionary cardiology failure. Ann N Y Acad Sci 2010;1188:58–67.

73. Kiss E, Ball NA, Kranias EG, et al. Differential changes in cardiac phospholamban and sarcoplasmic reticular Ca^{2+}-ATPase protein levels. Effects on Ca^{2+} transport and mechanics in compensated pressure overloaded hypertrophy and heart failure. Circ Res 1995;77:759–64.

74. Houser SR, Piacentino V, Weisser J. Abnormalities in calcium cycling in the hypertrophied and failing heart. J Mol Cell Cardiol 2002;32:1595–607.

75. Weber KT. Cardiac interstitium in health and disease: the fibrillar collagen network. J Am Coll Cardiol 1989;13:1637–52.

76. Brower GL, Gardner JD, Forman MF, et al. The relationship between myocardial extracellular matrix remodeling and ventricular function. Eur J Cardiothorac Surg 2006;30:604–10.

77. DeSimone G, DeDivitiis O. Extracellular matrix and left ventricular mechanics in overload hypertrophy. Adv Clin Path 2002;6:3–10.

78. Re RN. The intracellular renin-angiotensin system: the tip of intracrine physiology iceberg. Am J Physiol Heart Circ Physiol 2007;293:H905–6.

79. Kumar R, Singh VP, Baker KM. The intracellular rennin-angiotensin system: implication in cardiovascular remodeling. Curr Opin Nephrol Hypertens 2008;17:168–73.

80. Xu J, Carretero OA, Liao TD, et al. Local angiotensin II aggravates cardiac remodeling in hypertension. Am J Physiol Heart Circ Physiol 2010; 299:H1304–6.

81. Kehat I, Molkentin JD. Molecular pathways underlying cardiac remodeling during pathophysiological stimulation. Circulation 2010;122:2727–35.

82. Bache RJ. Effects of hypertrophy on the coronary circulation. Prog Cardiovasc Dis 1988;30:403–40.

83. Marcus ML, Harrison DG, Chilian WM, et al. Alterations in the coronary circulation in hypertrophied ventricles. Circulation 1987;75(Suppl 1):I19–25.

84. Levy AS, Chung JCS, Kroetsch JT, et al. Nitric oxide and coronary vascular endothelium adaptations in hypertension. Vasc Health Risk Manag 2009;5:1075–87.

85. Susic D, Francischetti A, Frohlich ED. Prolonged L-arginine on cardiovascular mass and myocardial hemodynamics and collagen in aged SHR and normal rats. Hypertension 1999;33(1 Pt 2):451–5.

86. Mancini GB, Dahlöf B, Díez J. Surrogate markers for cardiovascular disease. Structural markers. Circulation 2004;109(25 Suppl 1):IV22–30.

87. Ruilope LM, Schmieder RE. Left ventricular hypertrophy and clinical outcomes in hypertensive patients. Am J Hypertens 2008;21:500–8.

88. Koren MJ, Devereux RB, Casale PN, et al. Relation of left ventricular mass and geometry to morbidity and mortality in uncomplicated essential hypertension. Ann Intern Med 1991;114:345–52.

89. Levy D, Garrison RJ, Savage DD, et al. Prognostic implications of echocardiographically determined left ventricular mass in the Framingham Heart Study. N Engl J Med 1990;322:1561–6.

90. Kahan T, Bergfeldt L. Left ventricular hypertrophy in hypertension: its arrhythmogenic potential. Heart 2005;91:250–6.

91. Kaplinsky E. Do we understand why regression of left ventricular hypertrophy is beneficial? Cardiovasc Res 2003;60:463–4.

92. Devereux RB, Wachtell K, Gerdts E, et al. Prognostic significance of left ventricular mass change during treatment of hypertension. JAMA 2004; 292:2350–6.

93. Okin PM, Devereux RB, Jern S, et al. Regression of electrocardiographic left ventricular hypertrophy during antihypertensive treatment and the prediction of major cardiovascular events. JAMA 2004; 292:2343–9.

94. Verma A, Solomon SD. Diastolic dysfunction as a link between hypertension and heart failure. Med Clin North Am 2009;93:647–64.

95. Kannel WB. Incidence and epidemiology of heart failure. Heart Fail Rev 2000;5:167–73.

96. Chinnaiyan KM, Alexander D, Maddens M, et al. Curriculum in cardiology: integrated diagnosis and management of diastolic heart failure. Am Heart J 2007;153:189–200.

97. Hamdani N, Paulus WJ. Treatment of heart failure with normal ejection fraction. Curr Treat Options Cardiovasc Med 2011;13:26–34.

98. Gradman AH, Alfayoumi F. From left ventricular hypertrophy to congestive heart failure: management of hypertensive heart disease. Prog Cardiovasc Dis 2006;48:326–41.

99. Lionetti V, Recchia FA. New therapies for the failing heart: trans-genes versus trans-cells. Transl Res 2010;156:130–5.

100. Bolli P, Chaudhry HW. Molecular physiology of cardiac regeneration. Ann N Y Acad Sci 2010; 1211:113–26.

101. Guyette JP, Cohen IS, Gauchette GR. Strategies for regeneration of heart muscle. Crit Rev Eukaryot Gene Expr 2010;20:2035–50.

102. Hannenhalli S, Putt ME, Gimore JM, et al. Transcriptional genomics associates FOX transcription factors with human heart failure. Circulation 2006; 114:1269–76.

103. Meijs MF, deWindt LJ, deJonge N, et al. Left ventricular hypertrophy: a shift in paradigm. Curr Med Chem 2007;14:157–71.

104. Luedde M, Katus HA, Frey N. Novel molecular targets in the treatment of cardiac hypertrophy. Recent Pat Cardiovasc Drug Discov 2006;1:1–20.

105. Samuel JL, Swynghedauw B. Is cardiac hypertrophy a required compensatory mechanism in pressure-overloaded heart. J Hypertens 2008;26: 857–8.

106. Diez J. Towards a new paradigm about hypertensive heart disease. Med Clin North Am 2009;93: 637–46.

107. Beer M, Seyfarth T, Sandestede J, et al. Absolute concentrations of high-energy phosphate metabolites in normal, hypertrophied, and failing human myocardium measured noninvasively with (31) P-SLOOP magnetic resonance spectroscopy. J Am Coll Cardiol 2002;40:1267–74.

108. Wende AR, Abel ED. Lipotoxicity in the heart. Biochim Biophys Acta 2010;1801:311–9.

109. Gonzales A, Lopez B, Ravassa S, et al. Stimulation of apoptosis in essential hypertension: potential role of angiotensin II. Hypertension 2002;39:75–80.

110. Rothermal BA, Hill JA. Autophagy in load-induced heart disease. Circ Res 2008;103:1363–9.

111. Berk BC, Fujiwara K, Lehoux S. ECM remodeling in hypertensive heart disease. J Clin Invest 2007;117:568–75.

112. McLenachan JM, Dargie JH. Ventricular arrhythmias in hypertensive left ventricular hypertrophy. Relation to coronary artery disease, left ventricular dysfunction, and myocardial fibrosis. Am J Hypertens 1990;3:735–40.

113. Feihl F, Liaudet L, Waeber B. The macrocirculation and microcirculation of hypertension. Curr Hypertens Rep 2009;11:182–9.

114. Susic D, Nunez E, Hosoya K, et al. Coronary hemodynamics in aging spontaneously hypertensive (SHR) and normotensive Wistar-Kyoto (WKY) rats. J Hypertens 1998;16:231–7.

115. Isoyama S, Ito N, Satoh K, et al. Collagen deposition and the reversal of coronary reserve in cardiac hypertrophy. Hypertension 1992;20:491–500.

116. Lapu-Bula R, Ofili E. From hypertension to heart failure: role of nitric oxide- mediated endothelial dysfunction and emerging insights from myocardial contrast echocardiography. Am J Cardiol 2007;99:7D–14D.

Volume Overload

Blase A. Carabello, MD[a,b],*

KEYWORDS

• Cardiac volume overload • Hypertrophy

The heart's major task is to perfuse the rest of the body with enough blood to provide the body with adequate oxygen and nutrients. This cardiac output is equal to the stroke volume × heart rate. Many normal and pathologic conditions require increased cardiac output to maintain adequate perfusion and it follows that increased output is accomplished in part by an increase in stroke volume. Because stroke volume = end-diastolic volume–end-systolic volume, increased stroke volume is predicated on an increase in total heart volume. Bodily growth, exercise, anemia, and thyrotoxicosis are a few such conditions that place a metabolic demand on the volume pumping capabilities of the heart. Structural abnormalities of the heart valves or the presence of intracardiac shunts, however, create a different kind of volume demand on the left ventricle (LV) and/or right ventricle (RV). These abnormalities create flow inefficiencies requiring increased stroke volume just to maintain normal resting forward cardiac output. It is these structural defects that place a chronic volume overload on the heart that are the subject of this article. Although all share the commonality of a cardiac demand for increased stroke volume, each presents a unique type of volume overload with unique cardiac consequences.

ETIOLOGY OF DIFFERENT VOLUME OVERLOADS AND RELATION TO PATHOPHYSIOLOGY
Structural (Primary) Mitral Regurgitation: A Pure Left Ventricular Volume Overload

In most LV volume overloads, the extra volume is ejected into the high pressure of the aorta, increasing stroke volume and LV systolic pressure, in turn increasing afterload. Thus in a sense these lesions are combined pressure and volume overloads. Mitral regurgitation (MR) is unique in generating a pure volume overload because the extra volume ejected by LV is ejected into the low pressure of the left atrium (LA).[1] Accordingly, the LV remodeling that attends MR is also specific for this disease. In experimental animals and in humans, MR gives way to a thin-walled enlarged ventricle with modest eccentric LV hypertrophy (LVH).[2,3] In 1973, Grossman and colleagues[4] proposed that the LV in valvular heart disease responded to the hemodynamic overloads placed on it in response to LV wall stress, where Laplace's law states that $\sigma = P \times r/2th$, where σ is stress, P is LV pressure, r is LV radius, and th is wall thickness. They proposed that the pressure overload of aortic stenosis, for example, induced concentric LV remodeling and/or LVH wherein sarcomeres were laid down in parallel so that myocyte thickness (and thus wall thickness) increased. An increase in the numerator of the Laplace equation from increased pressure is offset by increased wall thickness in the denominator, maintaining normal wall stress (afterload). Alternatively, volume overload was proposed as inducing an increase in diastolic stress, leading to sarcomeres being laid down in series, increasing myocyte length and increasing LV chamber volume, allowing the LV to increase stroke volume to accommodate volume lost to regurgitation. These changes have occurred in experimental MR where myocyte length increases substantially in concert with an increase in LV chamber volume.[5] Systolic blood pressure is usually normal or even slightly lower than normal in MR.[6] This high-volume, low-pressure set of hemodynamics leads to a nearly unique kind of LV remodeling, producing the enlarged thin-walled chamber (discussed previously).

a Department of Medicine, Baylor College of Medicine, Houston, TX, USA
b Michael E. DeBakey VA Medical Center, Medical Service (111), 2002 Holcombe Boulevard, Houston, TX 77401, USA
* Michael E. DeBakey VA Medical Center, Medical Service (111), 2002 Holcombe Boulevard, Houston, TX 77401.
E-mail address: blaseanthony.carabello@med.va.gov

Heart Failure Clin 8 (2012) 33–42
doi:10.1016/j.hfc.2011.08.013
1551-7136/12/$ – see front matter Published by Elsevier Inc.

The consequences of remodeling in MR on LV function

The eccentric remodeling of MR aids diastolic function, which is supernormal, unlike in almost any other form of heart disease in experimental animals and in patients with compensated disease.[7,8] The thin-walled MR ventricle is able to rapidly accept the large blood volume stored in the LA during systole and at a low filling pressure, helping patients avoid pulmonary

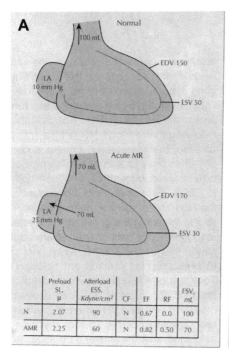

	Preload SL, μ	Afterload ESS, Kdyne/cm²	CF	EF	RF	FSV, mL
N	2.07	90	N	0.67	0.0	100
AMR	2.25	60	N	0.82	0.50	70

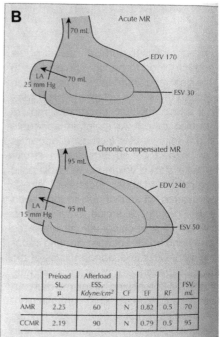

	Preload SL, μ	Afterload ESS, Kdyne/cm²	CF	EF	RF	FSV, mL
AMR	2.25	60	N	0.82	0.5	70
CCMR	2.19	90	N	0.79	0.5	95

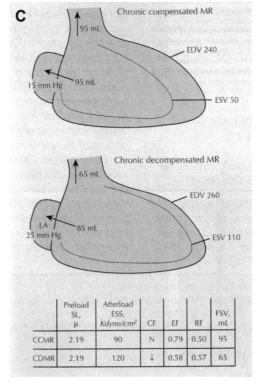

	Preload SL, μ	Afterload ESS, Kdyne/cm²	CF	EF	RF	FSV, mL
CCMR	2.19	90	N	0.79	0.50	95
CDMR	2.19	120	↓	0.58	0.57	65

congestion. Unfortunately this same remodeling is a hindrance to systolic function because it generates a high radius-to-thickness (r/th) ratio, a major portion of the Laplace equation. MR eccentric remodeling results in the highest r/th ratio of the left-sided valvular heart diseases.[1] MR is often viewed as a lesion that reduces LV afterload by affording a pathway for systolic ejection of blood into the low impedance of the LA. Although this concept has some validity, the LV geometry that develops with its increased r/th has the opposite effect of increasing systolic wall stress (afterload). Afterload is only reduced in acute MR, becomes normal in compensated MR, and actually is increased in advanced decompensated MR with LV dysfunction.[9] Thus, the remodeling induced by MR facilitates diastole but is detrimental to systolic function. The high r/th ratio not only tends to increase afterload but also leads the lowest mass-to-volume ratio in valvular heart disease so that there is the least amount of myocardium to generate stroke volume. When the increased stroke work from the volume overload of MR is matched to an equal amount of stroke work demanded by the pressure overload of aortic stenosis, LVH is far greater in pressure overload, emphasizing the lack of hypertrophy induced by MR.[10]

Protein synthesis in MR

The term, *hypertrophy*, indicates increased weight and differs from *remodeling*, the latter term indicating a change in geometry that may or may not be associated with hypertrophy. In MR, there is eccentric LVH. Increased LV weight occurs by a net gain in myocardial proteins, which in turn can only accrue from an increase in protein synthesis or by a decrease in protein degradation. The myocardial contractile proteins have a short half-life, turning over approximately every 10 days. Thus, synthesis rate can be calculated in experimental animals by measuring the rate that a tagged amino acid is incorporated into the myocardium in a short period of time (ie, 6 hours). After acute pressure overload, protein synthesis rate increases by 35% within 6 hours of institution of the overload.[11] After establishment of acute MR, however, no increase in protein synthesis rate can be detected.[11] Likewise no increased in protein synthesis rate can be detected at 2 weeks, 4 weeks, or 3 months after creation of severe MR.[12] This suggests that the LVH that develops in MR develops not from increased protein synthesis but rather is due to a reduction in degradation rate. This process could lead to older contractile proteins functioning in the MR ventricle, possibly making it susceptible to contractile dysfunction.

Heart failure in acute severe MR

In acute severe MR, 50% or more of the LV stroke is ejected into the LA, reducing forward stroke volume and cardiac output that cannot be compensated by the LV's limited preload reserve (**Fig. 1**).[2] At the same time, this volume overload on the unprepared LA increases LA pressure, resulting in pulmonary congestion. Thus, the major hemodynamic underpinnings of heart failure are present (increased filling pressure and decreased cardiac output) yet LV systolic function is completely normal or even supernormal, augmented by sympathetic nervous system reflexes that are activated by reduced cardiac output. Most patients cannot tolerate acute severe MR and require immediate surgical intervention. Other patients, however, may develop severe MR gradually as the MR increases incrementally over time. Such patients may enter a chronic compensated phase where eccentric hypertrophy and remodeling permit increased stroke volume to compensate that which is lost to MR (see **Fig. 1**B). At the same time, increased LA size accommodates the regurgitant volume at

Fig. 1. The stages of MR are demonstrated. (*A*) Normal physiology is compared with that of acute MR. In acute MR, end-diastolic volume (EDV) increases slightly as preload reserve (sarcomere length [SL] is maximized. Afterload (end systolic stress [ESS]) is reduced facilitating ejection so that end-systolic volume (ESV) is reduced. These changes act in concert with normal contractile function (CF) to increase total stroke volume, but because MR produces a regurgitant fraction (RF) of 0.5, forward stroke volume (FSV) is reduced. The excess volume displaced into the LA during systole increases LA pressure. Thus, despite normal CF, the elements of heart failure are present. (*B*) Acute MR is compared with chronic compensated MR. Eccentric hypertrophy has greatly increased EDV whereas a return to normal afterload has increased ESV slightly. The result is a large increase in FSV. At the same time a now enlarged LA can accommodate the regurgitant volume at nearly normal filling pressure. Despite severe MR, the elements of heart failure are compensated. (*C*) Chronic compensated MR is compared with chronic decompensated MR. Reduced CF and increased afterload cause a large increase in ESV, decreasing total, and forward stroke volume. LA pressure is again increased, reflecting the increased filling pressure of a failing LV. Despite the reduction in contractile function, increased preload maintains ejection fraction (EF) in the normal range. (*From* Carabello BA. Mitral regurgitation: basic pathophysiologic principles. Part 1. Mod Concepts Cardiovasc Dis 1988;57:53–8; with permission.)

a lower filling pressure, relieving pulmonary congestion, permitting patients to be asymptomatic despite the volume overload.

Heart failure in chronic MR

It was once believed that severe MR was tolerated for long periods of time before LV dysfunction ensued. Although this may be the case in some patients, in many others, decompensation occurs within 5 years of the onset of severe MR.[13,14] Afterload excess plays a role in decompensation but LV contractile dysfunction also ensues. Although reduced coronary blood flow reserve plays a role in the LV dysfunction of pressure overload,[15,16] coronary blood flow in MR is normal.[17] The contractile deficit of MR resides in the myocytes themselves.[18] At the myocyte level there is loss of contractile elements, especially in the endocardium and papillary muscles (**Fig. 2**).[5,18,19] There is also a severe shift in the force-frequency relation so that peak force is reduced, occurs at a much lower heart rate than normal, and falls off as heart rate increases.[19] This observation, coupled with forskolin reversing the observed contractile abnormalities, suggests that abnormalities in calcium handling are also operational in reducing contractility in MR. Reduced contractility is attended by sympathetic overactivity[20,21] and is reversed either by restoring mitral competence in experimental animals and in patients or by initiating beta-blockade.[22–24] A possible schema for the mechanisms of LV dysfunction in MR is shown in **Fig. 3**.

Correction of the volume overload: results of therapy

MR, like all valvular heart disease, is a mechanical problem that requires a mechanical solution. Although logical, pharmacologic attempts to reduce afterload in an effort to increase forward flow and decrease regurgitant flow have failed to improve outcome.[25–28] This may be because vasodilators reduce LV size, which could worsen mitral prolapse (the dominant cause of MR in the developed world) and might even increase rather than decrease MR. How vasodilators might work in rheumatic MR where the regurgitant orifice is less dynamic is unknown.

Alternatively, surgical correction of MR when performed in a timely manner leads to marked reverse remodeling and improved contractility (if it was reduced) preoperatively.[23,29] There is restoration in contractile element number and a return of diastolic function from supernormal to normal.[30] In correcting MR, it is crucial to allow the mitral valve and its apparatus to remain intact if LV function is to return to normal. The mitral valve apparatus not only prevents MR but also coordinates LV contraction and is a key element of LV performance. Its destruction leads to reduced postoperative LV ejection performance and longevity.[29,31–33] At some point the LV damage caused by MR becomes irreversible, and function and volume do not return to normal after surgery. The biology of such irreversibility is unknown but permanent damage can be avoided by operating before symptoms have become more than mild and/or before ejection falls to less than 0.60 or before the LV can no longer contract to an end-systolic diameter of 40 mm.[34]

Impact of functional MR: chicken or egg?

In primary (organic) MR (discussed previously), the volume overload caused by the MR lesion results in eventual myocardial damage, heart failure, and death. MR may also result, however, from the LV damage caused by myocardial infarction or dilated cardiomyopathy. In these diseases, regional wall motion abnormalities combine with papillary muscle displacement and annular dilitation to cause MR. But here the MR is the result of severe

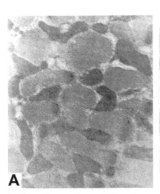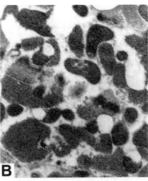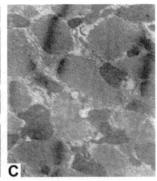

A   B   C

Fig. 2. The histology of normal canine myocardium (*A*) is compared with that of chronic MR (*B*) showing a loss of contractile elements. (*C*) Histology returns to normal after correction of the MR. (*From* Spinale FG, Ishihara K, Zile M, et al. Structural basis for changes in left ventricular function and geometry because of chronic mitral regurgitation and after correction of volume overload. J Thorac Cardiovasc Surg 1993;106(6):1147–57; with permission.)

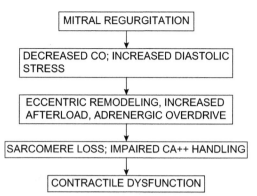

Fig. 3. A potential schema for the development of LV dysfunction in chronic MR is shown.

LV dysfunction rather than the cause of it. The presence of functional MR worsens prognosis (Fig. 4)[35] for which there are two different explanations. It may be that the presence of the MR adds an additional burden to the already damaged LV, further worsening outcome. Alternatively MR may simply reflect the degree of LV dysfunction—the worse the LV function, the worse the MR. In support of the latter explanation is that correction of functional MR has never been shown to prolong life, an outcome that might be expected if it were the MR itself that was the major culprit in worsening prognosis in functional MR.[36–39]

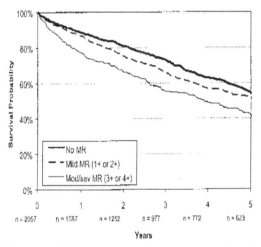

Fig. 4. Survival in patients with heart grouped by MR severity is demonstrated. Increasing MR is associated with but may not be the cause of worsened survival. (*From* Trichon BH, Felker GM, Shaw LK, et al. Relation of frequency and severity of mitral regurgitation to survival among patients with left ventricular systolic dysfunction and heart failure. Am J Cardiol 2003; 91(5):538–43; with permission.)

Chronic Aortic Regurgitation: A Combined Pressure and Volume Overload

For many years aortic regurgitation (AR) was classified together with MR as a volume-overloading lesion. AR does impart a volume overload on the LV as blood pumped from the LV during systole leaks back into the chamber during diastole. As in MR, the LV must enlarge to increase total stroke volume, in turn compensating forward stroke volume toward normal.[40] In AR, however, the interaction of the large total stroke volume with the inelasticity of the aorta increases systolic blood pressure. Although many AR patients are normotensive, systolic pressure in AR is approximately 50 mm Hg higher than it is in MR.[6] This combined pressure and volume overload of AR leads to unique remodeling that entails both eccentric and concentric hypertrophy,[41] producing the heaviest LV in valvular heart disease.[1] LVH in experimental animal models of AR is initiated by an increase in protein synthesis rate but maintained by a decrease in protein degradation rate.[42] The concentric component of the hypertrophy tends to offset the increased wall stress (afterload) produced by the increased systolic pressure. Because both terms in the numerator of the Laplace equation are elevated and the denominator is only modestly increased, systolic wall stress (afterload) increases substantially.[6,43,44] In many cases afterload in this so-called volume overload is as high as that found in the classic pressure overload lesion, aortic stenosis. As afterload excess increases, it progressively inhibits LV contraction, reducing ejection fraction and contributing to the heart failure syndrome. Unlike MR, chronic severe AR is tolerated for a prolonged period of time and may exist for many years before heart failure ensues.[45] In addition to afterload excess, myocardial changes contribute to both diastolic and systolic dysfunction.[46,47] Increased proliferation of collagen and noncollagen elements of the extracellular matrix stiffen the myocardium and also encroach on contractile elements. Reduced coronary blood flow reserve may lead to subendocardial ischemia, further worsening LV function.[48]

Therapy for aortic regurgitation

Because afterload is often excessive in AR, afterload reduction therapy seems apt. Unfortunately, trials of vasodilator therapy to reduce afterload have had disparate results. An early trial of hydralazine versus placebo found that active drug reduced LV volume, a potentially beneficial result.[49] A larger trial comparing nifedipine to digoxin, by Scognamiglio and colleagues,[50] found

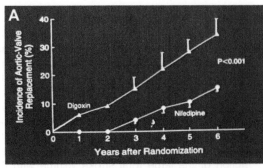
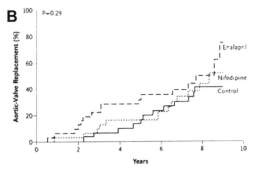

Fig. 5. (A) Patients with severe asymptomatic AR and normal LV function were randomized to receive digoxin or nifedipine and were then followed until early LV dysfunction or symptoms indicated the need for aortic valve replacement. Nifedipine seemed to delay the need for surgery. (B) Patients with severe asymptomatic AR and normal LV function were randomized to receive placebo, nifedipine, or enalapril and followed until the onset of symptoms or LV dysfunction indicated the need for valve replacement. Therapy in this study did not delay the need for surgery. ([A]From Scognamiglio R, Rahimtoola SH, Faoli G, et al. Nifedipine in asymptomatic patients with severe aortic regurgitation and normal left ventricular function. N Engl J Med 1994;331:689–94, with permission; and [B] Evangelista A, Tornos P, Samola A, et al. Long-term vasodilator therapy in patients with severe aortic regurgitation. N Engl J Med 2005;353:1342–9, with permission.)

that nifedipine seemed to forestall the need for AVR by approximately 2 years (**Fig. 5**A). A subsequent study comparing placebo with the same dose of nifedipine and with enalapril, however, found no benefit from the vasodilators and a trend toward harm for enalapril (see **Fig. 5**B).[51] In this study, systolic blood pressure was considerably lower than in the Scognogmilio study, suggesting that the difference in the 2 studies might be attributed to treatment of hypertension rather than of AR itself.

As with all valve lesions, AR is a mechanical problem that responds best to a mechanical solution (ie, AVR). After AVR, afterload is reduced dramatically and ejection performance improves if it was depressed preoperatively.[43,52–54] Although some improvement may be due to restoration of contractility, afterload reduction plays an important role in allowing EF to increase as reverse remodeling ensues fairly rapidly after AVR.

Acute Aortic Regurgitation

The hemodynamics of acute AR, as might occur in infective endocarditis with rapid destruction of the aortic, valve are remarkably different from those of chronic AR and much more dangerous. In acute AR, there is no time for compensatory development of ventricular hypertrophy; thus, there is a sudden volume overload on a small noncompliant LV.[55,56] This small LV in acute AR leads to several deleterious consequences. First the stroke volume lost to regurgitation cannot be compensated for by an increased end-diastolic volume; thus, forward stroke volume and cardiac output

are reduced, compromising organ perfusion. Next, diastolic LV volume overload causes high filling pressure leading to pulmonary congestion. As shown **Fig. 6**, a rapidly rising LV diastolic pressure in concert with a rapidly falling aortic diastolic pressure leads to equalization in mid-diastole. It is the gradient between aortic diastolic pressure and LV diastolic pressure, however, that is responsible for driving endocardial coronary blood flow, and this lack of gradient likely causes endocardial ischemia. It may be this constellation of hemodynamic events that leads to rapid deterioration of patients with acute AR, culminating in shock and pulmonary edema unless aortic valve replacement is undertaken urgently.[57]

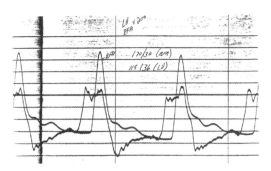

Fig. 6. Pressure tracings from a patient with severe acute AR are shown demonstrating augmentation of femoral artery systolic pressure (Hill sign), a rapid rise in LV diastolic pressure with equalization of aortic, and LV pressures in diastole. (*From* Carabello BA, Ballard WL, Gazes PC. Cardiology pearls. Sahn SA, Heffner JE, series editors. Philadelphia: Hanley & Belfus, Inc; 1994; with permission.)

Congenital Ventricular Septal Defect: A Combined Left and Right Ventricular Volume Overload

Ventricular septal defect (VSD) is usually a congenital anatomic abnormality in which LV volume is transferred to the RV through a hole in the septum that normally divides the 2 chambers. As such, LV volume and pressure are imposed on the RV. At the same time, the LV must pump the additional volume shunted to the RV, returning to the LV via the pulmonary circuit. LV remodeling in VSD often takes 2 distinct pathways.[58] In many children, LV enlargement is adequate to compensate for the LV volume overload; forward cardiac output is normal as are growth and development. In other children, normal growth and development are impaired. In these cases, cardiac output is subnormal. Reduced output seems the result of neither contractile failure nor abnormal LV loading. Rather there is inadequate eccentric hypertrophy to normalize forward stroke volume. This modest increase in LV mass in children with VSD and growth impairment is reminiscent of the pattern of remodeling seen in MR. In VSD and MR, blood is ejected early in systole into a low-pressure zone; thus, there is almost no period of isovolumic systole. Perhaps it is hemodynamic signaling during isovolumic systole that is part responsible for the induction of LVH, signaling that is curtailed when isovolumic systole is aborted.

Isolated Right Ventricular Volume Overload

The LV tolerates pressure overload well and patients may endure hypertension and aortic stenosis for many years before developing LV dysfunction and heart failure. Alternatively, the LV tolerates the pure volume overload of MR poorly, with most patients developing adverse sequelae within 5 years of onset of severe disease,[13,14] whereas the combined volume-pressure overload of AR is tolerated intermediately between aortic stenosis and MR.[46] Conversely, the RV tolerates a pressure overload poorly while tolerating the pure volume overloads of tricuspid regurgitation and atrial septal defect well. The nongeometric shape of the RV has not lent it to typical analysis of ventricular function. The advent of strain rate imaging, however, has allowed an easier assessment of RV function. In almost every case, strain rate is normal or enhanced in patients with atrial septal defect consistent with normal contractility and increased preload.[59–62]

Most cases of tricuspid regurgitation are secondary to pressure or volume overload placed on the RV by left-sided disease. In some cases of incurable infective endocarditis, however, the tricuspid valve was removed, a situation initially tolerated for several years, eventually culminating in heart failure.[63] Heart failure was probably more do to absence of the tricuspid valve than to myocardial failure because in a canine model of severe TR, contractility at the sarcomere level was well preserved.[64]

SUMMARY

Structural cardiac volume overload is comprised of a group of heterogeneous diseases, each creating a nearly unique set of loading conditions on the LV and/or RV. In turn the heart responds to each with unique patterns of remodeling, leading to both adaptive and maladaptive consequences. An understanding of these different patterns of hypertrophy and/or remodeling should be useful in developing strategies for the timing and correction of cardiac volume overload.

REFERENCES

1. Carabello BA. The relationship of left ventricular geometry and hypertrophy to left ventricular function in valvular heart disease. J Heart Valve Dis 1995; 4(Suppl 2):S132–8 [discussion: S138–9].
2. Carabello BA. Mitral regurgitation: basic pathophysiologic principles. Part 1. Mod Concepts Cardiovasc Dis 1988;57:53–8.
3. Kleaveland JP, Kussmaul WG, Vinciguerra T, et al. Volume overload hypertrophy in a closed-chest model of mitral regurgitation. Am J Physiol 1988; 254:H1034–41.
4. Grossman W, Jones D, McLaurin LP. Wall stress and patterns of hypertrophy in the human left ventricle. J Clin Invest 1975;53:332–41.
5. Spinale FG, Ishihara K, Zile M, et al. Structural basis for changes in left ventricular function and geometry because of chronic mitral regurgitation and after correction of volume overload. J Thorac Cardiovasc Surg 1993;106(6):1147–57.
6. Wisenbaugh T, Spann JF, Carabello BA. Differences in myocardial performance and load between patients with similar amounts of chronic aortic versus chronic mitral regurgitation. J Am Coll Cardiol 1984;3:916–23.
7. Zile MR, Tomita M, Nakano K, et al. Effects of left ventricular volume overload produced by mitral regurgitation on diastolic function. Am J Physiol 1991;261(5 Pt 2):H1471–80.
8. Corin WJ, Murakami T, Monrad ES, et al. Left ventricular passive diastolic properties in chronic mitral regurgitation. Circulation 1991;83(3):797–807.
9. Corin WJ, Monrad ES, Murakami T, et al. The relationship of afterload to ejection performance in

chronic mitral regurgitation. Circulation 1987;76: 59–67.

10. Carabello BA, Zile MR, Tanaka R, et al. Left ventricular hypertrophy due to volume overload versus pressure overload. Am J Physiol 1992;263:H1137–44.

11. Imamura T, McDermott PJ, Kent RL, et al. Acute changes in myosin heavy chain synthesis rate in pressure versus volume overload. Circ Res 1994; 75(3):418–25.

12. Matsuo T, Carabello BA, Nagatomo Y, et al. Mechanisms of cardiac hypertrophy in canine volume overload. Am J Physiol 1998;275(1 Pt 2):H65–74.

13. Enriquez-Sarano M, Avierinos JF, Messika-Zeitoun D, et al. Quantitative determinants of the outcome of asymptomatic mitral regurgitation. N Engl J Med 2005;352(9):875–83.

14. Rosenhek R, Rader F, Klaar U, et al. Outcome of watchful waiting in asymptomatic sever mitral regurgitation. Circulation 2006;113(18):2238–44.

15. Marcus ML, Doty DB, Hiratzka LF, et al. Decreased coronary reserve: a mechanism for angina pectoris in patients with aortic stenosis and normal coronary arteries. N Engl J Med 1982;307:1362–6.

16. Julius BK, Spillman M, Vassali G, et al. Angina pectoris in patients with aortic stenosis and normal coronary arteries: mechanisms and pathophysiological concepts. Circulation 1997;95:892–8.

17. Carabello BA, Nakano K, Ishihara K, et al. Coronary blood flow in dogs with contractile dysfunction due to experimental volume overload. Circulation 1991; 83:1063–75.

18. Urabe Y, Mann DL, Kent RL, et al. Cellular and ventricular contractile dysfunction in experimental canine mitral regurgitation. Circ Res 1992;70(1):131–47.

19. Mulieri LA, Leavitt BJ, Martin BJ, et al. Myocardial force-frequency defect in mitral regurgitation heart failure is reversed by forskolin. Circulation 1993; 88(6):2700–4.

20. Nagatsu M, Zile MR, Tsutsui H, et al. Native beta-adrenergic support of left ventricular dysfunction in experimental mitral regurgitation normalizes indexes of pump and contractile function. Circulation 1994; 89(2):818–26.

21. Mehta RH, Supiano MA, Oral H, et al. Relation of systemic sympathetic nervous system activation to echocardiographic left ventricular size and performance and its implications in patients with mitral regurgitation. Am J Cardiol 2000;86(11): 1193–7.

22. Tsutsui H, Spinale FG, Nagatsu M, et al. Effects of chronic β-adrenergic blockade on the left ventricular and cardiocyte abnormalities of chronic canine mitral regurgitation. J Clin Invest 1994; 93(6):2639–48.

23. Starling MR. Effects of valve surgery on left ventricular contractile function in patients with long-term mitral regurgitation. Circulation 1995;92(4):811–8.

24. Nakano K, Swindle MM, Spinale F, et al. Depressed contractile function due to canine mitral regurgitation improves after correction of the volume overload. J Clin Invest 1991;88(2):723.

25. Harris KM, Aeppli DM, Carey CF. Effects of angiotensin-converting enzyme inhibition on mitral regurgitation severity, left ventricular size, and functional capacity. Am Heart J 2005;150(5): 1106.

26. Wisenbaugh T, Sinovich V, Dullabh A, et al. Six month pilot study of captopril for mildly symptomatic, severe isolated mitral and isolated aortic regurgitation. J Heart Valve Dis 1994;3(2):197–204.

27. Marcotte F, Honos GN, Walling AD, et al. Effect of angiotensin-converting enzyme inhibitor therapy in mitral regurgitation with normal left ventricular function. Can J Cardiol 1997;13(5):479–85.

28. Dujardin KS, Enriquez-Sarano M, Bailey KR, et al. Effect of losartan on degree of mitral regurgitation quantified by echocardiography. Am J Cardiol 2001; 87(5):570–6.

29. Rozich JD, Carabello BA, Usher BW, et al. Mitral valve replacement with and without chordal preservation in patients with chronic mitral regurgitation: mechanisms for differences in postoperative ejection performance. Circulation 1992;86(6):1718–26.

30. Zile MR, Tomita M, Ishihara K, et al. Changes in diastolic function during development and correction of chronic LV volume overload produced by mitral regurgitation. Circulation 1993;87:1378–88.

31. Horskotte D, Schultz HD, Bircks W, et al. The effect of chordal preservation on late outcome after mitral valve replacement: a randomized study. J Heart Valve Dis 1993;2(2):150–8.

32. David TE, Uden DE, Strauss HD. The importance of the mitral apparatus in left ventricular function after correction of mitral regurgitation. Circulation 1983; 68(3 Pt 2):II76–82.

33. Enriquez-Sarano M, Schaff HV, Orszulak TA, et al. Valve repair improves the outcome of surgery for mitral regurgitation: a multivariate analysis. Circulation 1995;91(4):1022–8.

34. American College of Cardiology/American Heart Association Task Force on Practice Guidelines, Society of Cardiovascular Anesthesiologists, Society for Cardiovascular Angiography and Interventions, Society of Thoracic Surgeons, Bonow RO, Carabello BA, Kanu C, et al. ACC/AHA 2006 guidelines for the management of patients with valvular heart disease: a report of the American College of Cardiology/American Heart Association Task Force on Practice Guidelines (writing committee to revise the 1998 Guidelines for the Management of Patients with Valvular Heart Disease): developed in collaboration with the Society of Cardiovascular Anesthesiologists: endorsed by the Society of Cardiovascular Angiography and Interventions and the Society

of Thoracic Surgeons. Circulation 2006;114(5): e84–231.

35. Trichon BH, Felker GM, Shaw LK, et al. Relation of frequency and severity of mitral regurgitation to survival among patients with left ventricular systolic dysfunction and heart failure. Am J Cardiol 2003; 91(5):538–43.

36. Wu AH, Aaronson KD, Bolling SF, et al. Impact of mitral valve annuloplasty on mortality risk in patients with mitral regurgitation and left ventricular systolic dysfunction. J Am Coll Cardiol 2005;45(3):381–7.

37. Benedetto U, Melina G, Roscitano A, et al. Does combined mitral valve surgery improve survival when compared to revascularization alone in patients with ischemic mitral regurgitation? a meta-analysis on 2479 patients [review]. J Cardiovasc Med (Hagerstown) 2009;10(2):109–14.

38. Mihaljevic T, Lam BK, Rajeswaran J, et al. Impact of mitral valve annuloplasty combined with revascularization in patients with functional ischemic mitral regurgitation. J Am Coll Cardiol 2007; 49(22):2191–201.

39. Harris KM, Sundt TM 3rd, Aeppli D, et al. Can survival of patients with moderate ischemic mitral regurgitation be impacted by intervention on the valve? Ann Thorac Surg 2002;74(5):1468–75.

40. Carabello BA. Aortic regurgitation: hemodynamic determinants of prognosis. In: Cohn LH, DiSesa VJ, editors. Aortic regurgitation: medical and surgical management. New York: Marcel Dekker; 1986 . p. 89–103.

41. Feiring AJ, Rumberger JA. Ultrafast computed tomography analysis of regional radius-to-wall thickness ratios in normal and volume-overloaded human left ventricle. Circulation 1992;85(4):1423–32.

42. Magid NM, Wallerson DC, Borer JS. Myofibrillar protein turnover in cardiac hypertrophy due to aortic regurgitation. Cardiology 1993;82(1):20–9.

43. Taniguchi K, Nakano S, Kawashima Y, et al. Left ventricular ejection performance, wall stress, and contractile state in aortic regurgitation before and after aortic valve replacement. Circulation 1990;82(3): 1051–3.

44. Sutton M, Plappert T, Spiegel A, et al. Early postoperative changes in left ventricular chamber size, architecture, and function in aortic stenosis and aortic regurgitation and their relation to intraoperative changes in afterload: a prospective two-dimensional echocardiographic study. Circulation 1987;76(1):77–89.

45. Bonow RO, Lakatos E, Maron BJ, et al. Serial long-term assessment of the natural history of asymptomatic patients with chronic aortic regurgitation and normal left ventricular systolic function. Circulation 1991;84(4):1625–35.

46. Schwarz F, Flameng W, Schaper J, et al. Myocardial structure and function in patients with aortic valve disease and their relation to postoperative results. Am J Cardiol 1978;41(4):661–9.

47. Krayenbuehl HP, Hess OM, Monrad ES, et al. Left ventricular myocardial structure in aortic valve disease before, intermediate, and late after aortic valve replacement. Circulation 1989;79(4):744–55.

48. Gascho JA, Mueller TM, Eastham C, et al. Effect of volume-overload hypertrophy on the coronary circulation in awake dogs. Cardiovasc Res 1982;16(5):288–92.

49. Greenberg B, Massie B, Bristow JD, et al. Long-term vasodilator therapy of chronic aortic insufficiency. A randomized double-blinded, placebo-controlled clinical trial. Circulation 1988;78(1):92–103.

50. Scognamiglio R, Rahimtoola SH, Faoli G, et al. Nifedipine in asymptomatic patients with severe aortic regurgitation and normal left ventricular function. N Engl J Med 1994;331:689–94.

51. Evangelista A, Tornos P, Samola A, et al. Long-term vasodilator theraphy in patients with severe aortic regurgitation. N Engl J Med 2005;353:1342–9.

52. Bonow RO, Rosing DR, Maron BJ, et al. Reversal of left ventricular dysfunction after aortic valve replacement for chronic aortic regurgitation: influence of duration of preoperative left ventricular dysfunction. Circulation 1984;70(4):570–9.

53. Bonow RO, Dodd JT, Maron BJ, et al. Long-term serial changes in left ventricular function and reversal of ventricular dilatation after valve replacement for chronic aortic regurgitation. Circulation 1988;78(5 Pt 1):1108–20.

54. Borer JS, Bonow RO. Contemporary approach to aortic and mitral regurgitation. Circulation 2003; 108:2432–8.

55. Mann T, McLaurin L, Grossman W, et al. Assessing the hemodynamic severity of acute aortic regurgitation due to infective endocarditis. N Engl J Med 1975;293(3):108–13.

56. Carabello BA, Ballard WL, Gazes PC. In: Sahn SA, Heffner JE, editors. Cardiology pearls. Philadelphia: Hanley & Belfus, Inc; 1994. p. 45–6.

57. Sareli P, Klein HO, Schamroth CL, et al. Contribution of echocardiography and immediate surgery to the management of severe aortic regurgitation from active infective endocarditis. Am J Cardiol 1986; 57(6):413–8.

58. Corin WJ, Swindle MM, Spann JF Jr, et al. Mechanism of decreased forward stroke volume in children and swine with ventricular septal defect and failure to thrive. J Clin Invest 1988;82:544–51.

59. Pauliks LB, Chan KC, Chang D, et al. Regional myocardial velocities and isovolumic contraction acceleration before and after device closure of atrial septal defects: a color tissue Doppler study. Am Heart J 2005;150(2):294–301.

60. Jategaonkar SR, Scholtz W, Butz T, et al. Two-dimensional strain and strain rate imaging of the right ventricle in adult patients before and after

percutaneous closure of atrial septal defects. Eur J Echocardiogr 2009;10(4):499–502.

61. Van De Bruaene A, Buys R, Vanhees L, et al. Regional right ventricular deformation in patients with open and closed atrial septal defect. Eur J Echocardiogr 2011;12(3):206–13.

62. Eyskens B, Ganame J, Claus P, et al. Ultrasonic strain rate and strain imaging of the right ventricle in children before and after percutaneous closure of an atrial septal defect. J Am Soc Echo 2006; 19(8):994–1000.

63. Arbulu A, Asfaw I. Management of infective endocarditis: seventeen years' experience. Ann Thorac Surg 1987;43(2):144–9.

64. Ishibashi Y, Rembert JC, Carabello BA, et al. Normal myocardial function in severe right ventricular volume overload hypertrophy. Am J Physiol Heart Circ Physiol 2001;280(1):H11–6.

Ischemia/Infarction

Bodh I. Jugdutt, MD, DM

KEYWORDS

- Infarct expansion • Infarct size • Remodeling
- Reperfusion injury • Extracellular matrix

Myocardial infarction (MI) accounts for most incidences of heart failure (HF) and low ejection fraction (**Fig. 1**). Acute MI, usually preceded by myocardial ischemia, leads to early cardiac remodeling, with changes in ventricular geometry and structure that in turn lead to a vicious cycle of progressive ventricular dilation, increased wall stress, hypertrophy and more ventricular dilation and dysfunction, and worsening of HF.[1–8] Depending on the extent of early damage and severity of early remodeling, some patients with acute MI may die in the first few days from arrhythmias or mechanical complications, whereas many others may survive with or without symptoms of HF. Evidence suggests that the early geometric and structural changes contribute to not only early mechanical complications but also the subsequent progressive ventricular remodeling and the development of chronic HF.[1–8] A clear understanding of the underlying mechanisms is helpful in developing optimal preventive and therapeutic strategies for HF.

FACTORS CONTRIBUTING TO STRUCTURAL ABNORMALITIES POST-MI

Over nearly 3 decades since the late 1970s, a vast amount of experimental and clinical research data has mapped out the pathway leading from cardiovascular risk factors to MI, and thence to dilative left ventricular (LV) remodeling and heart failure with a low ejection fraction (see **Fig. 1**). Two key events contribute to this progression to heart failure. First is the coronary artery occlusion and thrombosis that lead to myocardial ischemic injury and infarction. Second is the early infarct

remodeling and ventricular dilation that lead to subsequent progressive ventricular dilation and dysfunction. Many studies have identified the potential factors that contribute to the structural and functional abnormalities during acute MI (**Table 1**), with evidence pointing to infarct size and collateral blood flow as the two major determinants of adverse remodeling, ventricular dysfunction, and outcome.

INFARCT SIZE, TRANSMURALITY, AND EARLY VENTRICULAR REMODELING

Data in the canine model showed that coronary artery occlusion reduces downstream perfusion and renders myocardium at risk for infarction.[9] Infarct size correlates with the gradient of nutrient flow from central to border regions of the area at risk and from the endocardium to the epicardium in the early hours postocclusion.[10] The progression to infarction in that study correlated spatially and temporally with the changes in collateral blood flow.[10] Regional ventricular dysfunction develops within seconds in myocardium within the distribution of the infarct-related artery,[11] and its severity correlates with the transmural extent of ischemic injury and eventual infarction.[12] In a canine model of reperfused MI, Reimer and Jennings[13] showed that coronary occlusion triggers a march to necrosis that begins within 40 minutes, spreads as a wavefront from the endocardium to the epicardium, and is completed by 3 hours.

INFARCT EXPANSION

Concurrent studies at the bench and bedside showed that transmural MIs (now termed *ST*

This work was supported in part by grant IAP99003 from the Canadian Institutes of Health Research, Ottawa, Ontario.

The author has nothing to disclose.

Division of Cardiology, Department of Medicine, 2C2 Walter MacKenzie Health Sciences Centre, University of Alberta and Hospital, 8440-112 Street, Edmonton, Alberta, T6G 2R7, Canada

E-mail address: bjugdutt@ualberta.ca

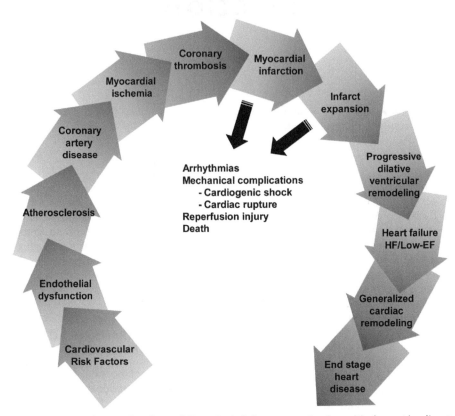

Fig. 1. Schematic showing the march to heart failure. Early infarct expansion is a critical event leading to progressive ventricular enlargement and systolic dysfunction. EF, ejection fraction; HF, heart failure.

segment elevation MIs [STEMIs]) result in significant early infarct remodeling, with expansion (ie, stretching, thinning, and dilation) of the infarct area within minutes to hours after coronary artery occlusion.[1–8] This early complication of acute MI contributes significantly to morbidity and mortality, and differed from infarct extension, implying additional myocardial necrosis.[14] Although infarct expansion was first described in autopsied hearts of patients who died within approximately 10 days after transmural MI,[14] subsequent studies using two-dimensional echocardiographic imaging established that infarct expansion is an early event that is detectable while patients are still alive, thus making early diagnosis possible.[15] Other serial two-dimensional echocardiographic studies showed that the early regional infarct expansion was a major cause of global LV dilation and impaired functional status in patients post-MI.[16,17] In the pathologic study, 50% of the patients who died within 30 days had infarct expansion, which was most severe in those with large, transmural, and anterior MI.[14] In the first clinical study, 50% of the patients with early infarct expansion on echocardiography died by 8 weeks.[15]

Other pathologic and experimental studies suggested that severe infarct expansion preceded fatal free wall cardiac rupture in patients,[18] and was linked to infarct transmurality in the canine model[19] and to infarct size and late aneurysm formation in the rat model.[20,21] An important finding in one rat study was that the regional and aneurysmal shape change occurred early and did not change significantly thereafter.[20] Taken together with the findings in the echocardiographic studies, the data suggested that the aneurysmal shape change resulted from early infarct expansion during the infarction process rather than from later scar expansion during the subsequent healing process. The studies also led to the concept that the spared epicardial rim in subendocardial infarcts (now termed non–ST segment elevation MIs [NSTEMIs]) provided a protective scaffold that prevented regional infarct dilation in acute MI.

Subsequent studies using echocardiographic imaging reinforced the concepts that early infarct expansion predicted ventricular septal rupture[22]; large transmural MIs were prone to early infarct expansion, LV dilation, and dysfunction in patients[23]; infarct expansion was more severe

Table 1
Factors in structural ventricular remodeling after acute myocardial infarction

Infarct characteristics	Size and transmural extent (STEMI; NSTEMI) Location (anterior vs inferior) Type (eg, reperfused; nonreperfused)
Physiologic reactions	Collateral reserve; changes in collateral blood flow post-occlusion Responses to reperfusion; reperfusion injury; no-reflow Previous LV hypertrophy (eg, history of hypertension) Previous ischemia and infarction Patient age and changes with cardiovascular aging
Molecular/cellular and biochemical reactions	Activation of pathways for apoptosis, oncosis, autophagy, and necrosis Response to reperfusion; reperfusion injury with progressive necrosis Activation of inflammatory pathway (cytokines and cells) Activation of ECM-proteolytic pathways (extracellular and intracellular) Activation of bioactive molecules (eg, Ang II, ROS, NOSs, TGF-β, TNF-α) Extracellular collagen matrix degradation
Mechanical forces	Intracavitary distending forces (preload, afterload, wall stress) Intramural traction forces (contractility, wall stress) External restraining forces (pericardium, extracardiac structures)
Progressive LV dilation (first 48 h)	Imbalance between distending and restraining forces Imbalance between matrix proteinases (MMPs) and inhibitors (TIMPs) Imbalance between inflammatory and antiinflammatory cytokines Regional blood flow (infarct and noninfarct regions) ECM remodeling LV shape, size, and systolic/diastolic function Remodeling of the right ventricle and atria Remodeling of vascular structures and vascular damage with no-reflow

Abbreviations: Ang II, angiotensin II; ECM, extracellular matrix; MMP, matrix metalloproteinase; NOS, nitric oxide syn-thases; NSTEMI, non–ST segment elevation myocardial infarction; ROS, reactive oxygen species; STEMI, ST segment eleva-tion myocardial infarction; TGF-β, transforming growth factor β; TIMP, tissue inhibitor of MMP; TNF-α, tumor necrosis factor α.

after anterior than inferior transmural MI[23]; and transmural infarct extension was a major factor in infarct expansion and aneurysmal dilation.[24,25] A study in the rat model suggested that cardiomyo-cyte slippage might mediate the regional dilation of the infarct area.[26] A large clinical study showed that early infarct remodeling with infarct zone expansion after STEMIs sets the stage for progressive global LV enlargement, dysfunction, and poor clinical outcome in patients post-MI.[4] In that study, expanders with more infarct dilation were more frequently anterior STEMI and had more severe LV dysfunction, more septal and free wall rupture, and more in-hospital deaths.[4]

Collectively, the findings of temporal and spatial correlates among regional collateral blood flow, myocardial damage, severity of mechanical dysfunc-tion, and infarct expansion in these early studies strongly suggested that acute STEMIs result in profound early changes in ventricular structure, shape, size, and systolic function that negatively impact subsequent outcome beyond just the infarction phase. These studies prompted testing of potential therapeutic strategies for preventing

infarct expansion during progression of myocardial damage and thereafter (**Table 2**).[2–8,27–29] Several strategies were aimed at reducing the mechanical remodeling forces that act on the infarct and no-infarct regions during acute and subacute MI (**Fig. 2**).[5–8]

TRANSLATION OF ANIMAL DATA TO HUMANS

Four pertinent points should be considered in translating animal data to the bedside in the context of acute infarction and the early remodel-ing processes. First, in contrast to the canine and other animal models, coronary occlusion is usually less abrupt in humans, and the progression to necrosis is more prolonged, estimated to occur within up to 14 hours for nonreperfused MI[7,29] and longer for MI with late reperfusion.[7] Second, in the clinical setting, the new definition of acute coro-nary syndrome includes patients with unstable angina, NSTEMI, and STEMI[30,31]; acute coronary syndromes result from atherosclerotic plaque disruption leading to thrombus formation[32]; and

Table 2
Potential approaches for limitation of early postinfarct ventricular remodeling

Target	Approach
Infarction	Reduce infarct size (increase oxygen supply, reduce demand) Interrupt transmural march of necrosis; early reperfusion of STEMI Provide epicardial scaffold to restrain dilation; early reperfusion Maintain external restraint to dilation by other devices Reduce reperfusion injury through early reperfusion Therapies to reduce apoptosis, oncosis, and necrosis; enhance autophagy
Blood flow	Restore flow (antegrade via IRA patency; collateral via NIRA patency) Vasodilators; angiogenic therapy Protect and preserve collagen matrix Collagen synthesis promoters Avoid collagen synthesis inhibitors Avoid collagen disrupters
Wall stress	Reduce wall stress and mechanical deformation forces Reduce contractile pull on infarct segment (eg, ß-blockers) Reduce intracavitary distending forces (preload, afterload) LV unloading (RAS inhibitors, NO donors, other vasodilators)
Oxidative stress	Early inhibition of ROS (eg, specific gene and RAS inhibitors)
Inflammation	Early inhibition of inflammation (eg, specific gene and RAS inhibitors)
Extracellular matrix	Protect and preserve collagen matrix that provided support Early inhibition of ECM degradation (eg, MMP, RAS inhibitors)
Intracellular matrix	Early inhibition of intracellular matrix degradation (eg, MMP inhibitors)

Abbreviations: ECM, extracellular matrix; IRA, infarct-related artery; MMP, matrix metalloproteinase; NIRA, non–infarct-related artery; NO, nitric oxide; RAS, renin-angiotensin system; ROS, reactive oxygen species.

most patients with STEMI have an occlusive thrombus and develop a Q wave MI (previously termed *transmural MI*), whereas most patients with an NSTEMI have a nonocclusive or mural thrombus and develop non-Q wave MI (previously termed *nontransmural* or *subendocardial MI*).[33–35]

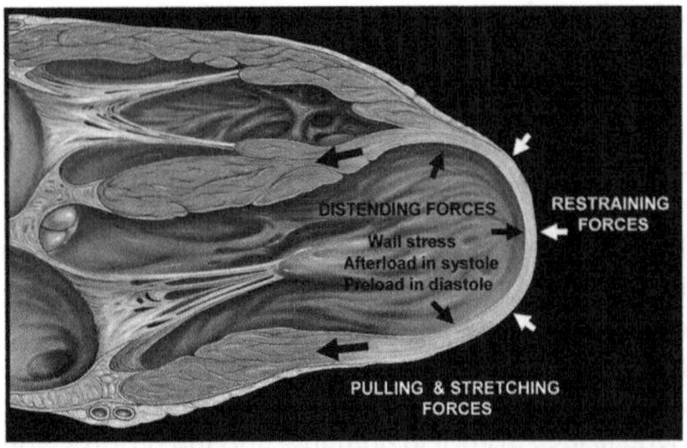

Fig. 2. Schematic showing the remodeling forces after myocardial infarction. The forces act on the infarct segment and noninfarct segments on a beat-to-beat basis during the early infarction phase and the subsequent healing phase, setting the stage for aneurysm formation and progressive ventricular enlargement. Arrows indicate the direction of force. (*From* Dhalla N, Beamish ER, Takeda N, et al, editors. The failing heart. New York: Lippincott-Raven Press; 1995; with permission.)

Third, the times to completion of infarction differ across species, occurring within approximately 30 minutes in mice, 30 to 90 minutes in rats, 2 to 6 hours in dogs, and 6 to 14 hours in humans.[5,36] Fourth, the rate of infarct healing and extracellular collagen matrix deposition also differ across species, being longer for higher species and humans.[7,36]

CORONARY REPERFUSION, INFARCT SIZE, AND EARLY REMODELING

Advances in the biology of MI have established that coronary artery occlusion triggers several biochemical, molecular, and cellular reactions that participate in early structural ventricular remodeling and dysfunction. Early biochemical abnormalities, including increased lactate, acidosis, ionic pump failure, and reactive oxygen species (ROS), and ATP depletion, set in motion events that led to a rapid loss of cellular homeostasis and progressive cardiomyocyte cell death. In the mid-1970s, Braunwald[37] identified the major determinants of infarct size, and pioneered the concept of improving the balance between myocardial oxygen supply and demand during the early hours after coronary occlusion to limit ischemic injury and infarct size, and in turn reduce post-MI mortality and morbidity. Vasodilator therapy was tested during MI and shown to effectively improve collateral blood flow (ie, supply), decrease hemodynamic load (ie, demand), decrease infarct size, limit infarct expansion and complications, and improve function.[27–29] However, the benefits were jeopardized by excessive reduction of blood pressure, resulting in impaired perfusion.[38,39]

Reimer and Jennings'[13] finding of transmural progression of necrosis during MI suggested that coronary reperfusion might interrupt this progression to necrosis, and thereby reduce infarct size and transmurality, which in turn might salvage an epicardial rim that would buttress against dilation of the infarct area. Studies in the rat model suggested that early or late reperfusion might limit infarct expansion.[40,41] In the dog model, reperfusion made 2 hours after coronary occlusion, which was relatively late during infarct progression, reduced infarct expansion.[42,43] Although reperfusion is widely used in patients with acute MI and has its benefits, it can be a two-edged sword.[44,45] In large MI, reperfusion is often associated with significant reperfusion damage and persistent LV dysfunction,[44,45] microvascular damage leading to no-reflow,[44,45] a surge of ROS,[44,45] calcium overload,[44,45] apoptosis and oncosis,[46,47] progression of necrosis,[48] enhanced degradation of the extracellular matrix (ECM),[49,50] increased activity of matrix metalloproteinases (MMPs) that degrade ECM,[51–53] enhanced inflammation,[54–56] early infarct expansion,[1–8,42,43] and persistent LV remodeling and dysfunction.[56–58]

Although aggressive reperfusion of STEMI using percutaneous coronary intervention (PCI) or thrombolytic agents is more beneficial if achieved within 90 minutes, this is not always clinically feasible. Reperfusion after 90 minutes, a more common clinical scenario, is often problematic because of reperfusion damage. Thus, survivors with persistent postischemic LV dysfunction remain at risk for progressive remodeling and its consequences (infarct expansion and thinning, LV aneurysm, dilation, rupture, heart failure, and death).[57,58] In older patients, more severe remodeling may aggravate outcome,[59] and reperfusion may increase the risk of rupture.[60,61]

NEW INSIGHTS INTO MECHANISMS OF EARLY REMODELING POSTREPERFUSION

Recent evidence in the canine model[56] suggests that reperfusion of STEMI after 90 minutes of ischemia induces early regional increases in markers of ECM remodeling (including various matrix proteases, matrix metalloproteinase

[MMP]-9, MMP-2, and a disintegrin and metalloproteinase [ADAM]-10 and -17); other bioactive molecules, such as inducible nitric oxide synthase; and markers of inflammation, including proinflammatory (ie, tumor necrosis factor-α and interleukin [IL]-6) and antiinflammatory cytokines (ie, transforming growth factor [TGF]-β1 and IL-10). Aging augments these changes, and early angiotensin II type 1 (AT$_1$) receptor blockade therapy, initiated at the onset of reperfusion in a non–blood-pressure-lowering dose, attenuated these changes, supporting the upstream regulatory role of angiotensin II and the renin-angiotensin system.

Other corroborative experimental and clinical data support the concept that, during acute reperfused STEMI, increased circulating and tissue angiotensin II results in enhanced inflammation (from an imbalance between inflammatory and noninflammatory cytokines) and ECM damage (from an imbalance between MMPs and tissue inhibitors of MMPs [TIMPs], with increased MMP/TIMP ratio and increase in other ECM proteinases), that in turn modulate matrix and ventricular remodeling and dysfunction.[56] For example, early MMP-9/TIMP-3 imbalance with a surge in MMP-9 during canine acute reperfused STEMI is associated with adverse LV remodeling and dysfunction,[51] and pretreatment with an AT$_1$ receptor blocker suppresses the MMP-9 surge, normalizes the MMP-9/TIMP-3 ratio, and limits the LV early remodeling and dysfunction.[51] However, pretreatment before STEMI or treatment from the onset of STEMI are not clinically feasible. Moreover, treatment at the onset of reperfusion might be feasible.[56]

Previous studies established that early ECM remodeling with cardiomyocyte slippage is a major mechanism for early LV remodeling.[7,8] ECM degradation after MI is mainly from MMPs, whereas TIMPs provide posttranslational control of MMP activity.[8] MMPs such as MMP-2 and MMP-9 were shown to play a major role in adverse LV remodeling.[8] The MMP/TIMP balance is critical for normal ECM remodeling.[8] A sharp rise in MMPs post-MI, with a high MMP/TIMP ratio, induces rapid ECM proteolysis, decreased collagen, and adverse ECM and LV remodeling and dysfunction.[7,8,51] However, recent evidence suggests that important interactions between ECM-proteolytic pathways (including several matricellular and other matrix proteases, and MMPs/TIMPs) and inflammatory pathways contribute to early ECM and LV remodeling.[56]

Other emerging evidence suggests that, besides oxidative stress and the early surge of ROS post-reperfusion, inflammation plays an important role in reperfusion damage (**Fig. 3**). It is

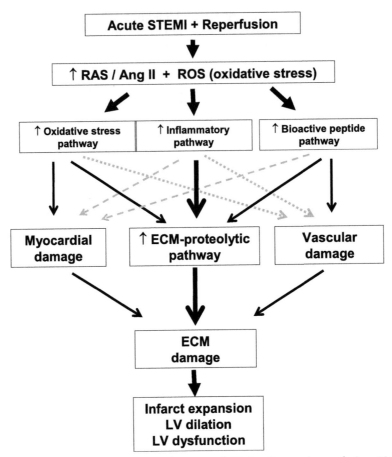

Fig. 3. Schematic depicting pathways during early myocardial infarction and reperfusion. Multiple pathways interact and converge on ECM damage and early infarct expansion. Up arrow indicates upregulated and down arrow indicates downregulated. Ang II, angiotensin II.

known that MI triggers the healing process that involves early acute inflammation with infiltration of neutrophils and monocytes.[5–8,55] The author and others have shown that post-MI healing involves a timed sequence of three sets of molecular and cellular events: (1) inflammation: acute and chronic; (2) tissue repair: with fibroblast proliferation, deposition of ECM (mostly collagen) by fibroblasts and myofibroblasts, and formation of a "live" scar; and (3) structural and functional remodeling of both infarcted and noninfarcted myocardium through dilation, hypertrophy, and angiogenesis.[5–8,55] However, acute inflammation begins very early after coronary occlusion, with an increase in inflammatory cytokines and influx of inflammatory cells.[5–8,55] Neutrophil depletion was shown to reduce reperfusion damage and infarct size.[55]

Recently, the toll-like receptor-4 (TLR4) of the inflammation pathway was suggested as a potential target. TLR4 is a known cell surface receptor

and inducer of inflammation via activation of signaling mediators.[62] Activation of TLR4 increases expression of proinflammatory cytokines and activates nuclear factor kappaB (NF-κB) signaling. Absence of TLR4 was shown to suppress early inflammation and reperfusion injury/damage.[62,63] TLR4 was also correlated with expression of proinflammatory cytokines in the rat model of reperfused STEMI.[64] Pretreatment with a TLR4 antagonist was shown to reduce reperfusion injury and markers of inflammation,[65] implicating activation of the TLR4-mediated pathway in the inflammatory response to ischemia-reperfusion injury.

Other pathways have also been implicated in ischemia-reperfusion injury/damage,[66] such as AMP-activated protein kinase[67] and Akt-secreted frizzled-related protein 2.[68] In addition, the inflammatory cytokines and ECM proteases can participate in the early myocardial damage.[56,69] For example, TGF-β exerts antiinflammatory effects during early healing (repression of inflammation, macrophage deactivation, resolution of inflammatory infiltrate), and early TGF-β activation protects against early myocardial damage.[70]

Recent evidence also suggests that, besides their well-known effects on degradation of the ECM, MMPs may also have intracellular effects and participate in early LV dysfunction after reperfusion.[70] For example, MMP-2 contributes to degradation of specific intracellular sarcomeric and cytoskeletal proteins such as troponin I, myosin light chain, α-actinin, and titin, and thereby participate in ischemia-reperfusion injury.[70]

AGING

Researchers recognize that the burden of STEMI and HF is greatest in the elderly population.[69] Although clinical studies found that age is a strong predictor of adverse events after MI and that elderly cohorts are at high risk for heart failure and adverse remodeling,[59] recommended therapies do not target these issues in the elderly.[69] Evidence suggests that the age-related increase in post–reperfused MI mortality involves cardiac rupture.[60] Studies in young mice, in which post-MI rupture is common, suggest that ECM damage through MMPs mediates rupture.[53] In humans, thrombolytic therapy has been implicated in rupture after reperfused MI.[61] The author and colleagues[22,23] previously reported rupture and significant early LV remodeling in patients with transmural MI, suggesting that infarct size is a significant factor.

SUMMARY

Despite advances in cardiovascular therapeutics, early management of acute STEMI remains a medical challenge, especially in elderly patients. The collective evidence suggests that early structural alterations play a significant role in early and subsequent outcome. Rather than single molecules and pathways, multiple molecules and pathways and intersecting pathways and overlapping mechanisms seem to participate in the early pathophysiologic processes, leading to early structural remodeling and dysfunction after MI. More research is needed to develop optimal preventive and therapeutic strategies to minimize early structural remodeling and the progression to HF.

ACKNOWLEDGMENTS

This work was supported in part by grant IAP99003 from the Canadian Institutes of Health Research, Ottawa, Ontario. The author thanks Catherine Jugdutt for her assistance.

REFERENCES

1. Pfeffer MA, Braunwald E. Ventricular remodeling after myocardial infarction. Experimental observations and clinical implications. Circulation 1990;81:1161–72.
2. Michorowski B, Senaratne PJM, Jugdutt BI. Myocardial infarct expansion. Cardiovasc Rev Rep 1987;8:42–7.
3. Michorowski B, Senaratne PJM, Jugdutt BI. Deterring myocardial infarct expansion. Cardiovasc Rev Rep 1987;8:55–62.
4. Jugdutt BI. Identification of patients prone to infarct expansion by the degree of regional shape distortion on an early two–dimensional echocardiogram after myocardial infarction. Clin Cardiol 1990;13:28–40.
5. Jugdutt BI. Prevention of ventricular remodeling post myocardial infarction: Timing and duration of therapy. Can J Cardiol 1993;9:103–14.
6. Jugdutt BI. Prevention of ventricular remodeling after myocardial infarction and in congestive heart failure. Heart Fail Rev 1996;1:115–29.
7. Jugdutt BI. Ventricular remodeling post-infarction and the extracellular collagen matrix. When is enough enough? Circulation 2003;108:1395–403.
8. Jugdutt BI. Remodeling of the myocardium and potential targets in the collagen degradation and synthesis pathways. Curr Drug Targets Cardiovasc Haematol Disord 2003;3:1–30.
9. Jugdutt BI, Hutchins GM, Bulkley BH, et al. Myocardial infarction in the conscious dog: Three dimensional mapping of infarct, collateral flow and region at risk. Circulation 1979;60:1141–50.
10. Jugdutt BI, Becker LC, Hutchins GM. Early changes in collateral blood flow during myocardial infarction in conscious dogs. Am J Physiol 1979;237:H371–80.
11. Tennant R, Wiggers CJ. The effect of coronary occlusion on myocardial contraction. Am J Physiol 1935;112:351–6.
12. Lieberman AN, Weiss JL, Jugdutt BI, et al. Two-dimensional echocardiography and infarct size: relationship of regional wall motion and thickening to the extent of myocardial infarction in the dog. Circulation 1981;63:739–46.
13. Reimer KA, Jennings RB. The "wavefront phenomenon" of myocardial ischemic cell death. II. Transmural progression of necrosis within the framework of ischemic bed size (myocardium at risk) and collateral flow. Lab Invest 1979;40:633–44.
14. Hutchins GM, Bulkley BH. Infarct expansion versus extension: two different complications of acute myocardial infarction. Am J Cardiol 1978;41:1127–32.
15. Eaton LW, Weiss JL, Bulkley BH, et al. Regional cardiac dilation after acute myocardial infarction: Recognition by two-dimensional echocardiography. N Engl J Med 1979;300:57–62.

16. Erlebacher JA, Weiss JL, Eaton LW, et al. Late effects of acute infarct dilation on heart size: a two-dimensional echocardiographic study. Am J Cardiol 1982;49:1120–6.

17. Erlebacher JA, Weiss JL, Weisfeldt ML, et al. Early dilation of the infarcted segment of acute transmural myocardial infarction: Role of infarct expansion in acute left ventricular enlargement. J Am Coll Cardiol 1984;4:201–8.

18. Schuster EH, Bulkley BH. Expansion of transmural myocardial infarction: A pathophysiological factor in cardiac rupture. Circulation 1979;60:1532–8.

19. Eaton LW, Bulkley BH. Expansion of acute myocardial infarction: Its relationship to infarct morphology in a canine model. Circ Res 1981;49:80–8.

20. Hochman JS, Bulkley BH. Expansion of acute myocardial infarction: an experimental study. Circulation 1982;65:1446–50.

21. Hochman JS, Bulkley BH. Pathogenesis of left ventricular aneurysms: an experimental study in the rat model. Am J Cardiol 1982;50:83–8.

22. Jugdutt BI, Michorowski B. Role of infarction expansion in rupture of the ventricular septum after acute myocardial infarction. A two-dimensional echocardiography study. Clin Cardiol 1987;10:641–52.

23. Jugdutt BI, Basualdo CA. Myocardial infarct expansion during indomethacin and ibuprofen therapy for symptomatic post-infarction pericarditis: Effect of other pharmacologic agents during early remodeling. Can J Cardiol 1989;5:211–21.

24. Jugdutt BI, Khan MI. Impact of increased infarct transmurality on remodeling and function during healing after anterior myocardial infarction in the dog. Can J Physiol Pharmacol 1992;70:949–58.

25. Jugdutt BI, Tang SB, Khan MI, et al. Functional impact on remodeling during healing after non-Q-wave versus Q-wave anterior myocardial infarction in the dog. J Am Coll Cardiol 1992;20:722–31.

26. Weisman HF, Bush DE, Mannisi JA, et al. Cellular mechanisms of myocardial infarct expansion. Circulation 1988;78:186–201.

27. Jugdutt BI, Becker LC, Hutchins GM, et al. Effect of intravenous nitroglycerin on collateral blood flow and infarct size in the conscious dog. Circulation 1981;63:17–28.

28. Jugdutt BI, Sussex BA, Warnica JW, et al. Persistent reduction in left ventricular asynergy in patients with acute myocardial infarction with infusion of nitroglycerin. Circulation 1983;68:1264–73.

29. Jugdutt BI, Warnica JW. Intravenous nitroglycerin therapy to limit myocardial infarct size, expansion and complications: effect of timing, dosage and infarct location. Circulation 1988;78:906–19.

30. Alpert JS, Thygesen K, Antman E, et al. Myocardial infarction redefined–a consensus document of the Joint European Society of Cardiology/American College of Cardiology Committee for the redefinition of myocardial infarction. J Am Coll Cardiol 2000;36:959–69.

31. Thygesen K, Alpert JS, White HD. Joint ESC/ACCF/AHA/WHF task force for the redefinition of myocardial infarction. Universal definition of myocardial infarction. Eur Heart J 2007;28:2525–38.

32. Libby P. Current concepts of the pathogenesis of the acute coronary syndromes. Circulation 2001;104:365–72.

33. DeWood MA, Stifter WF, Simpson CS, et al. Coronary arteriographic findings soon after non-Q-wave myocardial infarction. N Engl J Med 1986;315:417–23.

34. The TIMI III Investigators Early effects of tissue-type plasminogen activator added to conventional therapy on the culprit coronary lesion in patients presenting with ischemic cardiac pain at rest. Results of the Thrombolysis in Myocardial Ischemia (TIMI IIIA) Trial. Circulation 1993;87:38–52.

35. Boersma E, Mercado N, Poldermans D, et al. Acute myocardial infarction. Lancet 2003;361:847–58.

36. Jugdutt BI. Extracellular matrix and cardiac remodeling. In: Villarreal FJ, editor. Interstitial fibrosis in heart failure. New York: Springer; 2004. p. 23–55.

37. Braunwald E. Protection of ischemic myocardium. Introductory remarks. Circulation 1976;53:I1–2.

38. Jugdutt BI. Myocardial salvage by intravenous nitroglycerin in conscious dogs: loss of beneficial effect with marked nitroglycerin-induced hypotension. Circulation 1983;68:673–84.

39. Jugdutt BI. Intravenous nitroglycerin unloading in acute myocardial infarction. Am J Cardiol 1991;68:52D–63D.

40. Hochman JS, Choo H. Limitation of myocardial infarct expansion by reperfusion independent of myocardial salvage. Circulation 1987;75:299–306.

41. Boyle MP, Weisman HF. Limitation of infarct expansion and ventricular remodeling by late reperfusion. Study of time course and mechanism in a rat model. Circulation 1993;88:2872–83.

42. Jugdutt BI, Khan MI, Jugdutt SJ, et al. Impact of left ventricular unloading after late reperfusion of canine anterior myocardial infarction on remodeling and function using isosorbide-5-mononitrate. Circulation 1995;92:926–34.

43. Jugdutt BI. Effect of reperfusion on ventricular mass, topography and function during healing of anterior infarction. Am J Physiol 1997;272:H1205–11.

44. Braunwald E, Kloner RA. The stunned myocardium: prolonged, postischemic ventricular dysfunction. Circulation 1982;66:1146–9.

45. Kloner RA, Ellis SG, Lange R, et al. Studies of experimental coronary artery reperfusion: Effects on infarct size, myocardial function, biochemistry, ultrastructure and microvascular damage. Circulation 1983;68(2 Pt 2):I8–15.

46. Fliss H, Gattinger D. Apoptosis in ischemic and re-perfused rat myocardium. Circ Res 1996;76:949–56.

47. Ohno M, Takemura G, Ohno A. 'Apoptotic' myocytes in infarct area in rabbit hearts may be oncotic myocytes with DNA fragmentation: analysis by immunogold electron microscopy combined with In situ nick end-labeling. Circulation 1998;98:1422–30.

48. Matsumura K, Jeremy RW, Schaper J, et al. Progression of myocardial necrosis during reperfusion of ischemic myocardium. Circulation 1998;97:795–804.

49. Zhao MJ, Zhang H, Robinson TF, et al. Profound structural alterations of the extracellular collagen matrix in postischemic dysfunctional ("stunned") but viable myocardium. J Am Coll Cardiol 1987;10:1322–34.

50. Charney RH, Takahashi S, Zhao M, et al. Collagen loss in the stunned myocardium. Circulation 1992;85:1483–90.

51. Sawicki G, Menon V, Jugdutt BI. Improved balance between TIMP-3 and MMP-9 after regional myocardial ischemia-reperfusion during AT_1 receptor blockade. J Card Fail 2004;10:442–9.

52. Cleutjens JP, Kandala JC, Guarda E, et al. Regulation of collagen degradation in the rat myocardium after infarction. J Mol Cell Cardiol 1995;27:1281–92.

53. Heymans S, Luttun A, Nuyens D, et al. Inhibition of plasminogen activators or matrix metalloproteinases prevents cardiac rupture but impairs therapeutic angiogenesis and causes cardiac failure. Nat Med 1999;5:1135–42.

54. Vinten-Johansen J. Involvement of neutrophils in the pathogenesis of lethal myocardial reperfusion injury. Cardiovasc Res 2004;61:481–97.

55. Frangogiannis NG, Smith CW, Entman ML. The inflammatory response in myocardial infarction. Cardiovasc Res 2002;53:31–47.

56. Jugdutt BI, Jelani A, Palaniyappan A, et al. Aging-related changes in markers of ventricular and matrix remodeling after reperfused ST-segment elevation myocardial infarction in the canine model. Effect of early therapy with an angiotensin II type 1 receptor blocker. Circulation 2010;122:341–51.

57. Kim CB, Braunwald E. Potential benefits of late reperfusion of infarcted myocardium. The open artery hypothesis. Circulation 1993;88:2426–36.

58. Bolognese L, Neskovic AN, Parodi G, et al. Left ventricular remodeling after primary coronary angioplasty: patterns of left ventricular dilation and long-term prognostic implications. Circulation 2002;106:2351–7.

59. St John Sutton M, Pfeffer MA, Moye L, et al. Cardiovascular death and left ventricular remodeling two years after myocardial infarction: baseline predictors and impact of long-term use of captopril: information from the Survival and Ventricular Enlargement (SAVE) trial. Circulation 1997;96:3294–9.

60. Maggioni AP, Maseri A, Fresco C, et al. Age-related increase in mortality among patients with first myocardial infarctions treated with thrombolysis. The investigators of the Gruppo Italiano per lo Studio della sSupravvivenza nell'Infarcto Miocardico (GISSI-2). N Engl J Med 1993;329:1442–8.

61. Honan MB, Harrell FE Jr, Reimer KA, et al. Cardiac rupture, mortality and the timing of thrombolytic therapy: a meta-analysis. J Am Coll Cardiol 1990;16:359–67.

62. Oyama J, Blais C Jr, Liu X, et al. Reduced myocardial ischemia-reperfusion injury in toll-like receptor 4-deficient mice. Circulation 2004;109:784–9.

63. Chong AJ, Shimamoto A, Hampton CR, et al. Toll-like receptor 4 mediates ischemia/reperfusion injury of the heart. J Thorac Cardiovasc Surg 2004;128:170–9.

64. Yang J, Yang J, Ding JW, et al. Sequential expression of TLR4 and its effects on the myocardium of rats with myocardial ischemia-reperfusion injury. Inflammation 2008;31:304–12.

65. Shimamoto A, Chong AJ, Yada M, et al. Inhibition of Toll-like receptor 4 with eritoran attenuates myocardial ischemia-reperfusion injury. Circulation 2006;114(Suppl 1):I270–4.

66. Nakagawa M, Takemura G, Kanamori H, et al. Mechanisms by which late coronary reperfusion mitigates postinfarction cardiac remodeling. Circ Res 2008;103:98–106.

67. Shinmura K, Tamaki K, Saito K, et al. Cardioprotective effects of short-term caloric restriction are mediated by adiponectin via activation of AMP-activated protein kinase. Circulation 2007;116:2809–17.

68. Mirotsou M, Zhang Z, Deb A, et al. Secreted frizzled related protein 2 (Sfrp2) is the key Akt-mesenchymal stem cell-released paracrine factor mediating myocardial survival and repair. Proc Natl Acad Sci U S A 2007;104:1643–8.

69. Jugdutt BI. Aging and remodeling during healing of the wounded heart: current therapies and novel drug targets. Curr Drug Targets 2008;9:325–44.

70. Ali MA, Cho WJ, Hudson B, et al. Titin is a target of matrix metalloproteinase-2. Implications in myocardial ischemia/reperfusion injury. Circulation 2010;122:2039–47.

Cardiomyopathies: Classification, Diagnosis, and Treatment

Bernhard Maisch, MD, FESC[a],*, Michel Noutsias, MD[b],
Volker Ruppert, PhD[b], Anette Richter, MD[b],
Sabine Pankuweit, PhD[b]

KEYWORDS

- Cardiomyopathies • Myocarditis
- Hypertrophic cardiomyopathy
- Right ventricular cardiomyopathy
- Restrictive cardiomyopathy

By their historic definition, cardiomyopathies or myocardiopathies were defined as genuine heart muscle diseases. This definition excluded such causes as hypertension, congenital or valvular disease, a purely pericardial manifestation without epicardial inflammation, and also ischemic cardiovascular disease. In the eighteenth century, the only heart muscle disease known in medicine was myocarditis, as in these ancient times even coronary artery sclerosis and infarction were unknown and if they occurred they were put into the basket of myocarditides. Around 1900, heart muscle diseases were mentioned as such, but it was not until 1960 that the term cardiomyopathy or myocardiopathy was used for the first time.[1–3] Until 1980, several definitions for the term cardiomyopathies or myocardiopathies were in use until the World Health Organization/International Society and Federation of Cardiology (WHO/ISFC) Task Force defined it as "heart muscle diseases of unknown cause."[4] The WHO/ISCF classification of 1996

expanded the term cardiomyopathies to all heart muscle diseases that lead to functional disturbances of the heart.[5] Both classifications described 4 main phenotypes, which can be assessed by invasive and noninvasive imaging methods: dilated cardiomyopathy (DCM), hypertrophic cardiomyopathy (HCM), restrictive cardiomyopathy (RCM), and unclassified forms. In 1996, right ventricular cardiomyopathy, previously right ventricular dysplasia (ARVCM), was added (**Fig. 1**). These phenotypes were at that time thought to be primary cardiomyopathies, that is, heart muscle diseases of unknown cause. As secondary cardiomyopathies, heart muscle diseases of known causes, the task force included inflammatory heart muscle diseases (myocarditis, perimyocarditis), hypertensive cardiomyopathy, ischemic cardiomyopathy, and other forms of heart failure. Ischemic cardiomyopathy was defined as cardiac dysfunction of the nonischemic part of the heart muscle owing to overload following adverse

This work was supported by a grant of the Bundesministerium für Wissenschaft und Forschung (BMBF) in the German Competence Net of Heart Failure (KNHI), by the Prof. Dr Reinfried Pohl Stiftung, by the Marburg Heart Foundation (VFDK) and the UKGM Foundation.
The authors have nothing to disclose.
[a] Division of Cardiology, Department of Internal Medicine, Faculty of Medicine, Philipps University, UKGM GmbH, Baldinger Street, 35043 Marburg, Germany
[b] Division of Cardiology, Department of Internal Medicine, UKGM GmbH, Baldinger Street, 35043 Marburg, Germany
* Corresponding author.
E-mail addresses: maisch@staff.uni-marburg.de; bermaisch@aol.com

Heart Failure Clin 8 (2012) 53–78
doi:10.1016/j.hfc.2011.08.014
1551-7136/12/$ – see front matter © 2012 Elsevier Inc. All rights reserved.

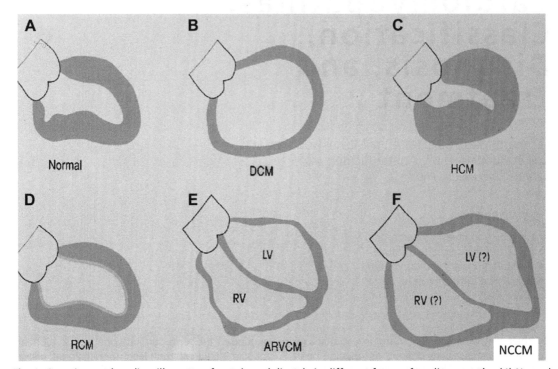

Fig. 1. Superimposed cardiac silhouette of systole and diastole in different forms of cardiomyopathy. (*A*) Normal systole and diastole in a ventricle without dilatation and no segmental wall motion abnormality. (*B*) DCM: dilated cardiomyopathy with enlarged systolic and diastolic volumes and decreased ejection fraction. Diastolic parameters are also pathologic in most cases. (*C*) HCM: Hypertrophic cardiomyopathy with (hyper)normal systolic contraction, in infiltrative or storage disease diastolic compliance is disturbed. (*D*) RCM: restrictive cardiomyopathy. (*E*) ARVCM: arrhythmogenic right ventricular cardiomyopathy. (*F*) NCCM: nonclassified cardiomyopathy.

remodeling of the noninfarcted area. Inflammatory cardiomyopathy as a new and distinct entity was defined histologically as myocarditis, in association with cardiac dysfunction. Infectious and autoimmune forms of inflammatory cardiomyopathy were recognized. Viral cardiomyopathy was defined as viral persistence in a dilated heart without ongoing inflammation. If it was accompanied by myocardial inflammation, it was termed inflammatory viral cardiomyopathy (or viral myocarditis with cardiomegaly). This entity was specified in a World Heart Federation consensus meeting in 1999 by quantitative immunohistological criteria for inflammation ($\geq$14 infiltrating cells/mm^2). These infiltrating cells could be lymphocytes (CD3-, CD4-[Helper T cells], CD8-[Suppressor T cells]) or CD45R0 activated T cells and incorporate up to 4 monocytes/macrophages/mm^2. The causative microbial agent present in the myocardial tissue was defined by molecular biologic methods (eg, polymerase chain reaction [PCR]) as viral, bacterial, or autoimmune (= nonmicrobial).[6,7] The appropriate terms derived from this classification are as follows: viral myocarditis, if inflammation by biopsy was associated with a positive test for viral RNA or

DNA; viral inflammatory cardiomyopathy, if a positive PCR on microbial agents in the biopsy was associated with a dilated and inflamed heart; or viral heart disease, if dilated cardiomyopathy was associated with viral persistence with inflammation. Autoreactive myocarditis or autoreactive inflammatorycar diomyopathy was defined as an inflamed heart with 14 or more infiltrating cells but with no detectable microbial agent.[6,7]

With the discovery of a genetic background in several forms of cardiomyopathies previously alluded to as "of unknown origin," a new genomic classification was proposed taking the underlying gene mutations and the cellular level of expression of encoded proteins into consideration for the respective classification.[8–12] Thus, DCM or ARVC were attributed to cytoskeletal mutations, HCM and RCM to sarcomeric mutations, and modified ion channels (channelopathies, eg, long or short QT syndrome and Brugada syndrome) were introduced into the classification of cardiomyopathies in 2006 by the American Heart Association (AHA), the latter even without hemodynamic dysfunction.[13] The ESC (European Society of Cardiology) Working Group on Myocardial and Pericardial Diseases deliberately took a different approach: their clinically oriented classification of heart muscle disorders was still grouped according to morphology and function, as in previous classifications. Only in a second step was familial from nonfamilial/acquired disease labeled.[14] This obviously remains the clinically most useful approach for the diagnosis and management of patients and families with heart muscle disease.[15] In the ESC position statement of 2008,[14] cardiomyopathies were defined as myocardial disorders in which the heart muscle is structurally and functionally abnormal, and in which coronary artery disease, hypertension, and valvular and congenital heart disease are absent or do not sufficiently explain the observed myocardial abnormality. The aim was to help clinicians look beyond generic diagnostic labels to reach more specific diagnoses. For this purpose, we proposed a clinical pathway for the diagnosis and treatment of dilated cardiomyopathy with or without inflammation.[16] One year later, a scientific statement on the role of endomyocardial biopsy in the management of cardiovascular disease was published,[17] making useful recommendations for clinical practice and providing an understanding for the use of endomyocardial biopsy in an individual patient by different clinical scenarios. Taking the classification of cardiomyopathies and the recommendations for endomyocardial biopsies in different clinical situations, the clinician is now able to identify genetic, autoimmune, and viral causative factors by using a thorough and logical approach to reach a diagnosis in patients with familial and nonfamilial forms of the underlying structural heart muscle diseases in the perspective of a treatment option (**Tables 1**A, B and **2**A, B).[16]

HYPERTROPHIC CARDIOMYOPATHIES
Definition

Hypertrophic cardiomyopathy is defined phenotypically by left ventricular hypertrophy, which cannot be explained by hypertension, valvular disease, or storage diseases. A hypertrophic obstructive cardiomyopathy (HOCM) is present when the left ventricular (LV) outflow tract is narrowed by the mitral valve opposing the interventricular septum (SAM = septal anterior motion) or as a consequence of a Venturi effect. Hypertrophic nonobstructive cardiomyopathy is hypertrophy without obstruction, which may be found as an apical, a midventricular isolated septal form, or as hypertrophy of the papillary muscles.

Genetics

HCM was the first cardiomyopathy in which a monogenetic cause in the beta-myosin gene

was shown. Later on, other sarcomeric genes with mostly autosomal mutations followed. At present, we find a genetic link in about 60% of patients.[8,18] HCM is primarily a sarcomeric disease with more than 450 mutations in 21 different genes (**Table 3**). This may in part explain the highly variable clinical phenotype.[19]

Further screening of families with index patients led to the concept that many cardiomyopathies are consequences of one or more gene defects.

Noninvasive Imaging

Noninvasive imaging relies primarily on echocardiography and magnetic resonance imaging (MRI), by which hypertrophy, the presence of an outflow tract obstruction (SAM), and the different forms of apical, a midventricular isolated septal form, or as hypertrophy of the papillary muscles can be assessed (**Fig. 2**). It was recently shown that localized apical and anterolateral hypertrophies are underdiagnosed applying echo.[20] Both methods give hints for the differential diagnosis to an infiltrative disorder, particularly amyloidosis, by its characteristic impression of the septum in echocardiography and the characteristic pattern of late gadolinium enhancement (LGE). "Hypertrophy," as assessed by echocardiography, contrasts in many cases with the low-voltage electrocardiogram (EKG) because of the amyloid deposits, which may mimic hypertrophy.[21]

Biomarkers

Biomarkers of heart failure (BNP, nt-pro BNP, ANP) may be increased. Markers of necrosis (troponins) are missing except in the case of accompanying necrosis. Presence of the hepatitis C genome has been reported only in patients from South East Asia.

Heart Catheterization

Heart catheterization is warranted to exclude coronary artery disease in cases with a pseudo-infarction–like EKG, to demonstrate the obstruction in LV angiography, verify or provoke the gradient by a Valsalva maneuver (**Fig. 3**A) or Brockenbrough phenomenon, and to perform percutaneous transfemoral septal ablation (PTMSA), which is able to reduce the outflow gradient effectively and also is demonstrable by the missing obstruction in LV angiography thereafter (see **Fig.3**B).

Endomyocardial Biopsy

Endomyocardial biopsy, either from the left ventricle or septum, should be performed in nonfamilial and nonobstructive forms, when the

Table 1
Classification of cardiomyopathies according to the American Heart Association 2006[13] with commentary

A. Primary Cardiomyopathies (Predominantly Involving the Heart)

Genetic	Mixed	Acquired
HCM	DCM	Inflammatory (myocarditis)
ARVC/D	RCM (nonhypertrophied, nondilated)	Tako-Tsubo (stress provoked)
LVNC		Peripartum
Glycogen storage		Tachycardia-induced
Conduction defects		Infants of insulin-dependent diabetic mothers

Mitochondrial myopathies

Ion channel disorders (LQTS, Brugada, SQTS, CVPT, Asian SUNDS)

Commentaries:
1. Patients come to the physician not with a genetic analysis of their cardiovascular disorder but with symptoms (eg, dyspnea, arrhythmia, angina, cardiomegaly, hypertrophy)
2. A mixed form may relate to fact that dilatation and restriction can be observed in both the genetic and acquired forms. It refers to the dilemma describe in 1.
3. Many ion channel disorders show no hemodynamic dysfunction (=cardiomyopathy). They should be listed as cardiopathies but not as cardiomyopathies.

B. Secondary Cardiomyopathies (Systemic Disorders Involving the Heart)

Infiltrative (accumulation between the myocytes)	Amyloidosis (primary, familial autosomal dominant, senile, secondary forms), Gaucher,[a] Hurler,[a] Hunter[a] diseases
Storage (accumulation within the myocytes)	Hemochromatosis, Fabry disease,[a] glycogen storage disease (Pompe),[a] Niemann-Pick disease[a]
Toxicity	Drugs, heavy metals, chemical agents
Endomyocardial	Endomyocardial fibrosis (EMF), hypereosinophilic syndrome (HES), eg, Löffler's endocarditis
Inflammatory granulomatous	Sarcoidosis
Endocrine	Diabetes mellitus,[a] hyperthyroidism, hypothyroidism, hyperparathyroidism, pheochromocytoma, acromegaly
Cardiofacial	Noonan syndrome,[a] lentiginosis[a]
Neuromuscular/neurologic	Friedreich ataxia,[a] Duchenne-Becker muscular dystrophy,[a] Emery-Dreifuss muscular dystrophy,[a] myotonic dystrophy,[a] neurofibromatosis,[a] tuberous sclerosis[a]
Nutritional deficiencies	Beriberi(thiamine), pellagra, scurvy, selenium, carnitine, Kwashiokor
Autoimmune/collagen	Systemic lupus erythematosus, dermatomyoxitis, rheumatoid arthritis, polyarteritis nodosa
Electrolyte imbalance	
Consequence of cancer therapy	Anthracyclines (doxorubicin, daunorubicin), cyclophosphamide, radiation

Commentary: The distinction between primary and secondary cardiomyopathy in the AHA classification 2006 is similar to the differentiation in the 1996 classification of the WHO/ISFC classification, in which primary was labeled of "unknown cause"(=idiopathic) and secondary as specific cardiomyopathies with an established etiopathogenetic origin. The dilemma lies in the use of primary and secondary for different meanings in cardiomyopathy classifications, which causes misunderstandings, which could have been otherwise avoided.

Abbreviations: ARVC/D, arrhythmogenic right ventricular cardiomyopathy or dysplasia; CVPT, cardiac ventricular periodic tachycardia; DCM, dilated cardiomyopathy; HCM, hypertrophic cardiomyopathy; LQTS, Long QT-syndrome; LVNC, left ventricular noncompaction; RCM, restrictive cardiomyopathy; SQTS, short QT-syndrome; Asian SUNDS, sudden unexpected nocturnal death syndrome.

[a] Genetic or familial origin.

Data from Maron BJ, Towbin JA, Thiene G, et al. Contemporary definitions and classification of the cardiomyopathies: an American Heart Association scientific statement from the Council on Clinical Cardiology, Heart Failure and Transplantation Committee; Quality of Care and Outcomes Research and Functional Genomics and Translational Biology Interdisciplinary Working Groups; and Council on Epidemiology and Prevention. Circulation 2006;113:1807–16.

Table 2
Classification of cardiomyopathies according to the ESC Scientific Statement 2008

A. Functional classification and clinical phenotype precedes genetic and disease subtypes

Phenotypes	HCM	DCM	ARVC	RCM	Unclassified
Genetics	a. Familial/ Genetic b. Nonfamilial/ Nongenetic	a. Familial/ Genetic b. Nonfamilial/ Nongenetic	a. Familial/ Genetic b. Nonfamilial/ Nongenetic	a. Familial/ Genetic b. Nonfamilial/ Nongenetic	a. Familial/ Genetic b. Nonfamilial/ Nongenetic

For the familial/genetic forms of each phenotype, either an already specified disease subtype or an unidentified gene defect is assumed.
For the nonfamilial/nongenetic forms of each phenotype, either an already specified disease subtype or an idiopathic form is assumed.

B. Examples of specified subtypes (known genes) of familial/genetic forms of cardiomyopathies

Phenotype	HCM (Hypertrophic Cardiomyopathy)	Commentary
a. Familial/Genetic	Sarcomeric protein disease: β-myosin heavy chain, cardiac myosin binding protein C, cardiac troponin I, troponin I, a-tropomyosin, essential myosin light chain, regulatory myosin light chain, cardiac actin, a-myosin heavy chain, titin, troponin c, muscle LIM protein. Glycogen storage disease: eg, GSDII (Pompe disease), GSD III (Forbe disease), AMP kinase (WPW), HCM, conduction disease, Danon disease). Lysosomal storage diseases: eg, Anderson-Fabry disease, Hurler syndrome. Disorders of fatty acid metabolism Carnitine deficiency Phosphorylase B kinase deficiency Mitochondrial cytopathies: eg, MELAS, MERFF, LHON Syndromic HCM: Noonan, LEOPARD syndromes, Friedreich's ataxia, Beckwith-Wiedermann, Sawyer's syndromes (pure gonadal dysgenesis) Other: Familial Amyloid, Phospolamban promoter	Originally thought to be a sarcomeric protein disease, which it still is, not the overlap with DCM for sarcomeric protein mutations and with RCM for storage diseases with an HCM phenotype. Clinically important are amyloidosis and Anderson-Fabry disease
b. Nonfamilial/Nongenetic	Obesity, infants of diabetic mothers, athletic training, Amyloid (AL/prealbumin)	

(continued on next page)

Table 2
(continued)

Phenotype	DCM (Dilated Cardiomyopathy)	Commentaries
a. Familial/Genetic	Sarcomeric protein disease (see HCM): β-myosin heavy chain, cardiac myosin binding protein C, cardiac troponin I, troponin I, a-tropomyosin, essential myosin light chain, regulatory myosin light chain, cardiac actin, a-myosin heavy chain, titin, troponin c, Z-band: muscle LIM protein, TCAP Cytoskeletal gene mutations: dystrophin, desmin, metavinculin, sarcoglycan complex, CRYAB, epicardin Nuclear membrane: Lamin A/C, emerin Mildly dilated cardiomyopathy Intercalated disc protein mutations (see ARVC): plakoglobin, desmoplakin, plakophilin, desmoglein, desmocollin Mitochondrial cytopathy	1. Genetic/familial DCM was originally thought to be primarily caused by cytoskeletal gene mutation. But there is overlap in the same families to HCM with sarcomeric mutations and ARVC with intercalated disc protein mutations 2. For some cases of myocarditis, a genetic predisposition has been described, which is particularly relevant in rheumatic forms or collagen diseases 3. Viral persistence as assessed by PCR can sometimes in the acute disease state show little or no hemodynamic dysfunction. This is applicable particularly to Parvovirus B19 and human herpesvirus 6 infection with little or no inflammation
b. Nonfamilial/ Nongenetic	Myocarditis: infective, toxic, immune Kawasaki disease Eosinophilic (Churg Strauss syndrome) Viral persistence Drugs Pregnancy Endocrine Nutritional: thiamine, carnitine, selenium, hypophatemia Alcohol Tachycardiomyopathy	

Phenotype	ARVC (Arrhythmogenic Right Ventricular Cardiomyopathy)	Commentary
a. Familial/Genetic	Intercalated disc protein mutations: plakoglobin, desmoplakin, plakophilin, desmoglein, desmocollin Cardiac ryanodine receptor (RyR2) Transforming growth factor-β3(TGβ3)	1. The intercalated disc protein mutations are also rarely found in the DCM phenotype. There is remarkable extension of ARVC also to the left ventricle in up to 70% of cases
b. Nonfamilial/ Nongenetic	Inflammation (see myocarditis with preselection of the right heart)	2. In the nonfamilial form, myocarditis primarily of the right ventricle has been a phenocopy of ARVC. Fatty cells in the right heart are a common phenomenon of a postinflammatory state

Phenotype	RCM (Restrictive Cardiomyopathy)	Commentary
a. Familial/Genetic	Sarcomeric protein mutations: Troponin I (RCM ± HCM), essential light chain of myosin Familial amyloidosis: Transthyretin (RCM + neuropathy), apolipoprotein (RCM + nephropathy) Desminopathy, Pseudoxanthoma elasticum Hemochromatosis Anderson-Fabry disease Glycogen storage disease (see also HCM)	1. A restrictive filling pattern is also the correlate of diastolic heart failure or heart failure with normal ejection fraction, eg, in hypertension or in diabetic cardiomyopathy
b. Nonfamilial/Nongenetic	Amyloid (AL/prealbumin) Scleroderma Endomyocardial fibrosis: hypereosinophilic syndrome, idiopathic, chromosomal cause, drugs (serotonin, methysergide, ergotamine, mercurial agents, busulfan) Carcinoid heart disease Metastatic cancers Radiation Drugs (eg, anthracyclines)	

Phenotype	Unclassified	Commentary
a. Familial/Genetic	Left ventricular noncompaction (LVNC), Barth syndrome Lamin A/C ZASP a-dystrobrevin	1. Tako Tsubo cardiomyopathy can be a mixed bag in which toxic (transient ultra high adrenalin concentration) and inflammation may interact. Its reversibility within a few days to weeks is indirect evidence of a stress-induced cardiomyopathy, which could be also listed under dilated cardiomyopathy
b. Nonfamilial/Nongenetic	Tako Tsubo cardiomyopathy	2. LVNC is still a matter of definition with respect to the amount of noncompacted areas. It can also fit into the subgroup of familial DCM

Abbreviations: GSD, glycogen storage disease; LHON, Leber hereditary optic neuropathy; MELAS, mitochondrial encephalomyopathy, lactic acidosis, and stroke-like episodes; MERFF, myoclonic epilepsy with ragged red fibers; PRC, polymerase chain reaction; WPW, Wolff-Parkinson-White syndrome.

Data from Elliott P, Andersson B, Arbustini E, et al. Classification of the cardiomyopathies: a position statement from the European Society of Cardiology Working Group on Myocardial and Pericardial Diseases. Eur Heart J 2008;29:270–6.

Table 3
Causal genes for hypertrophic cardiomyopathy (HCM)

Gene	Symbol	Frequency	Associated Phenotype
β-Myosin heavy chain	MYH7	25%–35%	Mild or severe HCM
Myosin binding protein C	MYBPC3	20%–30%	Mild or severe HCM, late onset
Cardiac troponin T	TNNT2	~3%–5%	Mild hypertrophy, sudden death
Cardiac troponin I	TNNI3	~3%–5%	Extreme intrafamilial heterogeneity, no sudden death without severe disease
α-tropomyosin	TPM1	~1%	Variable prognosis, sudden death
Myozenin 2 (calsarcin 1)	MYOZ2	Rare	Typical HCM
Myosin light chain 1	MYL3	Rare	Skeletal myopathy
Myosin light chain 2	MYL2	Rare	Skeletal myopathy
α-actin	ACTC1	Rare	Apical hypertrophy
Titin	TTN	Rare	Typical HCM
Telethonin	TCAP	Rare	Typical HCM, variable penetrance
Myosin light chain kinase 2	MYLK2	Rare	Early Onset
α-Myosin heavy chain	MYH6	Rare	Late onset
Cardiac troponin C	TNNC1	Rare	Typical HCM
Muscle LIM protein	CSRP3	Rare	Late onset, variable penetrance
Phospholamban	PLN	Rare	Typical HCM, variable penetrance
Vinculin/metavinculin	VCL	Rare	Obstructive midventricular hypertrophy
a-Actinin 2	ACTN2	Rare	Mainly sigmoidal HCM
LIM binding domain 3	LDB3	Rare	Mainly sigmoidal HCM
Junctophilin 2	JHP2	Rare	Typical HCM
Caveolin 3	CAV3	Rare	Unclear

Data from Keren A, Syrris P, McKenna WJ. Hypertrophic cardiomyopathy: the genetic determinants of clinical disease expression. Nat Clin Pract Cardiovasc Med 2008;5(3):158–68; and Marian AJ. Hypertrophic cardiomyopathy: from genetics to treatment. Eur J Clin Invest 2010;40(4):360–9.

differential diagnosis to storage diseases and amyloidosis has to be clarified.

The histologic hallmark of hypertrophic cardiomyopathy is myofiber hypertrophy, which often may be bizarre, with myocyte degeneration and abnormal branching and curling of myocytes and interstitial fibrous depositions found regularly (see **Fig. 3**D, E). The latter are thought to be the morphologic correlate for ventricular arrhythmias in these patients.

DILATED CARDIOMYOPATHY
Definition

Dilated cardiomyopathies are commonly defined by a dilatation of the left (or both) ventricles and LV contractile dysfunction, which cannot be explained by coronary artery disease, hypertension, or valvular disease. Its prevalence is 1 per 2500 subjects, and mortality at 5 years is 30% to 50%, depending on current treatment. Echocardiographic criteria are commonly a reduced ejection fraction (EF) of less than 55%, in some studies less than 45%, and a LV end diastolic diameter (LVEDD) greater than 117% of normal value predicated to age and body surface area. Similarly, an increased end diastolic volume greater than 100 mL/m^2 with a decreased EF fits the criteria.

Familial Dilated Cardiomyopathies and Genetics

The etiology of the clinical phenotype of dilated cardiomyopathy comprises genetic, autoimmune, and viral factors. Most likely, all 3 factors interplay to a different extent.[8–12,22] Familial forms make up to 30%.[10,12,22] Not all mutations, polymorphisms, and modifier genes have yet been identified. The phenotype in monogenetic forms is determined by mutation itself, but it can be modified also by transmission mode, penetrance, environmental influence, current or changing immune status, polymorphisms, modifier genes, and other confounders and thus explains in part the different functional status. Genotype-phenotype correlations are not so strict as originally thought.

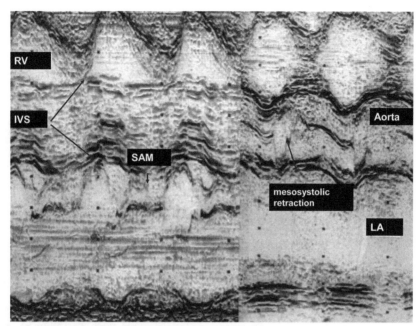

Fig. 2. Time motion echocardiogram in HOCM: hypertrophy of the interventricular septum (IVS) of 24 mm (normal: up to 11 mm); systolic anterior motion of anterior and posterior mitral valve leaflet (SAM). RV, right ventricle; LA, left atrium. Note the mesosystolic retraction of the opening of the aortic valve cusps due to decreased flow by outflow obstruction. (*Adapted from* Classen M, Diehl, Kochsiek. Innere Medizin. Urban & Fischer Verlag/Elsevier GmbH; 2006; with permission.)

Mutations in the same gene can also code for a hypertrophic phenotype. In families, the clinical and functional phenotype can vary considerably. For details see **Tables 1**B and **2**B and **Table 4**.

The Inflammatory and Postinfective Subtype

Inflammatory and postinfective cardiomyopathies have been considered secondary heart muscle diseases[5] or special subtypes[14] of dilated cardio-myopathy, whereby inflammation in the myocardium was defined by a World Heart Federation (WHF) expert panel as 14 or more lymphocytes (eg, CD3, CD4 + CD 8, or CD 45 R0) and macro-phages/mm^2 (CD14, CD11c, CD68) and the etiology of the inflammation was determined from the presence of microbial RNA or DNA by PCR, in situ hybridization, or dot blot.[6,7] The most frequent etiologies in Europe have shown an epidemiologic shift that has occurred in the past 15 years from enteroviral and adenoviral infections to Parvovirus B19, human herpesvirus 6 (HHV 6), and cytomega-lovirus (CMV).[9,15,23,24] To what extent, or if at all, the persistence of a viral genome's DNA, such as Parvovirus B19 or HHV 6, found in a cardiac tissue specimen contributes to the cardiac pathology is still a matter of discussion.[25–27] Our own clinical evidence favors a role of these 2 viruses in the cardiomyopathic process via a microvascular patho-genesis,[28–30] because Parvovirus B19 as an erythrovirus docks to the respective receptor at the vascular wall in the myocardium. The largest group of patients with myocarditis is still the autor-eactive (virus-negative) form. Depending on the respective underlying infection, the inflammatory process, the hemodynamic compromise, the New York Heart Association classification, and the effect of specific heart failure and antiarrhythmic treatment, the prognosis of DCM can be as poor as in patients with cancer or much better.[29–31] Of note, the clinical phenotype of dilated cardiomy-opathy can be expressed through single or multi-factorial etiopathogenesis with or without viral persistence, with or without inflammation.

Key questions in the etiology, pathogenesis, and clinical management of inflammatory cardiomyop-athy and myocarditis follow.

How to Diagnose Myocarditis Clinically?

Acute and chronic myocarditis may have many clinical faces or phenotypes. Phenotypes (faces) may vary in different phases of the same etiological disease. Acute myocarditis can present as a fulmi-nate deterioration of heart failure, life-threatening ventricular arrhythmia, or sudden death. The more frequent chronic forms may present as heart failure of unknown etiology after exclusion of rele-vant coronary artery disease, uncontrolled hyper-tension, or valvular disorders. Angina pectoris is

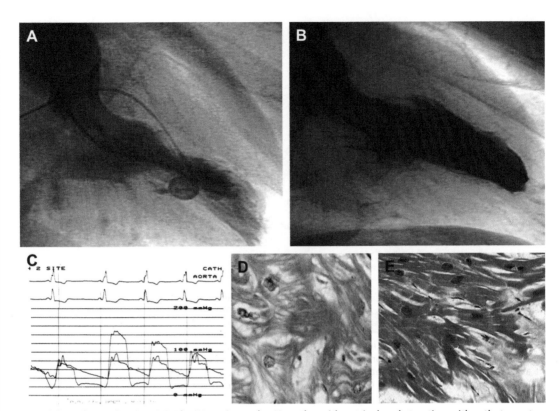

Fig. 3. (*A*) LV obstruction in HOCM by LV angiography. Note the midventricular obstruction with catheter entrapment. (*B*) After PTSMA obstruction has disappeared. (*C*) During the Valsalva maneuver in HOCM the gradient can increase dramatically. (*D*) Endomyocardial biopsy of the same patient as in *A* and *B* with hypertrophy and whirling of fibers, branching and enlargement of nuclei. (*E*) The same patient as in (*D*) showing degeneration, fiber hypertrophy, and branching (*D, E*: H&E staining, original magnification ×250).

a feature found frequently in patients with Parvovirus B19–associated heart disease with or without inflammation; precordial discomfort can also be caused by accompanying pericarditis. Atrial rhythm disturbances and atrial fibrillation in particular can be associated with any form of heart failure or cardiomyopathy and myocarditis.

Table 5 gives a clinical classification that was initially proposed by Liebermann and colleagues[32] in 1991 and has been adjusted to histologic and immunohistological findings by Maisch and colleagues[29] in 2002 and to an integrated biomarker approach.[21]

How to Diagnose Inflammation in a Diseased Heart?

Inflammation in myocarditis can be diagnosed noninvasively and indirectly by a set of serologic biomarkers (see Table 5),[21,29] by imaging biomarkers, such as cardiac MRI[21,33–37] and echocardiography for segmental wall motion abnormality or dilatation, and an accompanying pericardial effusion and specifically by

endomyocardial biopsy.[6,7,9,10,15,17,21,23,28,35] Cardiospecific serologic biomarkers, which are useful for the assessment of myocardial necrosis are Troponin I and CK-MB. These biomarkers are elevated in myocardial infarction, and may be in the gray zone or above it in hypertension with heart failure or in myocarditis. So, infarction and hypertensive emergencies have to be excluded before myocarditis should be suspected.

MRI criteria for the diagnosis of myocarditis have been proposed by several groups,[21,33–36] which all incorporated LGE, which is by itself noncharacteristic because it can mean fibrosis as well. In the Journal of the American College of Cardiology (JACC) white paper, an international consortium agreed on a set of MRI criteria: LGE, gRE, and the T2-weighted comparison between myocardial and skeletal muscle. Our own criteria incorporated these 3, and added pericardial effusion as an additional criterion of inflammation of the epicardium and pericardium. Two of these 4 criteria have to be positive to make the diagnosis of suspected myocardial inflammation a feasible working hypothesis. We have tested these criteria

Table 4
Monogenetic forms of dilated cardiomyopathy (DCM)

Gene	Locus	Gene Product	Frequency	Allelic Disorders/Phenotypes
LMNA	1q21.2-.3	lamin A/C	4%–8%	Lipodystrophy, Charcot-Marie-Tooth 2B1, Emery-Dreifuss muscular dystrophy, Hutchinson-Gilford progeria syndrome, limb girdle muscular dystrophy (LGMD) 1B
MYH7	14q12	β-myosin heavy chain	4%–6%	Laing distal myopathy, HCM
TNNT2	1q32	cardiac troponin T	3%	HCM
SCN5A	3p21	sodium channel	2%–3%	Long QT syndrome type 3, Brugada syndrome, idiopathic ventricular fibrillation, sick sinus syndrome, cardiac conduction system disease
MYH6	14q12	α-myosin heavy chain	? 2%–3%	HCM, dominantly inherited atrial septal defect
DES	2q35	desmin	<1%–1%	desminopathy, myofibrillar myopathy
VCL	10q22.1–23	metavinculin	<1%–1%	HCM
LDB3	10q22.2–23.3	LIM binding protein 3	<1%–1%	HCM, myofibrillar myopathy
TCAP	17q12	titin-cap or telethonin	<1%–1%	LGMD2G, HCM
PSEN1/PSEN2	14q24.3/1q31–q42	presenilin 1/2	<1%–1%	Early-onset Alzheimer disease/Early- and late-onset Alzheimer disease
ACTC	15q14	cardiac actin	<1%	HCM
TPM1	15q22.1	α-tropomyosin	<1%	HCM
SGCD	5q33–34	δ-sarcoglycan	<1%	Delta sarcoglycanopathy (LGMD2F)
CSRP3	11p15.1	muscle LIM protein	<1%	HCM
ACTN2	1q42–q43	α-actinin-2	<1%	N/A
ABCC9	12p12.1	SUR2A	<1%	N/A
TNNC1	3p21.3-p14.3	cardiac troponin C	<1%	N/A
TNNI3	19q13.4	cardiac troponin I	<1%	HCM, restrictive cardiomyopathy
ANKRD1	10q23.31	ankyrin repeat domain 1 (cardiac muscle)	?	N/A
CRYAB	11q22.3–q23.1	crystallin	?	HCM
DMD	Xp21.2	dystrophin	?	Dystrophinopathies (Duchenne muscular dystrophy, Becker muscular dystrophy)
EMD	Xq28	emerin		N/A
EYA4	6q23	eyes-absent 4	?	N/A
FHL2	2q12.2	Four-and-a-half LIM protein-2		N/A
FKTN	9q31–q33	fukutin		N/A
MYBPC3	11p11.2	myosin-binding protein C	?	HCM
MYPN	10q21.3	myopalladin	?	N/A

(continued on next page)

Table 4
(continued)

Gene	Locus	Gene Product	Frequency	Allelic Disorders/Phenotypes
PLN	6q22.1	phospholamban	?	N/A
TAZ/G4.5	Xq28	tafazzin	?	Barth syndrome, endocardial fibroelastosis type 2, familial isolated non-compaction of the left ventricular myocardium
TMPO	12q22	thymopoietin	?	N/A
TTN	2q31	titin	?	Udd distal myopathy; HCM; Edstrom myopathy; early-onset myopathy with fatal cardiomyopathy

Abbreviations: HCM, hypertrophic cardiomyopathy; N/A, not available; ?, unknown.
Data from Hershberger RE, Cowan J, Morales A, et al. Progress with genetic cardiomyopathies: screening, counseling, and testing in dilated, hypertrophic, and arrhythmogenic right ventricular dysplasia/cardiomyopathy. Circ Heart Fail 2009;2(3):253–61; and Kimura A. Molecular aetiology and pathogenesis of hereditary cardiomyopathy. Circ J 2008;72(Suppl A):A-38–48.

recently and found a fair sensitivity if 2 of 4 criteria are positive and a satisfying specificity when 3 or 4 criteria are positive and matched with the results of endomyocardial biopsy.[38] A correlation between a certain MRI pattern by identification of preferential sites for certain viruses has been attempted by Mahrhold and colleagues,[35] but could not be confirmed by others. Our own data show in addition that MRI is able to show abnormalities in severe cardiac inflammation (**Fig. 4**A) but is unable to be associated with viral infection without or with little inflammation.[38] A correlation with adjacent pericardial and epicardial inflammation can also be assessed by echocardiography[39] and classified according to the criteria from Horowitz and colleagues[40] and by MRI as well.

Endomyocardial biopsy is still the method of choice to diagnose inflammation in endomyocardial biopsies. The Dallas criteria are still widely applied to conventional hematoxylin and eosin (H & E) staining,[41] although they have been declared obsolete.[42] Therefore, meanwhile the quantitative WHF criteria of 14 or more infiltrating cells/mm² were accepted. It appears from our own data that increased attention has to be paid under current conditions to reparative processes with a predominance of macrophages in Parvovirus B19 virus and HHV 6 myocarditis or persistence (Bernhard M, personal observation), whereas classical enteroviral or adenoviral infection causes lymphocytic inflammation. Indications for endomyocardial biopsy in suspected myocarditis, which have been long disregarded in the United States after the myocarditis treatment trial, have now also been accepted in the USA by a stagewise and individual approach.[17] Our own criteria for endomyocardial biopsy have been less case oriented. They were

designed many years ago as criteria suited best for the European Study of Epidemiology and Treatment of Cardiac Inflammatory Disease (ESETCID) trial,[43] but they largely coincide with the scenarios proposed by AHA and ESC (**Table 6**). **Fig. 4** gives examples of H & E staining in a case with cardiac sarcoidosis (see **Fig. 4**B), immunohistological staining of lymphocytic myocarditis by CD45R0 (see **Fig. 4**C) and CD4 (see **Fig. 4**D), and immunoglobulin staining to the sarcolemma and vascular endothelium (see **Fig. 4**E) by direct immunofluorescence in autoreactive myocarditis. The underlying microbial etiology in a large cohort of patients with suspected myocarditis, who underwent LV endomyocardial biopsy, histology, immunohistology, and molecular biopsy testing of the 10 most common cardiotropic pathogens in the biopsy specimens, can be seen in **Table 7**.

How to Diagnose and Interpret the Underlying Pathogenic Process?

As could be derived from animal models of enteroviral myocarditis, one could elaborate at least 3 different phases and 2 major pathogenic pathways that are not mutually exclusive.

The pathogenic mechanisms are as follows:

1. The direct cytopathic effect of the virus, which corresponds roughly to phase 1.
2. The virus-induced anticardiac immune response, which comprises molecular mimicry between virus and heart cells. Both cross-reactive autoantibodies and the response of the innate immune system and primed T cells participate. The subacute phase 2 and the autoimmune phase 3 parallels them as clinical faces (phenotypes) 2 and 3.

Table 5
Clinical phenotypes of inflammatory dilated cardiomyopathy (DCM) and myocarditis

Clinical Phenotype	Fulminant Myocarditis	Acute Myocarditis	Chronic Active Myocarditis	Chronic Persistent Myocarditis
Symptoms	Shock, heart failure, rhythm disturbance	Heart failure, reduced EF with near normal LV dilatation, pericardial effusion (up to 20%), angina in Parvo B19 m.	Heart failure, variable EF with LV dilatation, pericardial effusion (up to 10%); angina in Parvo B19 m.	Heart failure, variable EF with LV dilatation, pericardial effusion (up to 10%); angina in Parvo B19 m.
Dallas criteria	Infiltrate (active myocarditis or giant cells), necrosis	Active, often focal lymphocytic myocarditis	Borderline myocarditis, focal small infiltrates	Borderline or persistent myocarditis
World Heart Federation criteria[a]	≥50 infiltrating cells/mm², necrosis, possibly giant cells	≥14 infiltrating cells, mostly lymphocytes, necrosis, necrosis likely	≥14 infiltrating cells, lymphocytes and macrophages, necrosis and apoptosis not obligatory	≥14 infiltrating cells, lymphocytes and macrophages, necrosis and apoptosis not obligatory
Immuno-histology	Immunglobulin binding mostly IgM to sarcolemma and fibrils & complement fixation	Immunglobulin (IgM, IgA, and IgG) binding to sarcolemma and fibrils	Immunglobulin (IgG) binding to sarcolemma and fibrils	Immunglobulin (IgG) binding to sarcolemma and fibrils
PCR on microbial pathogens	Negative in giant cell or autoreactive myocarditis, positive in up to one third	Negative in autoreactive lymphocytic myocarditis, positive in up to one-third of cases	Negative in autoreactive lymphocytic myocarditis, positive in up to one-third of cases	Negative in autoreactive lymphocytic myocarditis, positive in up to one-third of cases
Course	Variable—from lethal to spontaneous healing	Variable—from deterioration to defective healing	Chronic heart failure	Chronic heart failure
Treatment	Immunosuppression in PCR-negative cases, assist device, ICDs	Immunosuppression in PCR-negative cases, assist device, ICDs. In viral m. ivIg in trials	Immunosuppression in PCR-negative cases, prophylactic ICDs, when EF<35%. In viral m. ivIg or IFN in trials	Immunosuppression in PCR-negative cases, prophylactic ICDs, when EF<35%. In viral m. ivIg or IFN in trials

Abbreviations: EF, ejection fraction; ICD, implantable cardioverter defibrillator; IFN, interferon; LV, left ventricular; PCR, polymerase chain reaction.
From Refs.[21,29,32]

Phase 1 would correspond to the initial viral infection, which could heal with little damage, or lead to heart failure or to death,[44,45] or transform to phase 2.

ENTEROVIRAL MYOCARDITIS

In phase 1, the virus exerts its direct cytopathic effect. High titers of Coxsackie B viruses are found

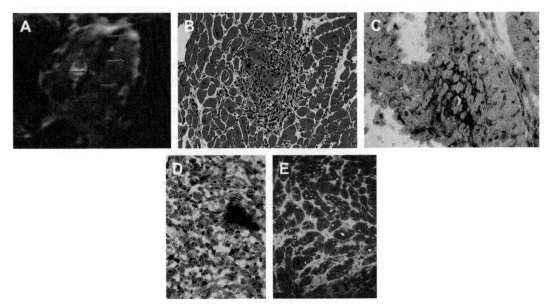

Fig. 4. Dilated cardiomyopathy (DCM). (*A*) MRI with late gadolinium enhancement in a patient with lymphocytic, active myocarditis. (*B*) Cardiac sarcoid (H & E staining) with giant cells within the granuloma. (*C*) CD45R0-positive interstitial infiltrate. (*D*) Focal infiltrate with CD4-positive cells. (*E*) IgG fixation to sarcolemma (ASA) and interstitial tissue and vascular endothelium in the EMB of the same patient as in *C* (*B–E*): H&E staining, magnification ×250. ((*B–E*) *From* Maisch B, Richter A, Koelsch S, et al. Management of patients with suspected (peri-)myocarditis and inflammatory dilated cardiomyopathy. Herz 2006;31:881–90; with permission.)

in blood, spleen, pancreas, and myocardium, consistent with systemic viremia. The clinical phenotype or face 1 would correspond to the very early and acute phase of myocarditis. This cytopathic effect of the infective virus was, of course, dependant on the susceptibility of the recipient mouse strain.[46] Myocarditic Balb/c mice could die rapidly, whereas amyocarditic DBA/2 mice would not and survived the infection.[47] The aggressive nature of the infecting enteroviral strain was of importance in inbred strains of mice: amyocarditic variants would do little or no harm, whereas myocarditic variants would.[48] The presence and expression of CAR (the coxsackie-adenoviral receptor) was a key discovery,[49] and less importantly of the earlier detected decay-accelerating factor (DAF or CD55),[50] which was a coreceptor for CVB serotypes B1, B2, and B5. The number of the infecting virus, the recovery of viral RNA copies in the tissue, and amount of detectable mRNA was considered a relative measure of later damage.[51,52] The virus itself was considered, at least in part, to cause damage directly,[53] as was its activity of producing mRNA, the upregulation of the adenoviral-receptor[54] and the preceding activation of STAT 1 transcription factor,[54] the influence of upregulated mediators[55,56] or their mRNA,[57] which could

contribute to necrosis or apoptosis.[58] The pathogenetic key to enteroviral infection was understood by the mechanisms of enteroviral protease 2A, which would also cleave dystrophin and thus cause a disrupture of the cytoskeleton.[59] In this stage, innate immunity and the myeloid differentiation factor-88 (MyD88) as an adaptor of toll-like receptors (TLR) of the innate immune system regulate cellular inflammation, infiltration, and cytokine expression.[60] The induction of TLR4 enhances the activation of antigen-presenting cells (APCs) and of proinflammatory cytokines and regulates T cells.[61,62]

Phase 2 is the period by which the immunologic effector systems play a major role. Its clinical correlate (face) is the subacute state of myocarditis. Apart from the release of progeny virus, it is characterized by the activation of natural killer (NK) cells, which may limit CVB replication,[63] the induction of cell adhesion molecules,[64–66] the infiltration by T cells and macrophages and their polarization,[67] cell-mediated heart cell lysis by cytotoxic T cells,[68,69] and the continuation of the innate immune response. Expression of costimulatory molecules like B7-1, B7-2, and CD40 on cardiomyocytes[70,71] is induced in the course of the attack of cytotoxic T cells (CTL) and NK cells. In this interplay, cytokines may determine the type of T-cell

Table 6
Case-oriented indication of endomyocardial biopsy and compared with the indications for the Marburg Registry and the European Study of Epidemiology and Treatment of Cardiac Inflammatory Disease (ESETCID) trial

No	Clinical Scenario	Class of Recommend JACC 2007[1]	Level of Evidence (A, B, C)[1]	Indications for Marburg Registry[2]	Comments/Clinical Suspicion
1	New-onset HF <2 weeks' duration	I	B	I, B	Giant-cell myocarditis (M)
2	New-onset HF 2 weeks' to 3 months' duration	I	B	I, B	Acute lymphocytic myocarditis
3	HF of <3 months with DCM, VA, 2nd- or 3rd degree AV-block or failure to respond to therapy	IIa	C	I, C	After exclusion of CAD, uncontrolled hypertension, or valvular disease
4	HF with DCM associated with eosinophilia/allergy	IIa	C	I, C	Allergic M, hypereosinophilic syndrome
5	HF with anthracycline DCM	IIa	C	IIa, C	All antineoplastic drug sequelae with DCM
6	HF with restrictive CM	IIa	C	IIa, C	Amyloid, Fabry, RCM, Fibroelastosis
7	Suspected cardiac tumors	IIa	C	I, C	If not otherwise diagnosed
8	Unexplained DCM in children	IIa	C	I, C	
9	New-onset HF <3 months without new VA, AV-block 2–3, responding to usual care	IIb	B	IIa, B	Suspected M
10	HF >3 months responding to usual care	IIb	B	IIa, B	Chronic M
11	HF associated with unexplained HCM	IIb	C	IIa, C	Storage disease
12	Suspected ARVC/D	IIb	C	IIa, C	RV myocarditis
13	Unexplained VA	IIb	C	IIa, C for Vtach and Vfib	Every unexplained ventricular tachycardia
14	Unexplained atrial fibrillation	III	C	IIb with DCM	Not otherwise explained
	Pericardial effusion with dilatation or wall motion abnormality or troponin release			IIa, C	Perimyocarditis is more often found than expected
	Troponin release not explained by CAD or decompensated H			IIa, C	
	HF with ≥2 myocarditis criteria by cardiac MRI			IIa, C	

Abbreviations: CAD, coronary artery disease; CM, cardiomyopathy; DCM, dilated cardiomyopathy; H, hypertension; HCM, hypertrophic cardiomyopathy; HF, heart failure; M, myocarditis; MRI, magnetic resonance imaging; RCM, restrictive cardiomyopathy; RV, right ventricular; VA, ventricular arrhythmia.
Data from Cooper LT, Baughman KL, Feldman AM, et al. The role of endomyocardial biopsy in the management of cardiovascular disease: a scientific statement from the American Heart Association, the American College of Cardiology, and the European Society of Cardiology. Circulation 2007;116:2216–33; and Maisch B, Hufnagel G, Schönian U, et al. The European study of epidemiology and treatment of cardiac inflammatory disease (ESETCID). Eur Heart J 1995;16(Suppl 0):173–5.

Table 7
Polymerase chain reaction–based microbial etiology in the Marburg registry in patients with suspected myocarditis or inflammatory dilated cardiomyopathy

Group	Inflammation (n = 1098)		No Inflammation (n = 2247)	
	1	2	3	4
Ejection fraction	>45%	<45%	>45%	<45%
No patients	816	282	1663	584
LVEDD, mm	54 ± 10	65 ± 7	51 ± 9	66 ± 11
Autoreactive(=no microbial agent)	70.2	55.9	69.5	77.8
Parvo B 19 virus[a]	20.4[b]	33.3[a/c]	23.9[b]	17.6[b]
Cytomegalovirus	3.1	3.9	2.0	0.8
Enterovirus	1.5	2.8	1.1	0.5
Adenovirus	1.5	2.1	1.4	1.2
Epstein-Barr virus	1.2	0.9	1.1	0.8
Human herpesvirus 6[a]	5.3	4.8	3.7	4.1
Borrelia Burgdorferi	0	0	0.1	0
Hepatitis C	0	0.1	0	0
HIV	0	0	0.1	0
Chlamydia pneumoniae	0.1	0	0.1	0
Rickettsia burnetii	0.1	0	0.1	0

[a] Double infection of Parvo B19 and HHV 6 were found in 2.4%–3.1%, for Parvo B19 and EBV in 0.6%–0.8% across the hemodynamic groups. Data are given for each virus as positive independent from double infection. Therefore, positivity for microbial agents add up higher than the difference between 100% - no microbial agent (=autoreactive group).
[b] $P<.05$ group 1 versus 2 or 3 versus 4.
[c] $P<.05$ group 2 versus 4.
Data from Pankuweit S, Moll R, Baandrup U, et al. Prevalence of the parvovirus B19 genome in endomyocardial biopsy specimens. Hum Pathol 2003;34:497–503.

response, the regulation of apoptosis and necrosis, and the remodeling of the extracellular matrix. Antiviral antibodies peak trying to eliminate or at least limit the viral destruction and consecutive inflammatory response. Myocarditis can in this phase heal or persist.

Phase 3 is the chronic phase, in which in BALB/c and DBA/2 mice, myocardial CVB infection is no longer detectable, whereas heart failure develops. The chronic inflammation leads to dilatation and impaired function and is particularly found in certain mice models (eg, SWR/J, A.BY/SnJ, A.CA/SnJ, A.SW/SnJ, C3H/HeJ, and NMRI mice). In mice, depending on the individual mouse strain, the hallmark (face) in chronic phase 3 is the anticardiac autoimmune response to various cardiac epitopes, such as surface molecules; receptors, such as the beta-receptor; intracellular proteins, such as the fibrils and their structural components myosin, actin, troponin, desmin, and laminin; and to mitochondrial and extracellular matrix proteins.[61,72,73] In humans, depending on the genetic background and the individual response of the immune system, molecular or antigenic mimicry plays a leading role in the production of anticardiac antibodies, whereas antibodies to surface molecules, such as the sarcolemma, the myolemma,[16,28,30,31,74–89] the beta-receptor,[90–98] laminin,[86] and even to cardiac conducting tissue[82,97] are considered to play a pathogenetic role,[99] whereas others could be just innocent bystanders or natural antibodies[74] or markers of a previous cardiac lesion. The role of antimitochondrial antibodies[100,101] and antibodies to the adenosine translocator (ANT) has been of interest because of their possible role in cardiac metabolism and function.[102,103]

At this stage, remodeling of the extracellular matrix, which can be observed by an imbalance of membrane metalloproteinases (MMPs) and their tissue inhibitors of metalloproteinase (TIMP)[104] expression, and scarring of the myocardial tissue occur. Here the clinical phenotype is cardiac dysfunction and heart failure.

PARVOVIRUS B19–ASSOCIATED HEART DISEASE

In the past 12 to 15 years, enteroviral and adenoviral myocarditis has almost disappeared in Europe, whereas Parvovirus B19 has emerged as a new important pathogen. Parvoviruses form small capsids of about 25 nm in diameter, which contain a genome of single-stranded DNA with about 5600 nucleotides. The viral genome encodes nonstructural protein 1 (NS1) and 2 structural proteins, VP1 and 2, which are identical with the exception of an additional 226 amino acids at its amino terminal.[105,106] Its infection is common in childhood, visible from erythem infectiosum, the fifth most common childhood exanthem. It continues during adult life, so that in elderly patients most patients are seropositive. In adults it may cause arthralgia and arthropathy, which can mimic rheumatoid arthritis and involve deposition of immune complexes. It can be associated with transient aplastic crises, persistent chronic anemia, hydrops fetalis with anemia,[105] purpura Schönlein-Henoch, myocarditis,[23,24,107–110] and heart failure.[23,24,107–110]

Parvoviruses need help from host cells or other viruses to replicate, this being one reason for the considerable amount of double infections noted in biopsied patients with suspected inflammatory cardiomyopathy (see **Table 7**). Animal models of Parvovirus B19–associated heart disease are not readily available. In humans, the pathogenesis is not so clearly structured as in enteroviral heart disease and the clinical phenotype is more variable. Parvovirus B19 as an erythrovirus has its P-receptor at the endothelial cell surface and not at the myocyte surface.[110] So, it is not surprising that symptoms resemble those of coronary artery or small vessel disease. Angina pectoris or diastolic dysfunction can prevail, and a chronic fatigue–like symptomatology is often described by individual patients. Viral persistence but not inflammation can be in the foreground of histology and molecular pathology (see **Table 7**). Often only a substantial viral load can be detected by PCR in the endomyocardial biopsy.

HUMAN HERPESVIRUS 6 HEART DISEASE

HHV 6 was first described in 1986 by Salahuddin.[111] It is a member of the herpesviridae-like human cytomegalovirus, which may become a serious pathogen in humans.[112] It commonly occurs early in life with lifelong persistence and is thus a candidate for opportunistic infections, which means it may cause overt clinical disease when reactivated in immunodeficient patients or occurs in coincidence with other reactivated viruses, such as Epstein-Barr or human cytomegalovirus (HCMV), with the possibility of mutual activation. The antibody prevalence of HHV 6 averages between 70% and 100% with variable mean titers in different countries.[112–116] It is also an emerging pathogen of myocardial disease in humans.

HHV 6 DNA can be incorporated in the genome. Approximately 0.8% of the population has a copy of the HHV 6 genome integrated into the chromosome of every cell. This "inherited" HHV 6 is passed through the germ line from parent to child, with a 50% chance of each child having the virus integrated. Individuals with chromosomally integrated or HHV 6 will always return positive results for PCR tested for whole blood.[112] It is apparently then hardly accessible to treatment (own observation).

CYTOMEGALOVIRUS MYOCARDITIS

Unrecognized infection with CMV is common in childhood, and most of the adult population has antibodies to CMV. Primary infection after the age of 35 years is uncommon, and generalized infection usually occurs only in immunosuppressed patients. The cardiovascular manifestations in adults are generally limited to asymptomatic and transient electrocardiographic abnormalities. Symptomatic cardiac involvement is rare, although a hemorrhagic pericardial effusion or myocarditis with left ventricular dysfunction and attendant congestive heart failure may occur. In our registry, CMV-associated myocarditis and DCM were detected in about 3% of patients with suspected myocarditis or inflammatory cardiomyopathy.[30,83,117,118] Cytomegalovirus DNA has been found in a limited but unchanging number of patients with inflammatory cardiomyopathy and myocarditis. CMV-DNA has been identified in the nuclei of myocytes, fibroblasts, and endothelial cells.[30,83,117,118]

HEPATITIS AND MYOCARDITIS

Clinical cardiac involvement in hepatitis is rare; however, there are contested data implicating hepatitis C virus (HCV) infection as an etiologic factor in at least some cases of human viral cardiomyopathy.[30,83] Fulminant myocarditis with congestive heart failure, hypotension, and death may occur in rare cases. Myocardial damage may be produced indirectly through an immune-mediated mechanism or directly by viral invasion of the heart. The characteristic pathologic changes in the myocardium associated with an infection with hepatitis C virus are minute foci of necrosis of isolated muscle bundles, often surrounded by lymphocytes and a diffuse serous inflammation. The ventricles may be dilated, with petechial hemorrhages. Among 106 hearts examined by Matsumori and colleagues,[119] HCV RNA was detected in 21.3%, and negative strands in 6.6%. HCV RNA was found in myocarditis in 33.3%, in DCM in 11.5%, and in hypertrophic cardiomyopathy in 26.0% of the patients; however, HCV RNA was not found in any of the patients with myocardial infarction or noncardiac disease. In contrast with the Japanese data, incidence of HCV-associated myocardial disease appears to be much less frequent in European patients (see **Table 7**), where it is less than 0.1%.[30,83]

HUMAN IMMUNODEFICIENCY VIRUS

Cardiac involvement has been described in 25% to 50% of HIV-infected patients, with clinically apparent heart disease in approximately 10%. Congestive heart failure, owing to LV dilatation and dysfunction, is the most common finding.[30,83] Barbaro and colleagues[120] have investigated endomyocardial biopsy specimens from 82 HIV-DCM and 80 idiopathic DCM patients for determination of the immunostaining intensity of tumor necrosis factor (TNF)-alpha and inducible nitric oxide synthetase (iNOS) and for virological examination. Negative controls were derived from autopsy myocardium specimens from 32 HIV-negative patients without known heart disease. The mean intensity of both TNF-alpha and iNOS staining was greater in patients with HIV-DCM (0.81 and 1.007, respectively) than in patients with idiopathic DCM (0.44 and 0.49, respectively) or controls (0.025 and 0.027, respectively). The staining intensity of both TNF-alpha and iNOS inversely correlated with CD4 count. The staining intensity of iNOS was greater in HIV-DCM patients with HIV/CVB3 or with HIV/CMV coinfection than in idiopathic DCM patients showing infection with CVB3 and adenovirus alone. The staining intensity of iNOS correlated with mortality rate (higher in HIV-DCM patients, in particular, in those with an optical density unit >1).[30,83] In the Marburg Registry, these patients are hardly represented (see **Table 7**).

INFECTIOUS MONONUCLEOSIS

Evident cardiac involvement in infectious mononucleosis is extremely rare, although nonspecific ST-segment and T-wave abnormalities may be seen. In rare cases, pericarditis and myocarditis (even simulating a myocardial infarction) may occur.[30,83]

INFLUENZA

Although clinically apparent myocarditis is rare in influenza, the presence of preexisting cardiovascular disease may increase the risk of morbidity and mortality.[121] During epidemics, 5% to 10% of infected patients may experience cardiac symptoms.[122] Postmortem findings in fatal cases include biventricular dilatation with evidence of a mononuclear infiltrate,[30,83] especially in perivascular areas. The prevalence of Influenza A, B, and C immunoglobulin G (IgG) antibodies is high in patients with DCM but also in age-matched controls and positive PCR findings in endomyocardial biopsies are very rare (<0.5% in our registry).

MUMPS

Myocardial involvement during the course of mumps is rarely recognized.[123,124] Histologically, there is diffuse interstitial fibrosis, with infiltration of mononuclear cells and areas of focal necrosis.[30,83,124] In our registry, incidence of PCR-positive endomyocardial biopsies was neglectable (see **Table 7**).

POLIOMYELITIS

Myocarditis occurs in about 5% to 10% of the cases during epidemics and is a frequent finding in fatal cases of poliomyelitis, occurring in half or more of all patients dying with this disease. Death may be sudden. Fortunately, this disease has been largely eliminated by immunization.[30,83]

RESPIRATORY SYNCYTIAL VIRUS

Although respiratory syncytial virus is an important cause of respiratory disease, particularly in children, it rarely results in cardiac involvement. Congestive heart failure and complete heart block have been seen on occasion.[30,83,125]

RUBELLA

Rare cases of postgestational myocarditis occur, with attendant conduction defects and heart failure (for details see Maisch and colleagues[31,86]).

VARICELLA

Clinical myocarditis is a rare finding in varicella, although unsuspected myocarditis is common in fatal varicella.[30,83] Histologic findings include rare but characteristic intranuclear inclusion. We have observed only 2 biopsy-proven cases in our registry.[30]

VARIOLA AND VACCINIA

Cardiac involvement following smallpox is rare, although several cases of myocarditis associated with acute cardiac failure and death have been reported. Myocarditis with pericardial effusion and congestive heart failure has also been observed as a complication of smallpox vaccination.[126,127] Dramatic responses to steroids have been reported. The histologic changes include a mixed mononuclear infiltrate, with interstitial edema and occasional degenerating or necrotic muscle bundles.[30,83,127]

ADENOVIRUS

Adenoviruses account for 3% to 5% of acute respiratory infections in children, but fewer than 2% of respiratory illnesses in civilian adults.[128] Nearly 100% of adults have serum antibody to multiple serotypes. Infections occur throughout the year, but are most common from fall to spring. This has been a frequently demonstrated virus by PCR in endomyocardial biopsies of patients with viral cardiomyopathy from 1989 to 2000.[23,30,83,128] In our registry, the incidence of positive PCRs in patients with myocarditis and DCM is up to 2.1% (see **Table 7**).

How to Assess Prognosis and How to Treat Inflammatory Cardiomyopathy Beyond Conventional Heart Failure and Antiarrhythmic Treatment?

Prognostic determinants put forth in the discussion of myocarditis have been the persistence of the inflammatory infiltrate, viral persistence, persistence of antimyolemmal,[30,31,83,92] antifibrillary[99] and anti-beta receptor antibodies.[27,92]

Obvious expectations are that apart from guideline-conforming heart failure treatment,[129,130] specific anti-inflammatory or antimicrobial treatment will influence prognosis by resolving the infiltrate and, if possible, also eradicate the cardiotropic microbial agents. The American Myocarditis trial using cyclosporine and corticoids[131] was underpowered to show benefit in the first randomized controlled trial. It did not differentiate viral from nonviral myocarditis and lacked immunohistochemistry and viral assessment in the biopsies.[132] Consequently, immunosuppressive treatment trials analyzed retrospectively or prospectively viral etiology and excluded viral myocarditis from immunosuppression.[16,39,133–136] Wojnicz and colleagues[134] and Frustaci and colleagues[135] retrospectively and also prospectively[136] demonstrated short-term benefit. The intermediate analysis of ESETCID, not yet published, aimed for a composite end point and a long-term prognostic impact.[39,133]

Interferon therapy was analyzed in the yet unpublished BICC trial,[137–139] which left the impression of treatment problems with Parvovirus B19 myocarditis, which represented a large part of the patient cohort.

Immunoglobulin treatment for viral, mostly Parvovirus B19 and CMV myocarditis, was based on preliminary promising results from uncontrolled and controlled trials and in experimental animal studies. We base our current treatment algorithm on the observation by Anthony and colleagues[140] that the anti-inflammatory activity of monomeric IgG is completely dependent on the sialylation of the N-linked glycan of the IgG Fc fragment. **Fig. 5**A, B illustrates the current management of patients with myocarditis and inflammatory dilated cardiomyopathy or DCM with viral persistence in our institution.[16] Other treatment options under investigation are immunoadsorption, stem cell transplantation, and virostatic treatment with ganciclovir or derivatives.

ARRHYTHMOGENIC RIGHT VENTRICULAR CARDIOMYOPATHY
Definition

Arrhythmogenic cardiomyopathy (ARVC) or dysplasia (ARVD) was originally thought to be primarily a right ventricular, inherited cardiomyopathy. William Osler in 1905 described it as "parchment-like thinning of the cardiac walls with dilation of all chambers. In places of the right auricle and ventricle, only the epicardium remains." Later on, sudden death was the focus of what later became the ARVC disease entity. In Japan, Inu in 1982 described it as Pokkuri disease, as "sudden death with a dreadful outcry during sleep." In the Philippines, this form of sudden death of unknown etiology was described in 1981 as Bangunjut. Marcus and colleagues[141] were the first to describe ARVC as an electrical abnormality and Thiene and colleagues[142,143] perceived it also as a histopathological entity, which in Europe was most frequently found in the Mediterranean area. ARVD 1 was first identified by Rampazzo 1994 (quoted from 147) as one of several in a series of autosomal mutations in the 14q23-14 chromosome. ARVD 2 with a mutation a locus in 1q42,1q43 and ARVD 4 with a mutation in 2q32 were also described by Rampazzo. The different chromosomal locations of the other ARVC-associated genes and the encoded proteins, which are located in the intercalated disk area, such as plakoglobin; plakophilin-2, desmoglein-1, -2, -4; Desmocolin; and Desmoplakin can be

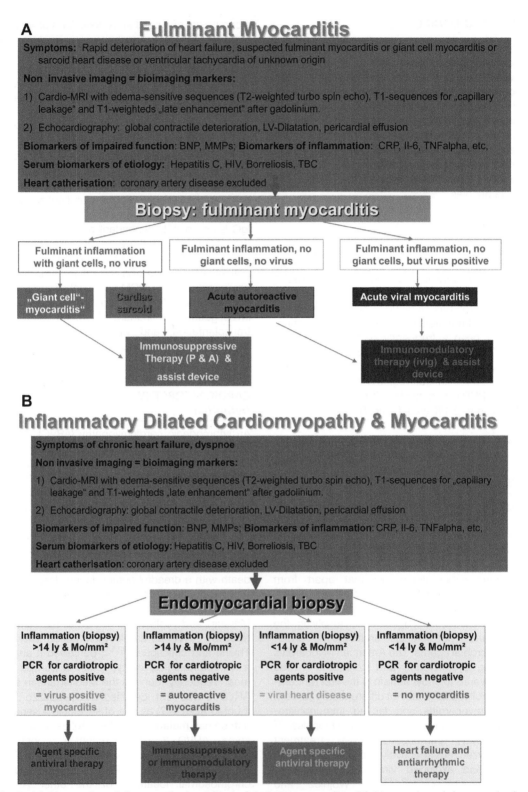

Fig. 5. (A) Diagnostic and therapeutic algorithm in fulminant myocarditis. (B) Diagnostic and therapeutic algorithm in inflammatory dilated cardiomyopathy and myocarditis. (*From* Maisch B, Richter A, Koelsch S, et al. Management of patients with suspected [peri-]myocarditis and inflammatory dilated cardiomyopathy. Herz 2006;31:881–90; with permission.)

Table 8
Desmosomal genes and encoded proteins implicated in inherited human disease

Gene Superfamily	Gene	Chromosomal Location	Encoded Protein	Mutation-Associated Phenotypes of ARVC
Armadillo	JUP	17q21	Plakoglobin	AR: Naxos disease arrhythmogenic cardiomyopathy with palmoplantar keratoderma and woolly hair AD: arrhythmogenic cardiomyopathy
	PKP1	1q32	Plakophilin-1	ARVC with ectodermal dysplasia and skin fragility syndrome
	PKP2	12p11	Plakophilin-2	AD: arrhythmogenic cardiomyopathy AR: arrhythmogenic cardiomyopathy
Desmosomal cadherin	DSG1	18q12	Desmoglein-1	palmoplantar keratoderma
	DSG2	18q12	Desmoglein-2	AD: arrhythmogenic cardiomyopathy AR: arrhythmogenic cardiomyopathy
	DSG4	18q12	Desmoglein-4	ARVC with Inherited hypotrichosis
Desmosomal cadherin	DSC2	18q12	Desmocollin	Arrhythmogenic cardiomyopathy with or without palmoplantar keratoderma and woolly hair
Plakin	DSP	6p24	Desmoplakin	ARVC with palmoplantar keratoderma

Abbreviations: AD, autosomal dominant; AR, autosomal recessive; ARVC, arrhythmogenic right ventricular cardiomyopathy.
Modified from Refs.[144–146]

derived from **Tables 1** and **2**, and **Table 8**.[144–146] The most recent task-force criteria with review of the previous ones are by Marcus and colleagues.[147]

Naxos disease is a very special autosomal variant of a 17q21variant mutation, which can already be identified by shaking hands with a patient with a keratosis pedoplantaris and curly hair, which are features found in addition to ARVC in inhabitants of the island of Naxos with a downregulation of the gap junction protein CX43 of plakoglobin.[144–146]

Management and Treatment

Treatment is focused on heart failure treatment and antiarrhythmic treatment, including the implantable defibrillator.[147]

REFERENCES

1. Kerr WW. Myocarditis. Cal State J Med 1904;2: 369–71.
2. Hickie JB, Hall GV. The cardiomyopathies: a report of fifty cases. Australas Ann Med 1960;9:258–70.
3. Goodwin JF, Gordon H, Hollman A, et al. Clinical aspects of cardiomyopathy. Br Med J 1961;1:69–79.
4. Report of the WHO/ISFC Task Force on the definition and classification of cardiomyopathies. Br Heart J 1980;44:672–4.
5. Richardson P, McKenna W, Bristow M, et al. Report of the 1995 World Health Organization/International Society and Federation of Cardiology Task Force on the Definition and Classification of Cardiomyopathies. Circulation 1996;93:841–2.
6. Maisch B, Bültman B, Factor S, et al. World Heart Federation consensus conference's definition of inflammatory cardiomyopathy (myocarditis): report from two expert committees on histology and viral cardiomyopathy. Heartbeat 1999;4:3–4.
7. Maisch B, Portig I, Ristic A, et al. Definition of inflammatory cardiomyopathy (myocarditis): on the way to consensus. Herz 2000;25:200–9.
8. Burkett EL, Hershberger RE. Clinical and genetic issues in familial dilated cardiomyopathy. J Am Coll Cardiol 2005;45:969–81.
9. Pankuweit S, Portig I, Eckhardt H, et al. Prevalence of viral genome in endomyocardial biopsies from patients with inflammatory heart muscle disease. Herz 2000;25:221–6.
10. Arbustini E, Morbini P, Pilotto A, et al. Familial dilated cardiomyopathy: from clinical presentation to molecular genetics. Am J Hum Genet 2001;69: 249–60.
11. Mason JW. Myocarditis and dilated cardiomyopathy: an inflammatory link. Cardiovasc Res 2003;60:5–10.
12. Shaw T, Elliot P, McKenna WJ. Dilated cardiomyopathy: a genetically heterogeneous disease. Lancet 2002;360:654–5.

13. Maron BJ, Towbin JA, Thiene G, et al. Contemporary definitions and classification of the cardiomyopathies: an American Heart Association scientific statement from the Council on Clinical Cardiology, Heart Failure and Transplantation Committee; Quality of Care and Outcomes Research and Functional Genomics and Translational Biology Interdisciplinary Working Groups; and Council on Epidemiology and Prevention. Circulation 2006; 113:1807–16.

14. Elliott P, Andersson B, Arbustini E, et al. Classification of the cardiomyopathies: a position statement from the European Society of Cardiology Working Group on Myocardial and Pericardial Diseases. Eur Heart J 2008;29:270–6.

15. Pankuweit S, Richter A, Ruppert V, et al. Classification of cardiomyopathies and indication for endomyocardial biopsy revisited. Herz 2009;34:55–62.

16. Maisch B, Richter A, Koelsch S, et al. Management of patients with suspected (peri-)myocarditis and inflammatory dilated cardiomyopathy. Herz 2006; 31:881–90.

17. Cooper LT, Baughman KL, Feldman AM, et al. The role of endomyocardial biopsy in the management of cardiovascular disease: a scientific statement from the American Heart Association, the American College of Cardiology, and the European Society of Cardiology. Circulation 2007;116:2216–33.

18. Keren A, Syrris P, McKenna WJ. Hypertrophic cardiomyopathy: the genetic determinants of clinical disease expression. Nat Clin Pract Cardiovasc Med 2008;5(3):158–68.

19. Marian AJ. Hypertrophic cardiomyopathy: from genetics to treatment. Eur J Clin Invest 2010; 40(4):360–9.

20. Rickers C, Wilke NM, Jerosch-Herold M, et al. Utility of cardiac magnetic resonance imaging in the diagnosis of hypertrophic cardiomyopathy. Circulation 2005;112:855–61.

21. Schulz-Menger J, Maisch B, Abdel-Aty H, et al. Integrated biomarkers in cardiomyopathies: cardiovascular magnetic resonance imaging combined with molecular and immunologic markers. A stepwise approach for diagnosis and treatment. Herz 2007; 32:458–72.

22. Mestroni L, Maisch B, McKenna WJ, et al. Guidelines for the study of familial dilated cardiomyopathies. Collaborative Research Group of the European Human and Capital Mobility Project on Familial Dilated Cardiomyopathy. Eur Heart J 1999;20(2):93–102.

23. Pankuweit S, Moll R, Baandrup U, et al. Prevalence of the parvovirus B19 genome in endomyocardial biopsy specimens. Hum Pathol 2003;34:497–503.

24. Kühl U, Pauschinger M, Noutsias M, et al. High prevalence of viral genomes and multiple viral infections in the myocardium of adults with "idiopathic" left ventricular dysfunction. Circulation 2005;11:887–93.

25. Küthe F, Lindner J, Matwschke K, et al. Prevalence of parvovirus B19 and human Bocavirus DNA in the heart of patients with no evidence of dilated cardiomyopathy or myocarditis. Clin Infect Dis 2009;49: 1660–6.

26. Stewart GC, Lopez-Molina J, Gottumukkala RV, et al. Myocardial parvovirus B19 persistence: lack of association with clinicopathologic phenotype in adults with heart failure. Circ Heart Fail 2011;4(1): 71–8.

27. Kindermann I, Kindermann M, Kandolf R, et al. Predictors of outcome in patients with suspected myocarditis. Circulation 2008;118:639–48.

28. Maisch B, Richter A, Sandmöller A, et al. BMBF-Heart Failure Network. Inflammatory dilated cardiomyopathy (DCMI). Herz 2005;30:535–44.

29. Maisch B, Ristic AD, Hufnagel G, et al. Dilated cardiomyopathies as a cause of congestive heart failure. Herz 2002;27:113–34.

30. Maisch B, Ristic AD, Portig I, et al. Human viral cardiomyopathy. Front Biosci 2003;8:S39–67.

31. Maisch B, Outzen H, Roth D, et al. Prognostic determinants in conventionally treated myocarditis and perimyocarditis—focus on antimyolemmal antibodies. Eur Heart J 1991;12(Suppl B):81–7.

32. Liebermann EB, Hutchin GM, Herskowitz A, et al. Clinico-pathologic description of myocarditis. J Am Coll Cardiol 1991;18:1617–26.

33. Friedrich MG, Strohm O, Schulz-Menger J, et al. Contrast media-enhanced magnetic resonance imaging visualizes myocardial changes in the course of viral myocarditis. Circulation 1998;97:1802–9.

34. Laissy JP, Messin B, Varenne O, et al. MRI of acute myocarditis: a comprehensive approach based on various imaging sequences. Chest 2002;122: 1638–48.

35. Mahrholdt H, Goedecke C, Wagner A, et al. Cardiovascular magnetic resonance assessment of human myocarditis: a comparison to histology and molecular pathology. Circulation 2004;109:1250–8.

36. Abdel-Aty H, Boye P, Zagrosek A, et al. Diagnostic performance of cardiovascular magnetic resonance in patients with suspected acute myocarditis: comparison of different approaches. J Am Coll Cardiol 2005;45:1815–22.

37. Friedrich MG, Sechtem U, Schulz-Menger J, et al. Cardiovascular magnetic resonance in myocarditis: a JACC White Paper. J Am Coll Cardiol 2009;53:1475–87.

38. Maisch B, Alter P, Romminger M, et al. MRI or EMB for the diagnosis of myocarditis and viral heart disease. Abstracts of the ESC Congress. 2011.

39. Maisch B, Seferovic PM, Ristic AD, et al. Task Force on the Diagnosis and Management of Pericardial Diseases of the European Society of Cardiology.

Guidelines on the diagnosis and management of pericardial diseases executive summary; The Task Force on the diagnosis and management of pericardial diseases of the European Society of Cardiology. Eur Heart J 2004;25(7):587–610.

40. Horowitz MD, Schultz CS, Stinson EB, et al. Sensitivity and specificity of echocardiographic diagnosis of pericardial effusion. Circulation 1974;50:239–45.

41. Aretz HT, Billingham M, Olsen E, et al. Myocarditis: the Dallas criteria. Hum Pathol 1987;18:619–24.

42. Baughman KL. Diagnosis of myocarditis: death of Dallas criteria. Circulation 2006;113:593–5.

43. Maisch B, Hufnagel G, Schönian U, et al. The European Study of Epidemiology and Treatment of Cardiac Inflammatory Disease (ESETCID). Eur Heart J 1995;16(Suppl 0):173–5.

44. Woodruff JF, Woodruff JJ. Involvement of T lymphocytes in the pathogenesis of coxsackie virus B3 heart disease. J Immunol 1974;113:1726–34.

45. Woodruff JF. Viral myocarditis. A review. Am J Pathol 1980;101:425–84.

46. Wolfgram LJ, Beisel KW, Herskowitz A, et al. Variations in the susceptibility to Coxsackievirus B3-induced myocarditis among different strains of mice. J Immunol 1986;136:1846–52.

47. Huber SA, Lodge PA. Coxsackievirus B-3-myocarditis. Identification of different pathogenic mechanisms in DBA/2 and Balb/c mice. Am J Pathol 1986;122:284–91.

48. Chow LH, Gauntt CJ, McManus BM. Differential effects of myocarditic variants of Coxsackievirus B3 in inbred mice. A pathologic characterization of heart tissue damage. Lab Invest 1991;64:55–64.

49. Bergelson JM, Cunningham JA, Droguett G, et al. Isolation of a common receptor for Coxsackie B viruses and adenoviruses 2 and 5. Science 1997;275:1320–3.

50. Bergelson JM, Chan M, Solomon KR, et al. Decay accelerating factor (CD55), a glycosylphosphatidylinositol-anchored complement regulatory protein, is a receptor for several echoviruses. Proc Natl Acad Sci U S A 1994;91:6245–9.

51. Klingel K, Kandolf R. The role of enterovirus replication in the development of acute and chronic heart muscle disease in different immunocompetent mouse strains. Scand J Infect Dis Suppl 1993;88:79–85.

52. Wessely R, Henke A, Zell R, et al. Low-level expression of a mutant coxsackieviral cDNA induces a myocytopathic effect in culture: an approach to the study of enteroviral persistence in cardiac myocytes. Circulation 1998;98:450–7.

53. McManus BM, Chow LH, Wilson JE, et al. Direct myocardial injury by enterovirus: a central role in the evolution of murine myocarditis. Clin Immunol Immunopathol 1993;68:159–69.

54. Ruppert V, Meyer T, Pankuweit S, et al. Activation of STAT1-transcription factor precedes up-regulation of coxsackievirus-adenovirus receptor during viral myocarditis. Cardiovasc Pathol 2008;17:81–92.

55. Li J, Schwimmbeck PL, Tschöpe C, et al. Collagen degradation in a murine myocarditis model: relevance of matrix metalloproteinase in association with inflammatory induction. Cardiovasc Res 2002;56:235–47.

56. Kishimoto C, Kawamata H, Sakai S, et al. Role of MIP-2 in coxsackievirus B3 myocarditis. J Mol Cell Cardiol 2000;32:631–8.

57. Seko Y, Takahashi N, Yagita H, et al. Expression of cytokine mRNAs in murine hearts with acute myocarditis caused by coxsackievirus b3. J Pathol 1997;183:105–8.

58. Huber SA, Budd RC, Rossner K, et al. Apoptosis in coxsackievirus B3-induced myocarditis and dilated cardiomyopathy. Ann N Y Acad Sci 1999;887:181–90.

59. Badorff C, Lee GH, Lamphear BJ, et al. Enteroviral protease2A cleaves dystrophin: evidence of cytoskeletal disruption in an acquired cardiomyopathy. Nat Med 1999;5:320–6.

60. Fuse K, Chan G, Liu Y, et al. Myeloid differentiation factor-88 plays a crucial role in the pathogenesis of Coxsackievirus B3-induced myocarditis and influences type I interferon production. Circulation 2005;112:2276–85.

61. Fairwheather D, Rose NR. Coxsackievirus-induced myocarditis in mice: a model of autoimmune disease for studying immunotoxicity. Methods 2007;41:118–22.

62. Frisancho-Kiss S, Davis SE, Nyland JF, et al. Cutting edge: cross-regulation by TLR4 and T cell Ig mucin-3 determines sex differences in inflammatory heart disease. J Immunol 2007;178:6710–4.

63. Godeny EK, Gauntt CJ. Murine natural killer cells limit coxsackievirus B3 replication. J Immunol 1987;139:913–8.

64. Seko Y, Tsuchimochi H, Nakamura T, et al. Expression of major histocompatibility complex class I antigen in murine ventricular myocytes infected with Coxsackievirus B3. Circ Res 1990;67:360–7.

65. Seko Y, Matsuda H, Kato K, et al. Expression of intercellular adhesion molecule-1 in murine hearts with acute myocarditis caused by coxsackievirus B3. J Clin Invest 1993;91:1327–36.

66. Seko Y, Yagita H, Okumura K, et al. T-cell receptor V beta expression in infiltrating cells in murine hearts with acute myocarditis caused by coxsackievirus B3. Circulation 1994;89:2170–5.

67. Li K, Xu W, Guo Q, et al. Differential macrophage polarization in male and female BALB/c mice infected with coxsackievirus B3 defines susceptibility to viral myocarditis. Circ Res 2009;105:353–64.

68. Huber SA, Feldman AM, Sartini D. Coxsackievirus B3 induces T regulatory cells, which inhibit cardiomyopathy in tumor necrosis factor-alpha transgenic mice. Circ Res 2006;99:1109–16.
69. Huber SA, Job LP. Cellular immune mechanisms in Coxsackievirus group B, type 3 included myocarditis in BALB/C mice. Adv Exp Med Biol 1983;161:491–508.
70. Seko Y, Takahashi N, Ishiyama S, et al. Expression of costimulatory molecules B7-1, B7-2, and CD40 in the heart of patients with acute myocarditis and dilated cardiomyopathy. Circulation 1998;97:637–9.
71. Takata S, Nakamura H, Umemoto S, et al. Identification of autoantibodies with the corresponding antigen for repetitive coxsackievirus infection-induced cardiomyopathy. Circ J 2004;68:677–82.
72. Latif N, Baker CS, Dunn MJ, et al. Frequency and specificity of antiheart antibodies in patients with dilated cardiomyopathy detected using SDS-PAGE and western blotting. J Am Coll Cardiol 1993;22:1378–84.
73. Latif N, Zhang H, Archard LC, et al. Characterization of anti-heart antibodies in mice after infection with coxsackie B3 virus. Clin Immunol 1999;91:90–8.
74. Maisch B, Drude L, Hengstenberg C, et al. Are antisarcolemmal (ASAs) and antimyolemmal antibodies (AMLAs) "natural" antibodies? Basic Res Cardiol 1991;86(Suppl 3):101–14.
75. Maisch B, Bauer E, Cirsi M, et al. Cytolytic cross-reactive antibodies directed against the cardiac membrane and viral proteins in coxsackievirus B3 and B4 myocarditis. Characterization and pathogenetic relevance. Circulation 1993;87(Suppl 5):IV49–65.
76. Maisch B, Berg PA, Kochsiek K. Autoantibodies and serum inhibition factors (SIF) in patients with myocarditis. Klin Wochenschr 1980;58(5):219–25.
77. Maisch B, Berg PA, Kochsiek K. Immunological parameters in patients with congestive cardiomyopathy. Basic Res Cardiol 1980;75:221–2.
78. Maisch B, Bülowius U, Schmier K, et al. Immunological cellular regulator and effector mechanisms in myocarditis. Herz 1985;10:8–14.
79. Maisch B, Dienesch CH, Wendl I. Effect of leukotrienes on isolated vital cardiac cells—an in vitro model of cardiocytotoxic mediators in inflammation? Eur Heart J 1997;8(Suppl J):463–5.
80. Maisch B, Drude L, Hengstenberg C, et al. Cytolytic anticardiac membrane antibodies in the pathogenesis of myopericarditis. Postgrad Med J 1992;68(Suppl 1):11–6.
81. Maisch B, Herzum M, Schönian U. Immunomodulating factors and immunosuppressive drugs in the therapy of myocarditis. Scand J Infect Dis Suppl 1993;88:149–62.
82. Maisch B, Lotze U, Schneider J, et al. Antibodies to human sinus node in sick-sinus syndrome. Pacing Clin Electrophysiol 1986;9(6 Pt 2):1101–9.
83. Maisch B, Ristic AD, Hufnagel G, et al. Pathophysiology of viral myocarditis: the role of humoral immune response. Cardiovasc Pathol 2002;11(2):112–22.
84. Maisch B, Trostel-Soeder R, Berg PA, et al. Assessment of antibody mediated cytolysis of vital adult cardiocytes isolated by centrifugation in a continuous gradient of Percoll TM in patients with acute myocarditis. J Immunol Methods 1981;44:159–69.
85. Maisch B, Trostel-Soeder R, Stechemesser E, et al. Diagnostic relevance of humoral and cell-mediated immune reactions in patients with acute viral myocarditis. Clin Exp Immunol 1982;48:533–45.
86. Maisch B, Wedeking U, Kochsiek K. Quantitative assessment of antilaminin antibodies in myocarditis and perimyocarditis. Eur Heart J 1987;8(Suppl J):223–35.
87. Maisch B. Autoreactivity to the cardiac myocyte, connective tissue and the extracellular matrix in heart disease and postcardiac injury. Springer Semin Immunopathol 1989;11:369–95.
88. Maisch B. Surface antigens of adult heart cells and their use in diagnosis. Basic Res Cardiol 1985;80(Suppl 1):47–52.
89. Maisch B. The sarcolemma as antigen in the secondary immunopathogenesis of myopericarditis. Eur Heart J 1987;8(Suppl J):155–65.
90. Magnusson Y, Wallukat G, Waagstein F, et al. Autoimmunity in idiopathic dilated cardiomyopathy. Characterization of antibodies against the beta1-adrenoceptor with positive chronotropic effect. Circulation 1994;89:2760–7.
91. Wallukat G, Wollenberg A, Morwinski R, et al. Anti-beta1-adrenoceptor autoantibodies with chronotropic activity from the serum of patients with dilated cardiomyopathy: mapping of epitopes in the first and second extracellular loops. J Mol Cell Cardiol 1995;27:397–406.
92. Jahns R, Boivin V, Siegmund C, et al. Autoantibodies activating human beta 1-adrenergic receptors are associated with reduced cardiac function in chronic heart failure. Circulation 1999;99:649–54.
93. Fu LX, Magnusson Y, Bergh CH, et al. Localization of a functional autoimmune epitope on the second extracellular loop of the human muscarinic acetylcholin receptor 2 in patients with idiopathic dilated cardiomyopathy. J Clin Invest 1993;91:1964–8.
94. Christ T, Wettwer E, Dobrev D, et al. Autoantibodies against the beta1-adrenoceptor from patients with dilated cadiomyopathy prolong action potential duration and enhance contractility in isolated cardiomyocytes. J Mol Cell Cardiol 2001;33:1515–25.
95. Christ T, Schindelhauer S, Wettwer E, et al. Interaction between autoantibodies against the beta1-adrenoceptor and isoprenaline in enhancing L-type Ca^{2+} current in rat ventricular myocytes. J Mol Cell Cardiol 2006;41:716–23.

96. Jahns R, Boivin V, Krapf T, et al. Modulation of beta1-adrenoceptor activity by domain-specific antibodies and heart failure associated autoantibodies. J Am Coll Cardiol 2000;36:1280–7.

97. Jahns R, Bovin V, Hein L, et al. Direct evidence for a beta1-adrenergic receptor directed autoimmune attack as a cause of idiopathic dilated cardiomyopathy. J Clin invest 2004;113:1419–29.

98. Lotze U, Maisch B. Humoral immune response to cardiac conducting tissue. Springer Semin Immunopathol 1989;11:409–22.

99. Caforio AL, Mahon NJ, Tona F, et al. Circulating cardiac autoantibodies in dilated cardiomyopathy and myocarditis: pathogenetic and clinical significance. Eur J Heart Fail 2002;4:411–7.

100. Klein R, Maisch B, Kochsiek K, et al. Demonstration of organ specific antibodies against heart mitochondria (anti M7) in sera from patients with some forms of heart diseases. Clin Exp Immunol 1984;58:283–92.

101. Pohlner K, Portig I, Pankuweit S, et al. Identification of mitochondrial antigens recognized by the antibodies in sera of patients with dilated cardiomyopathy by two-dimensional gel electrophoresis and protein sequencing. Am J Cardiol 1997;80:1040–5.

102. Schultheiss HP, Bolte HD. Immunological analysis of autoantibodies against the adenine nucleotide translocator in dilated cardiomyopathy. J Mol Cell Cardiol 1988;17:603–17.

103. Schulze K, Witzenbichler B, Christmann C, et al. Disturbance of myocardial energy metabolism in experimental virus myocarditis by antibodies against the adenin nucleotide translocator. Cardiovasc Res 1999;44:91–100.

104. Gluck B, Schmidtke M, Merkle I, et al. Persistent expression of cytokines in the chronic stage of CVB3-induced myocarditis in NMRI mice. J Mol Cell Cardiol 2001;33:1615–26.

105. Young NS, Brown KE. Mechanisms of disease. Parvovirus B19. N Engl J Med 2004;350:586–97.

106. Lamparter S, Schoppet M, Pankuweit S, et al. Acute parvovirus B19 infection associated with myocarditis in an immunocompetent adult. Hum Pathol 2003;34(7):725–8.

107. Saint-Martin I, Choulot JJ, Bonnau E, et al. Myocarditis caused by parvovirus. J Pediatr 1990;116:1007–8.

108. Nigro G, Bastianon V, Colloridl V, et al. Human parvovirus B19 infection in infancy associated with acute and chronic lymphocytic myocarditis and high cytokine levels: report of 3 cases and review. Clin Infect Dis 2000;13:65–9.

109. Schowengerdt KO, Ni J, Denfield SW, et al. Association of parvovirus B19 genome in children with myocarditis and cardiac allograft rejection: diagnosis using the polymerase chain reaction. Circulation 1997;96(10):3549–54.

110. Bock CT, Klingel K, Kandolf R. Human parvovirus B19-associated myocarditis. N Engl J Med 2010;362:213–4.

111. Salahuddin SZ. Isolation of a new virus, HBLV, in patients with lymphoproliferative disorders. Science 1986;234(4776):596–601.

112. Krueger GR, Ablashi DV. Human herpesvirus-6: a short review of its biological behavior. Intervirology 2003;46:257–69.

113. Buja LM. HHV-6 in cardiovascular pathology. In: Krueger GRF. In: Ablashi DV, editor. Human herpesvirus-6. 2nd edition. Amsterdam (London): Elsevier Science Publ; 2006. p. 137.

114. Fukae S, Ashizawa N, Morikawa S, et al. A fatal fulminant myocarditis with human herpesvirus-6 infection. Intern Med 2000;39:632–6.

115. De Ona M, Melon S, Rodriguez JL, et al. Association between human herpesvirus type 6 and type 7, and cytomegalovirus disease in heart transplant recipients. Transplant Proc 2002;34:75–6.

116. Komaroff AL. Is human herpesvirus-6 a trigger for chronic fatigue syndrome? J Clin Virol 2006;37(Suppl 1):S39–46.

117. Schönian U, Crombach M, Maisch B. Assessment of cytomegalovirus DNA and protein expression in patients with myocarditis. Clin Immunol Immunopathol 1993;68:229–33.

118. Schönian U, Crombach M, Maisch B. Does CMV infection play a role in myocarditis? New aspects from in-situ hybridization. Eur Heart J 1991;12(Suppl D):65–8.

119. Matsumori A, Yutani C, Ikeda Y, et al. Hepatitis C virus from the hearts of patients with myocarditis and cardiomyopathy. Lab Invest 2000;80(7):1137–42.

120. Barbaro G, Di Lorenzo G, Soldini M, et al. Intensity of myocardial expression of inducible nitric oxide synthase influences the clinical course of human immunodeficiency virus-associated cardiomyopathy. Gruppo Italiano per lo Studio Cardiologico dei pazienti affetti da AIDS (GISCA). Circulation 1999;100(9):933–9.

121. Sprenger MJ, Van Naelten MA, Mulder PG, et al. Influenza mortality and excess deaths in the elderly 1967–1982. Epidemiol Infect 1989;103:633–41.

122. Herskowitz A, Campbell S, Deckers J, et al. Demographic features and prevalence of idiopathic myocarditis in patients undergoing endomyocardial biopsy. Am J Cardiol 1993;71:982–6.

123. Ozkutlu S, Soylemezoglu O, Calikoglu AS, et al. Fatal mumps myocarditis. Jpn Heart J 1989;30:109–14.

124. Ward SC, Wiselka MJ, Nicholson KG. Still's disease and myocarditis associated with recent mumps infection. Postgrad Med J 1988;64:693–5.

125. Martin JT, Kugler JD, Gumbiner CH, et al. Refractory congestive heart failure after ribavirin in infants

with heart disease and respiratory syncytial virus. Nebr Med J 1990;75:23–6.

126. Matthews AW, Griffiths ID. Post-vaccinal pericarditis and myocarditis. Br Heart J 1974;36:1043–7.

127. Finlay-Jones LR. Fatal myocarditis after vaccinations for smallpox. N Engl J Med 1964;270:41–2.

128. Pauschinger M, Bowles NE, Fuentes-Garcia FJ, et al. Detection of adenoviral genome in the myocardium of adult patients with idiopathic left ventricular dysfunction. Circulation 1999;99:1348–54.

129. Hunt SA, Baker DW, Chin MH, et al. American College of Cardiology/American Heart Association Task Force on Practice Guidelines (Committee to Revise the 1995 Guidelines for the Evaluation and Management of Heart Failure); International Society for Heart and Lung Transplantation; Heart Failure Society of America. ACC/AHA guidelines for the evaluation and management of chronic heart failure in the adult: executive summary report of the American College of Cardiology/American Heart Association Task Force on Practice Guidelines (Committee to Revise the 1995 Guidelines for the Evaluation and Management of Heart Failure). Circulation 2001;104:2996–3007.

130. Dickstein K, Cohen-Solal A, Filippatos G, et al. ESC guidelines for the diagnosis and treatment of acute and chronic heart failure 2008: the task force for the diagnosis and treatment of acute and chronic heart failure of the European Society of Cardiology. Developed in collaboration with the Heart Failure Association of the ESC (HFA) and endorsed by the European Society of Intensive Care Medicine (ESICM). Eur J Heart Fail 2008;10:933–89.

131. Mason JW, O'Connell JB, Herskowitz A, et al. A clinical trial of immunosuppressive therapy for myocarditis. The Myocarditis Treatment Trial Investigators. N Engl J Med 1995;333:269–75.

132. Maisch B, Camerini F, Schultheiss HP. Immunosuppressive therapy for myocarditis [letter]. N Engl J Med 1995;333:1713.

133. Hufnagel G, Pankuweit S, Richter A, et al, for the ESETCID investigators. The European study of epidemiology and treatment of cardiac inflammatory diseases (ESETCID): first epidemiological results. Herz 2000;25(3):279–85.

134. Wojnicz R, Nowalany-Kozielska E, Wojciechowska C, et al. Randomized, placebo-controlled study for immunosuppressive treatment of inflammatory dilated cardiomyopathy: two-year follow-up results. Circulation 2001;104:39–45.

135. Frustaci A, Chimenti C, Calabrese F, et al. Immunosuppressive therapy for active lymphocytic myocarditis: virological and immunologic profile of responders versus nonresponders. Circulation 2003;107:857–63.

136. Frustaci A, Russo MA, Chimenti C. Randomized study on the efficacy of immunosuppressive therapy in patients with virus-negative inflammatory cardiomyopathy: the TIMIC study. Eur Heart J 2009;30:1995–2002.

137. Schultheiss HP, Noutsias M, Kuehl U. Antiviral interferon-ß treatment in patients with chronic viral cardiomyopathy. In: Schultheiß HP, Noutsias M, editors. Inflammatory cardiomyopathy (DCMi)—pathogenesis and therapy. Birkhäuser & Springer Basel AG; 2011. p. 265–78.

138. Takada H, Kishimoto C, Hiraoka Y. Therapy with immunoglobin suppresses myocarditis in a murine coxsackievirus B3 model. Antiviral and anti-inflammatory effects. Circulation 1995;92:1604–11.

139. McNamara DM, Holubkov R, Starling RC, et al. Controlled trial of intravenous immune globulin in recent-onset dilated cardiomyopathy. Circulation 2001;103:2254–9.

140. Anthony RM, Nimmerjahn F, Ashline DJ, et al. Recapitulation of IVIG anti-inflammatory activity with a recombinant Ig Fc. Science 2008;320:373–6.

141. Marcus FI, Fontaine GH, Guiraudon G, et al. Right ventricular dysplasia: a report of 24 adult cases. Circulation 1982;65:384–98.

142. Thiene G, Nava A, Corrado D, et al. Right ventricular cardiomyopathy and sudden death in young people. N Engl J Med 1988;318:129–33.

143. Nava A, Bauce B, Basso C, et al. Clinical profile and long-term follow-up of 37 families with arrhythmogenic right ventricular cardiomyopathy. J Am Coll Cardiol 2000;36:2226–33.

144. Delmar M, McKenna WJ. The cardiac desmosome and arrhythmogenic cardiomyopathies: from gene to disease. Circ Res 2010;107(6):700–14.

145. Herren T, Gerber PA, Duru F. Arrhythmogenic right ventricular cardiomyopathy/dysplasia: a not so rare "disease of the desmosome" with multiple clinical presentations. Clin Res Cardiol 2009;98(3):141–58.

146. Sen-Chowdhry S, Syrris P, McKenna WJ. Role of genetic analysis in the management of patients with arrhythmogenic right ventricular dysplasia/cardiomyopathy. J Am Coll Cardiol 2007;50(19):1813–21.

147. Marcus FI, McKennae WJ, Sherill D, et al. Diagnosis of arrhythmogenic right ventricular cardiomyopathy/dysplasia. Eur Heart J 2010;31:806–14.

Role of Apoptosis in Adverse Ventricular Remodeling

Antonio Abbate, MD, PhD, FESC[a],*,
Jagat Narula, MD, PhD, FRCP(Edin)[b]

KEYWORDS

- Apoptosis • Heart failure • Ventricular remodeling
- Caspase

Heart failure is a progressive disease. The substrate for symptomatic heart failure may exist long before the symptoms occur. Stage B heart failure refers to a condition in which the heart is structurally abnormal (such as after an acute myocardial infarction [AMI]), yet the clinical symptoms and signs of heart failure may not be present.[1,2] Unlike stage B, stage A refers to clinical conditions that predispose to heart failure but in which the heart is considered to be structurally normal. In stage C, structural heart disease is associated with symptoms of heart failure, and the disease is progressed to a point in which heart failure is considered refractory to conventional medical therapy in stage D. The classification of heart failure in stages A to D reflects very well the progressive nature of the disease.[1] The progressive changes in cardiac structure and function are referred to as adverse cardiac remodeling, a process in which heart chamber dilatation and wall thinning occur in association with systolic and diastolic dysfunction.[1,2]

Stage B heart failure therefore represents a transition between normal heart function and lack of symptoms (stage A) and abnormal heart structure/function and presence of heart failure symptoms (stage C). Independent of the etiology causing stage B heart failure, cardiac remodeling is characterized by changes in the size and number of cardiomyocytes; more specifically, in cell death (apoptosis) and hypertrophy of surviving cells (compensatory hypertrophy), as well as in qualitative changes in the type of cells, with a progressive increase in fibroblasts and myofibroblasts and an increase in extracellular matrix.[3] In this article, the authors review the role of apoptosis (or programmed cell death) in determining the evolution of symptomatic heart failure and particularly the adverse remodeling in the aftermath of AMI.

Myocardial dysfunction in the border zone extends to involve contiguous normal myocardium leading to a dilated cardiomyopathy in the weeks following AMI.[3–6] The border zone remodels as a small area circumferential to the infarct that is normally perfused but displays abnormal contractility and leads to increased circumferential stress and further involvement of adjacent normally contractile myocardial areas. The events occurring in the border zone are histopathologically characterized by patchy interstitial fibrosis and myofibrillarlytic or myocytolytic (vacuolized) cardiomyocytes, reflective of autophagy. The increased wall stress indeed alters the myocardium at biochemical and molecular levels that ultimately lead to loss of previously functional myocardium by nonischemic cell loss predominantly by the process of apoptosis (**Fig. 1**). The extent of remodeled myocardium is variable among patients and, in severe cases, may produce a gradually expanding dysfunction out of proportion to the initial ischemic insult.[6]

[a] VCU Pauley Heart Center, Virginia Commonwealth University, VCU Medical Center, 1200 East Broad Street, Richmond, VA, 23298, USA
[b] Cardiovascular Imaging Program, Zena and Michael A. Wiener Cardiovascular Institute, Marie-Josée and Henry R. Kravis Center for Cardiovascular Health, Mount Sinai School of Medicine, New York, NY, USA
* Corresponding author.
E-mail address: abbatea@yahoo.com

Heart Failure Clin 8 (2012) 79–86
doi:10.1016/j.hfc.2011.08.010
1551-7136/12/$ – see front matter © 2012 Elsevier Inc. All rights reserved.

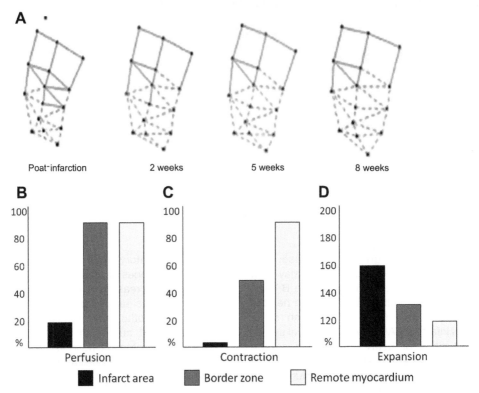

Fig. 1. (A) Geometrical changes in the infarct zone (*red*), the border zone (*blue*), and remote myocardium (*green*) over 8 weeks after AMI. (*B, C*) Changes in perfusion, contraction, and expansion (vs baseline) in the infarct area, border zone, and remote myocardium 8 weeks after experimental AMI in sheep. After AMI, the border zone becomes dysfunctional despite normal perfusion and expands parallel to the infarct area, extending to involve also the previously normocontracting myocardium. (*Data from* Jackson BM, Gorman JH, Moainie SL, et al. Extension of borderzone myocardium in postinfarction dilated cardiomyopathy. J Am Coll Cardiol 2002;40:1160–7.)

BIOCHEMICAL AND MOLECULAR ALTERATIONS OF THE REMODELED MYOCARDIUM

Numerous studies have focused on the remodeled myocardium in the border zone after AMI. The initial observations from light microscopy described findings of patchy interstitial fibrosis and cardiomyocytes filled with cytoplasmic vacuoles, and the severity of fibrosis and vacuolization predicted the severity of the cardiomyopathy.[6,7] The vacuolized cardiomyocytes have been described as degenerated, myofibrillarlytic, or cytolytic and were considered a prelude to cell death.[6–9] The vacuoles were further characterized by autophagosomes. Autophagy (self-eating) is now considered a cell survival program, a highly regulated process by which the cell uses cytoplasmic structures, which may be injured during stress, to provide fuel for the energy demand of the cell and substrates for cell repair and also allows for compartmentalization of injured mitochondria, which would otherwise have promoted cell death (mitophagy).[10] Myofibrillarlytic myocytes are therefore also called autophagic. Formation of autophagosomes and fusion with lysosomes is a physiologic process that is exaggerated in the remodeled myocardium. The formation of autophagosomes is, however, random, whereas, in response to cell injury, ubiquination occurs as the initial step wherein stressed or abnormal proteins are bound to ubiquitin and destined to degradation in the proteasomes. Although autophagy is generally protective, excessive proteolysis and excessive storage of ubiquitinated protein complexes lead to impaired cellular functions, primarily impaired contractility.[11] Further progression of cytolysis leads to blockade of protein synthesis and leads to the inability to save the injured cell, at which point cell death is inevitable via a unique form of autophagic cell death (or ubiquitin-related autophagic death).[11] Numerous studies have shown that ubiquitin-containing vacuolization and cell death are common in the border zones of recent infarcts.[11,12]

CASPASE 3: THE LINK BETWEEN DEGENERATION AND CELL DEATH

The mechanisms by which the functional proteolytic process in the injured cell fails leading to pathologic proteolysis and death are not completely understood. Caspase 3 has been consistently shown to be upregulated and activated in the remodeled myocardium.[12–16] Caspase 3 is an executor cysteine protease primarily involved in apoptotic cell death. Caspase 3 on one hand has been also shown to inhibit the proteasome leading to intracellular accumulation of ubiquitin conjugates, and, on the other hand, it induces cleavage of troponin I and other proteins in the sarcomere, leading to loss of the functional contractile apparatus. Caspase 3 is thought to mediate ischemic myocardial stunning.[16,17]

Activation of caspase 3 occurs through 2 distinct but not mutually exclusive pathways: caspase 8–mediated death receptor–dependent pathway and caspase 9–mediated mitochondrial pathway.[3] Although both pathways are activated in the remodeled myocardium, activation of the mitochondrial pathway seems to be predominant. Stressed cardiomyocytes consistently show elevated bax/bcl-2 ratios, known to regulate mitochondrial membrane permeability and decreased levels of mitochondrial cytochrome c, which impairs energy production, with consequently increased levels of cytoplasmic cytochrome c leading to activation of caspase 9. Caspase 9 activates caspase 3, which initiates the death program and ultimately leads to DNA fragmentation and cell condensation. The presence of activated caspase 3, DNA fragmentation, and cell condensation defines apoptosis (or apoptotic cell death) and differentiates it from other modalities of cell death, although overlap forms often occur.[18]

APOPTOSIS

Initially described in embryonic development and cancer, apoptosis has been rapidly found to have broad implications for tissue kinetics in health and disease.[18,19]

The interest in cardiac apoptosis is rather recent dating to the mid-1990s when the initial studies showed an increased rate of apoptosis in the hearts explanted from patients undergoing heart transplantation for end-stage heart failure.[13] The identification of a signaling cascade leading to cell death allows the definition of the molecular mechanisms and novel therapeutic strategies.

Transition toward stage C heart failure is characterized by a progressive decline in the number of cardiomyocytes in the heart,[20] later identified as cell death due to apoptosis.[21] Being an organ with low proliferation and turnover, if any, apoptosis was considered not to occur in the so-called postmitotic organs such as the heart. This assumption was not entirely appropriate. The initial studies of apoptosis in heart failure were substantially validated, and the concept that cell loss (by apoptosis) occurred in the heart, increases with age, and contributed to the development of cardiomyopathy became commonplace.

The observations in advanced heart failure, however, did not allow determining whether apoptosis was a consequence of heart failure or its cause. Subsequent studies showed that apoptosis occurs in many, if not all, stage B heart failure conditions that are prone to the development of heart failure, suggesting a causative role of apoptosis.[3,22–29] The cause-effect link was further validated by the use of experimental models in which the rate of apoptosis could be modulated.[24]

In the border zone of recent infarcts (remodeled myocardium), cardiomyocytes seem to be highly susceptible to proapoptotic insults and hence prone to apoptosis. Numerous studies have reported a marked increase in the rate of apoptosis in the border zone (by several folds) for several days to weeks after AMI and a gradual increase in apoptosis in the remote myocardium in the left and right ventricles.[14,25–27] The rate of apoptosis in the heart during the healing phases of AMI seems to be predictive of the severity of the adverse remodeling and the occurrence of heart failure. The greater the apoptosis in the border zone or in the remote myocardium, the worse the remodeling in both human and animal experimental studies.[3]

Although postmortem studies are not probative of a causal relationship, several studies have associated increased apoptosis with a pattern of more adverse cardiac remodeling progressing from uncomplicated AMI or compensated concentric hypertrophy to eccentric hypertrophy and to end-stage stages characterized by marked dilatation and thin walls.[25] In the most severe forms of adverse remodeling after AMI, dilatation of the right ventricle is also present (biventricular remodeling).[27,28]

The presence of a patent infarct-related artery indicating reperfusion is associated with a more favorable remodeling pattern and reduced apoptosis.[29] Neurohormonal blockers that prevent adverse remodeling, such as angiotensin-converting enzyme inhibitors and β-adrenergic blockers, also inhibit apoptosis after AMI.[3] Genetically modified animal models prone to apoptosis were shown to be prone also to heart failure and death, whereas animal models resistant to apoptosis were protected.[3]

Similar to ischemic cardiomyopathy, other cardiomyopathies, such as chronic pressure overload, volume overload, doxorubicin induced, and others, are also characterized by increased rate of apoptosis contributing to the transition between the compensated and decompensated stages of the disease.

APOPTOSIS INTERRUPTUS AND REMODELED MYOCARDIUM

The release of cytochrome c and activation of caspase 3 lead to increased incidence of apoptosis and progressive loss of cellular components and gradual increase in interstitial fibrosis. Many studies show that the degree of cell death by apoptosis or autophagic cell death and the degree of fibrosis predict the lack of functional recovery of hibernating myocardium after revascularization.[30–33] Activation of caspase 3, however, does not necessarily equate to cell death.[34,35] The finding of caspase 3 activation in cardiomyocytes is far more common than the finding of apoptotic cell death, and the presence of activated caspase 3 does not impede complete functional recovery of hibernating myocardium after revascularization.[11]

Such findings led to the concept of apoptosis interruptus.[36] This expression relates to the evidence of activation of the apoptotic cascade (namely caspase 3) in the absence of true apoptotic phenotype[35,36] and suggests that activation of the cascade does not necessarily accomplish cell death but denotes a relatively large area of myocardium at jeopardy in a fragile balance (**Fig. 2**).[35,36] This concept goes hand in hand with the concept of programmed cell survival. The injured or stressed cell responds by simultaneously activating a death pathway and a repair pathway; the balance or unbalance of these 2 pathways determines the outcome of the cell. Mitochondrial apoptosis pathways and the unfolded protein response are involved in this survival balance (see **Fig. 2**). Parallel to partial activation of inducer of apoptosis, such as *bid* and caspase 8, and the release of cytochrome c from mitochondria, caspase 9 and caspase 3 are also cleaved in heart failure, yet concomitant increase in inhibitors of apoptosis, such as XIAP, subdue the activation of caspase 3.[35] Survivin, an essential cellular antiapoptotic mechanism in control of the upstream initiation of mitochondrial-dependent apoptosis, is upregulated in the remodeled myocardium and promotes cell survival under stress.[37] Cellular stress is intimately related to stress of endoplasmic reticulum and the

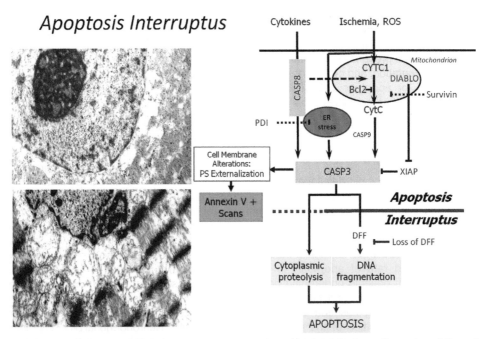

Apoptosis Interruptus

Fig. 2. In heart failure, the myocardium expresses proapoptotic and antiapoptotic mediators in a delicate balance between death and survival. Apoptosis interruptus refers to activation of the apoptotic cascade without the apoptotic phenotype. Caspase 3 activation occurs in the absence of DNA fragmentation. Cell membrane alterations secondary to caspase 3 activation lead to exposure of PS, which is recognized by annexin V.

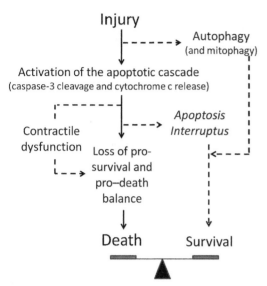

Fig. 3. A delicate balance exists between death and survival in the border zone after AMI (remodeled myocardium). Stretch and other form of injuries activate the apoptotic cascade, which eventually leads to cell death. Parallel to a cell death program, autophagy and natural inhibitors of apoptosis delay execution of cell death and prolong cell survival.

unfolded protein response, and failure to eliminate misfolded proteins leads to apoptotic cell death.[11,12] After AMI, endoplasmic reticulum stress occurs, yet upregulation of members of the unfolded protein response, such as protein disulfide isomerase, protects the cell from dying.[38] This survival instinct in the remodeled myocardium exemplifies as to why cardiomyocytes are

deserving of the supreme status of terminally differentiated cells (**Fig. 3**).[39]

The clinical implications of such observation are obvious, and it is likely that the strategies inhibiting cell death and/or promoting cell survival could help halt the progression of cardiomyopathy and prevent heart failure.

The recognition of the existence of a portion of the heart that is at jeopardy has generated the idea of rescuing the myocardium at risk. Most of the initial studies were focused on revascularization of ischemic myocardium, especially where there was evidence of hypoperfused hypocontractile myocardium (hibernating myocardium).[11] The recent multicenter Surgical Treatment for Ischemic Heart Failure trial has equated the benefits of medical therapy to that of revascularization and has emphasized the need to further strengthen medical therapy.[40] Based on the experimental evidence that the myocardium at risk in the border zone is often normally perfused yet hypocontractile and prone to apoptosis, it would be prudent that even revascularization is also abundantly supported by aggressive medical therapy.[6]

APOPTOSIS-TARGETED INTERVENTIONS IN HEART FAILURE

The observation that the activation of the apoptotic cascade and the actual rate of apoptotic cardiomyocytes correlate with prognosis and that apoptosis can be inhibited using pharmacologic inhibitors has led to a large number of studies addressing whether inhibition of apoptosis halts the progression of the cardiomyopathy.[3,41] Given the

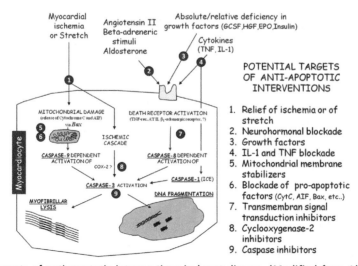

Fig. 4. Potential targets of antiapoptotic interventions in heart disease. (*Modified from* Abbate A, Bussani R, Amin MS, et al. Acute myocardial infarction and heart failure: role of apoptosis. Int J Biochem Cell Biol 2006;38:1837; with permission.)

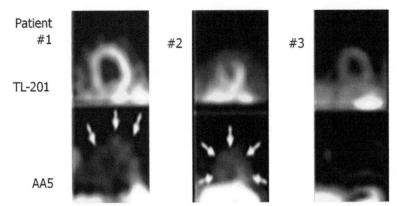

Fig. 5. Caspase 3 activation induces cell membrane alterations that lead to exposure of PS, which is recognized by annexin V. Annexin V scans have been performed in patients with nonischemic cardiomyopathy. Patients with annexin V uptake in the myocardium (*white arrows*) (approximately 50%, either patchy [as in patient #1] or diffuse [as in patient #2]) had further reduction in left ventricular systolic function compared with those with no myocardial uptake (as in patient #3). (*Modified from* Kietselaer BL, Reutelingsperger CP, Boersma HH, et al. Noninvasive detection of programmed cell loss with 99mTc-labeled annexin A5 in heart failure. J Nucl Med 2007;48:564; with permission.)

complexity of the apoptotic cascade, although multiple targets exist, only few may be viable in terms of targeted efficacy (**Fig. 4**). Treatment approaches vary from elimination of the triggers (ie, relief of ischemia and neurohormonal blockade and ventricular unloading with ventricular assist devices) to more focused inhibition of the apoptotic signaling. Although nonspecific apoptotic inhibitors have shown to be clinically effective (ie, angiotensin-converting enzyme inhibitors, β-adrenergic blockers, aldosterone antagonists), it remains unclear whether the benefit of such agents is through reduction of apoptosis. Animal studies with caspase inhibitors have shown promising results,[42,43] but clinical trials with targeted apoptotic inhibitors in heart disease are lacking.

MOLECULAR IMAGING OF CARDIAC APOPTOSIS

Most of the clinical studies on myocardial apoptosis are limited by the design being mostly cross-sectional. This is likely related to the challenges of detecting cell death in vivo because of the need of invasive procedure such as myocardial biopsies. The molecular imaging methods to detect apoptosis may offer means for adjunctive diagnostic or prognostic information. Proof of concept clinical studies has shown that annexin V–targeted nuclear scans identify cells in which the apoptotic cascade is activated. Caspase 3 leads to membrane abnormalities and redistribution of phosphatidylserine (PS) to the cell surface,

which is recognized by annexin V imaging. Annexin V uptake shows diffuse or patchy uptake in patients with heart failure.[32,43] An abnormal annexin V study in patients with decompensated heart failure predicted further worsening of left ventricular systolic function over time (**Fig. 5**).[32] It has been proposed that annexin V uptake represents the magnitude of caspase 3 activity and provides a noninvasive portal to identify the balance between proapoptotic and antiapoptotic factors in heart failure. However, whether annexin V imaging can guide management of patients remains to be tested.

SUMMARY

Apoptosis is a key feature in the progression of heart disease. Stage B heart failure is characterized by a structurally abnormal heart in which the remodeled myocardium is prone to apoptosis. Elimination of the proapoptotic stimuli or inhibition of the apoptotic cascade could presumably rescue the myocardium and halt the progression of adverse remodeling and heart failure.

REFERENCES

1. Jessup M, Abraham WT, Casey DE, et al. 2009 focused update: ACCF/AHA guidelines for the diagnosis and management of heart failure in adults. Circulation 2009;119:1977–2016.
2. Greenberg H, Mc Master P, Dwyer EM. Left ventricular dysfunction after acute myocardial infarction: results of a prospective multicenter study.

Multicenter Post-Infarction Research Group. J Am Coll Cardiol 1984;5:867–74.

3. Abbate A, Biondi-Zoccai GG, Baldi A. Pathophysiologic role of myocardial apoptosis in post-infarction left ventricular remodeling. J Cell Physiol 2002;193:145–53.

4. Reimer KA, Jennings RB. The "wave front phenomenon" of myocardial ischemic cell death. II. Transmural progression of necrosis within the framework of ischemic bed size (myocardium at risk) and collateral flow. Lab Invest 1979;40:633–42.

5. Hutchins GM, Bulkley BH. Infarct expansion versus extension: two different complications of acute myocardial infarction. Am J Cardiol 1978;41:1127–31.

6. Jackson BM, Gorman JH, Moainie SL, et al. Extension of borderzone myocardium in postinfarction dilated cardiomyopathy. J Am Coll Cardiol 2002;40:1160–7.

7. Dispersyn GD, Mesotten L, Meuris B, et al. Dissociation of cardiomyocyte apoptosis and dedifferentiation in infarct border zones. Eur Heart J 2002;23:849–57.

8. Canty JM, Suzuki G. Heterogeneity of apoptosis and myolysis in coronary microembolization: a competition between programmed cell death and programmed cell survival. Eur Heart J 2002;23:838–40.

9. Narula N, Narula J, Zhang PJ, et al. Is the myofibrillarlytic myocyte a forme frusta apoptotic myocyte? Ann Thorac Surg 2005;79:1333–7.

10. Gottlieb RA, Carreira RS. Autophagy in health and disease. Am J Physiol Cell Physiol 2010;299:C203–10.

11. Elsasser A, Vogt AM, Nef H, et al. Human hibernating myocardium is jeopardized by apoptotic and autophagic cell death. J Am Coll Cardiol 2004;43:2191–9.

12. Chandrashekhar Y, Narula J. Death hath a thousand doors to let out life. Circ Res 2003;92:710–4.

13. Narula J, Haider N, Virmani R, et al. Apoptosis in myocytes in end stage heart failure. N Engl J Med 1996;335:1182–9.

14. Narula J, Pandley P, Arbustini E, et al. Apoptosis in heart failure: release of cytochrome c from mitochondria and activation of caspase-3 in human cardiomyopathy. Proc Natl Acad Sci U S A 1999;96:8144–9.

15. Baldi A, Abbate A, Bussani R, et al. Apoptosis and post-infarction left ventricular remodeling. J Mol Cell Cardiol 2002;34:165–74.

16. Scheubel RJ, Bartling B, Simm A, et al. Apoptotic pathway activation from mitochondria and death receptors without caspase-3 cleavage in failing human myocardium: fragile balance of myocyte survival? J Am Coll Cardiol 2002;39:481–8.

17. Ruetten H, Badorff C, Ihling C, et al. Inhibition of caspase-3 improves contractile recover of stunned myocardium, independent of apoptosis-inhibitory effects. J Am Coll Cardiol 2001;38:2063–70.

18. Kroemer G, Galluzzi L, Vandenabeele P, et al. Classification of cell death: recommendations of the nomenclature committee on cell death 2009. Cell Death Differ 2009;16:3–11.

19. Kerr JF, Wyllie AH, Curie AR. Apoptosis: a basic biological phenomenon with wide ranging implications in tissue kinetics. Br J Cancer 1972;26:239–56.

20. Anversa P, Olivetti G, Capasso JM. Cellular basis of ventricular remodeling after myocardial infarction. Am J Cardiol 1991;68:7D–16D.

21. Olivetti G, Abbi R, Quaini F, et al. Apoptosis in the failing human heart. N Engl J Med 1997;336:1131–41.

22. Anselmi A, Gaudino M, Baldi A, et al. Role of apoptosis in pressure-overload cardiomyopathy. J Cardiovasc Med 2008;9:227–32.

23. Whelan RS, Kaplinskiy V, Kitsis RN. Cell death in the pathogenesis of heart disease: mechanisms and significance. Annu Rev Physiol 2010;72:19–44.

24. Wencker D, Chandra M, Nguyen K, et al. A mechanistic role for cardiac myocyte apoptosis in heart failure. J Clin Invest 2003;111:1497–504.

25. Abbate A, Biondi-Zoccai GG, Bussani R, et al. Increased myocardial apoptosis in patients with unfavorable left ventricular remodeling and early symptomatic post-infarction heart failure. J Am Coll Cardiol 2003;41:753–60.

26. Olivetti G, Quaini F, Sala R, et al. Acute myocardial infarction in humans is associated with activation of programmed myocyte cell death in the surviving portion of the heart. J Mol Cell Cardiol 1996;28:2005–16.

27. Abbate A, Bussani R, Sinagra G, et al. Right ventricular cardiomyocyte apoptosis in patients with acute myocardial infarction of the left ventricular wall. Am J Cardiol 2008;102:658–62.

28. Bussani R, Abbate A, Biondi-Zoccai GG, et al. Right ventricular dilatation after left ventricular acute myocardial infarction is predictive of extremely high peri-infarctual apoptosis at postmortem examination in humans. J Clin Pathol 2003;56:672–6.

29. Abbate A, Bussani R, Biondi-Zoccai GG, et al. Persistent infarct-related artery occlusion is associated with an increased myocardial apoptosis at postmortem examination in humans late after an acute myocardial infarction. Circulation 2002;106:1051–4.

30. Bondarenko O, Beek AM, Twisk JW, et al. Time course of functional recovery after revascularization of hibernating myocardium: a contrast-enhanced cardiovascular magnetic resonance study. Eur Heart J 2008;29:2000–5.

31. Saraste A, Pulkki K, Kallajoki M, et al. Cardiomyocyte apoptosis and progression of heart failure to transplantation. Eur J Clin Invest 1999;29:380–6.

32. Kietselaer BL, Reutelingsperger CP, Boersma HH, et al. Noninvasive detection of programmed cell loss with 99mTc-labeled annexin A5 in heart failure. J Nucl Med 2007;48:562–7.

33. Heusch G. Hibernating myocardium. Physiol Rev 1998;78:1055–85.

34. Communal C, Sumandea M, Solaro JR, et al. Functional consequences of apoptosis in cardiac myocytes: myofibrillar proteins are targets for caspase-3. Circulation (Abstract) 2001;104:2–162.

35. Haider N, Arbustini E, Gupta S, et al. Concurrent up-regulation of endogenous proapoptotic and antiapoptotic factors in failing human hearts. Nat Clin Pract Cardiovasc Med 2009;6:250–61.

36. Narula J, Arbustini E, Chandrashekhar Y, et al. Apoptosis and the systolic dysfunction in congestive heart failure. Story of apoptosis interruptus and zombie myocytes. Cardiol Clin 2001;19:113–26.

37. Santini D, Abbate A, Scarpa S, et al. Surviving acute myocardial infarction: survivin expression in viable cardiomyocytes after infarction. J Clin Pathol 2004; 57:1321–4.

38. Severino A, Campioni M, Straino S, et al. Identification of protein disulfide isomerase as a cardiomyocyte survival factor in ischemic cardiomyopathy. J Am Coll Cardiol 2007;50:1029–37.

39. Narula J, Young JB. Imaging heart failure: premonition to prevention in predisposed. Heart Fail Clin 2006;2:ix–x.

40. Velazquez EJ, Lee KL, Deja MA, et al. Coronary-artery bypass surgery in patients with left ventricular dysfunction. N Engl J Med 2011;364:1607–16.

41. Abbate A, Bussani R, Amin MS, et al. Acute myocardial infarction and heart failure: role of apoptosis. Int J Biochem Cell Biol 2006;38:1834–40.

42. Chandrashekhar Y, Sen S, Anway R, et al. Long-term caspase inhibition ameliorates apoptosis, reduces myocardial troponin-I cleavage, protects left ventricular function, and attenuates remodeling in rats with myocardial infarction. J Am Coll Cardiol 2004;43: 295–301.

43. Hofstra L, Liem IH, Dumont EA, et al. Visualisation of cell death in vivo in patients with acute myocardial infarction. Lancet 2000;356:209–12.

Neurohumoral Stimulation

Irving H. Zucker, PhD*, Kaushik P. Patel, PhD,
Harold D. Schultz, PhD

KEYWORDS

- Chronic heart failure • Neurohumoral activation • Baroreflex
- Sympathoexcitation • Carotid body chemoreflex

Neurohumoral activation has been recognized as one of the hallmarks in the compensatory response during the development of chronic heart failure (CHF), whatever its origin.[1–4] A large number of hormonal systems are activated in the CHF state, and virtually all vasoconstrictor substances are increased, including angiotensin II (Ang II), endothelin-1, vasopressin, and norepinephrine. In addition, it is now well accepted that potent vasodilator systems are downregulated in the CHF state. Nitric oxide and its downstream target, cGMP, are reduced and contribute to the general state of vasoconstriction in CHF. Furthermore, CHF has been viewed as a proinflammatory state and a condition characterized by high levels of oxidative stress.[5–7] In patients and animals with CHF, increased oxidative stress has been shown to occur in many tissues, including the heart and brain.[8–12]

Based on measures from techniques such as microneurography and norepinephrine spillover, sympathetic nerve activity is clearly elevated in CHF.[13,14] A clear indication of this phenomenon is illustrated in **Fig. 1**, in which a profound increase in muscle sympathetic nerve activity correlates with the severity of cardiac dysfunction. These data also suggest that sympathoexcitation occurs early in the progression of the heart failure syndrome. The central origin of this sympathoexcitation is also well established in both animal and human studies.[15] Although differences are seen in sympathetic outflow to various vascular beds in the CHF state, it is generally well accepted that sympathoexcitation is a global phenomenon.

The temporal relationship between the development of heart failure and activation of these neurohumoral systems has not been precisely defined. When a compensatory mechanism switches to a deleterious contributing factor in the progression of the disease is unclear. This article addresses these issues through evaluating the contribution of various cardiovascular reflexes and cellular mechanisms to the sympathoexcitation in CHF. It also sheds light on some of the important central mechanisms that contribute to the increase in sympathetic nerve activity in CHF.

ARTERIAL BAROREFLEXES

The primary and most powerful short-term modulators of arterial pressure are the arterial baroreflexes (ABRs). The sensory endings that mediate the ABR lie in the wall of the aortic arch and carotid sinus. This buffer reflex has been well characterized in humans and experimental animals. The maximum sensitivity of the ABR is defined by construction of full baroreflex curves in which the input (some parameter related to arterial pressure) is plotted against one of several output parameters (eg, heart rate, sympathetic nerve activity, peripheral resistance). The maximum of the first derivative of the negative slope of this relationship defines the peak sensitivity. Usually the peak negative slope occurs close to the ambient arterial pressure.

Some of the work shown in this paper was supported by a grant from the NIH; PO-1 HL62222.
Conflicts: None.
Department of Cellular and Integrative Physiology, University of Nebraska Medical Center, 985850 Nebraska Medical Center, Omaha, NE 68198-5850, USA
* Corresponding author.
E-mail address: izucker@unmc.edu

Heart Failure Clin 8 (2012) 87–99
doi:10.1016/j.hfc.2011.08.007

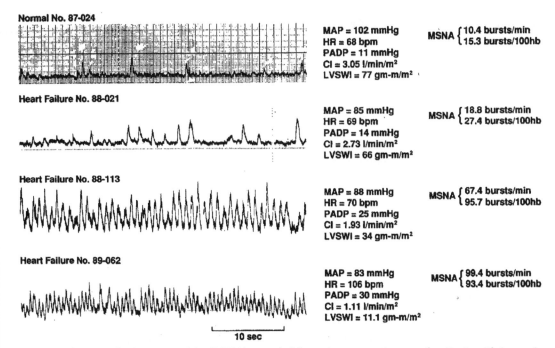

Fig. 1. Muscle sympathetic nerve activity (MSNA) recorded from the peroneal nerve of patients with increasing levels of cardiac dysfunction. (*Reprinted from* Ferguson DW, Berg WJ, Sanders JS, et al. Clinical and hemodynamic correlates of sympathetic nerve activity in normal humans and patients with heart failure: evidence from direct microneurographic recordings. CI, cardiac index; hb, heart beats; HR, heart rate; LVSWI, left ventricular stroke work index; MAP, mean arterial pressure; PADP, pulmonary artery diastolic pressure. J Am Coll Cardiol 1990;16: 1125–34; with permission.)

As in some forms of severe hypertension, ABR sensitivity is depressed in patients and animals with CHF.[16–18] This depression in baroreflex sensitivity in CHF occurs through several mechanisms. First, the sensitivity of baroreceptor endings to pressure is reduced.[19–21] This phenomenon can only be studied in experimental models. A reduced discharge sensitivity of single units dissected from the carotid sinus nerve has been shown in the dog model of pacing-induced CHF.[22] This decrease in sensitivity is mediated partly by an increase in Na^+-K^+-ATPase activity[21] in baroreceptor afferent endings. Aldosterone administered into the isolated carotid sinus reduced afferent discharge sensitivity through an apparent nongenomic effect.[23] Because aldosterone is elevated in CHF and mineralocorticoid receptor antagonists have been proven to be an effective and important therapy, aldosterone may contribute to baroreflex depression in the CHF state.

Clear evidence also shows that the central neural components that mediate ABRs are impaired in the CHF state. For instance, in dogs, stimulation of the carotid sinus nerve (thus bypassing the receptor endings) results in baroreflex responses that are impaired in CHF compared with normal animals.[24] These data suggest central

or efferent abnormalities in the control of baroreflex function in CHF.

Does ABR depression contribute to the sustained neurohumoral excitation in CHF or does it simply initiate this process at the beginning of the disease state? This question has been difficult to answer in humans. Grassi and colleagues[25] attempted to address this issue through evaluating muscle sympathetic nerve activity and ABR function in patients with mild (New York Heart Association [NYHA] class I and II) and severe (NYHA class III and IV) CHF. Although a gradation was seen in both resting muscle sympathetic nerve activity and ABR sensitivity, patients with mild CHF clearly exhibited significant sympathoexcitation and baroreflex depression compared with age-matched control subjects. In a subsequent study, these investigators[26] showed that angiotensin-converting enzyme inhibition (benazepril, 10 mg/d for 2 months) reduced sympathetic nerve activity in patients with mild CHF. Furthermore, benazepril treatment resulted in an enhancement in ABR sympathoinhibition in response to increasing arterial pressure.

Because activation of the renin-angiotensin system (RAS) is likely to occur early in the pathogenesis of CHF, and this activation may contribute to the central depression of ABR function, this raises the question of whether ABR depression a prerequisite of the chronic elevation of sympathetic tone in CHF. This question has also been difficult to answer definitively.

In studies performed in dogs with CHF and complete baroreceptor denervation, Brändle and colleagues[27] showed increases in plasma norepinephrine induced by CHF that were the same with or without intact ABR function. In a related study, Levett and colleagues[28] showed similar norepinephrine increases in dogs with CHF after chronic cardiac denervation. Therefore, although cardiovascular reflex function is impaired in the CHF state, it may not be the initiating factor responsible for early sympathoexcitation. In conscious rabbits with pacing-induced CHF, the authors observed a late increase in renal sympathetic nerve activity (RSNA) (Fig. 2). This increase was associated with an increase in plasma Ang II levels, suggesting a possible relationship between activation of the RAS and sympathoexcitation in CHF, at least in terms of late events.

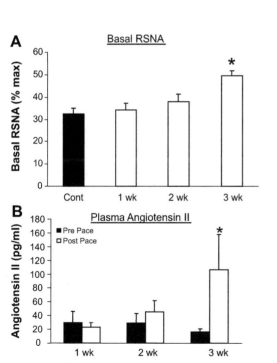

Fig. 2. (A) RSNA in conscious rabbits during the progression of pacing-induced CHF. A significant increase in RSNA was seen after 3 weeks of pacing; *P<.05 compared with control; n = 5. (B) Plasma Ang II concentration of groups of rabbits examined before (*black bars*) and after each week of cardiac pacing; *P<.05 compared with pre-pace; n = 5.

LOW PRESSURE REFLEXES
Evidence for Altered Volume Reflex in Heart Failure

Low pressure reflexes have been implicated in the control of salt and water balance in the normal state.[29,30] In addition to the ABR, cardiovascular reflexes emanating from the low pressure side of the circulation may be important in modulating fluid balance and sympathetic outflow in CHF. In normal humans, translocation of blood from the periphery to the thoracic circulation evokes a brisk diuresis and natriuresis.[31–34] Studies have shown that neural activity from sensory endings located in the atria and ventricles is markedly reduced in animals with CHF.[35–42] Data from humans with CHF also suggest that abnormal volume reflexes contribute to the chronic congestion and the sympathoexcitation of this disease.[43–45] Mechanical and chemical activation of atrial and ventricular reflexes have been shown to reduce sympathetic outflow and arginine vasopressin secretion.[41,46,47] Therefore, abnormalities in either the discharge characteristics of these endings or the central processing of neural information originating from these receptors may have profound effects on both sympathetic nerve activity and arginine vasopressin secretion.[41]

The volume reflex can be defined as the renal response to an acute volume challenge. An impaired ability to excrete a sodium load is a salient feature of the heart failure condition. The renal response (diuresis and natriuresis) to acute volume expansion (with isotonic saline) is clearly blunted in various animal models of CHF.[48–50] In addition to general sympathetic nerve activity, RSNA is also markedly elevated in CHF.[51,52] Several possible places in the volume reflex arc could be altered in CHF, including (1) the receptors (including electromechanical coupling factors), (2) mechanical properties of the cardiac tissue where the receptors are located, (3) cardiac vagal afferent fibers, (4) the central neural processing of afferent input (5) efferent renal sympathetic nerve fibers, (6) the end-organ response to transmitter release and (7) the release or action of humoral factors, such as atrial natriuretic peptide (ANP) and arginine vasopressin, on end-organ responses within the kidney.

Afferent limb of the volume receptor reflex
Even though the ABR is impaired in CHF, low pressure receptors more likely mediate the volume reflex. Studies in the authors' laboratory have addressed the hypothesis that the altered volume reflex in rats with CHF reflects reduced distensibility (compliance) of the right atrium and the

Relation between ΔCVP & ΔRSND

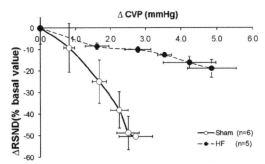

Fig. 3. Relationship between the change in renal sympathetic nerve discharge (RSND) and change in central venous pressure (CVP) in anesthetized sham-operated control rats and coronary artery–ligated rats with heart failure during acute volume expansion with isotonic saline. A significantly blunted renal sympathoinhibition was seen in rats with heart failure (P<.05).

venoatrial junction, structures known to possess a large number of volume (stretch) receptors.[50] The distensibility was assessed through measuring the stiffness constants of the pressure-volume curve (dP/dV) of the right atrium and venoatrial junction in CHF rats and sham rats. The results illustrate that the stiffness constant, the slope of the change in pressure versus change in volume of the right atrium and venoatrial junction, is significantly greater in CHF rats than in sham rats (**Fig. 3**). These data suggest that rats with CHF have stiffer right atria and venoatrial junctions, which may reduce stimulation of the volume receptors to a volume load. The decrease in diastolic compliance in the left atrium in CHF has been shown to limit the increase in receptor discharge as left atrial pressure increases during filling.[40] In addition, gross morphologic changes in atrial stretch receptors were observed in dogs with CHF.[42] Whether such a change in receptor discharge occurs in rats with CHF remains to be determined. Although the possibility of altered vagal afferent sensitivity in CHF has not been assessed in rats, available data indicate that an altered afferent limb of the volume reflex may contribute to the overall blunted diuretic and natriuretic response to volume load.

Central sites of integration for the volume receptor reflex

Anatomic, electrophysiologic, and histologic evidence have clearly identified the nucleus tractus solitarius (NTS) as the primary site of termination for afferent vagal fibers.[53] In addition, the forebrain has been examined thoroughly for its involvement in various aspects of fluid balance.[54]

The magnocellular subdivision of paraventricular nucleus (mPVN) and the supraoptic nucleus are known to produce arginine vasopressin, an important humoral factor involved in fluid balance.[55] In addition to these effects, the parvocellular subdivision of the paraventricular nucleus (pPVN) has been implicated in the control of sympathetic outflow. Specifically, the authors showed that lesioning the pPVN with kainic acid altered the renal sympathoinhibition produced in response to acute volume expansion.[56] Other areas in the forebrain, important in the control of fluid balance, are the subfornical organ and the organum vasculosum of the lamina terminalis.[57] In addition, neurons in the paraventricular nucleus (PVN) are known to function as integrators of autonomic outflow, particularly to the kidneys.[55]

Few studies have examined changes in the central structures of the brain associated with the volume reflex in CHF.[58] In previous studies the authors found that rats with CHF had significantly elevated hexokinase activity (an index of metabolic activity) in the pPVN and mPVN compared with sham rats.[59] Because the mPVN is a main site for arginine vasopressin–synthesizing neurons, these changes are in accord with findings of increased serum levels of arginine vasopressin reported in humans[60] and rats[61] with CHF. In addition, rats with CHF exhibit a resetting of the osmotic regulation of arginine vasopressin secretion in such a way that higher plasma arginine vasopressin levels were observed at lower levels of plasma sodium or osmolality.[61,62] This resetting of the osmotic regulation of arginine vasopressin secretion may also contribute to the blunted volume reflex in rats with CHF. The effectiveness of tolvaptan in the treatment of chronic hyponatremia in CHF may be related to this mechanism.[63] In addition, the increased neuronal activity in the pPVN of rats with CHF may contribute to the increased renal sympathoexcitation observed in this model of CHF.[59,64]

Finally, the neuronal isoform of nitric oxide synthase (nNOS) within the PVN has been shown to be an important contributor to the volume reflex–mediated renal sympathoinhibition in normal rats[65] and that nNOS within the PVN of rats with CHF is decreased.[66,67] Decreased nNOS within the PVN of rats with CHF may be partly responsible for the altered volume reflex in rats with CHF. Further studies are needed to elucidate the causal relationship between these parameters.

Efferent limb of the volume receptor reflex

The efferent mechanisms that regulate the reflex diuretic and natriuretic responses to volume expansion are neural and humoral.[48,50] The neural component of the diuretic and natriuretic response to volume expansion is known to be mediated partly by a decrease in RSNA.[48,50] Because increased RSNA produces retention of salt and water, decreased RSNA can contribute to diuresis and natriuresis.[50] Several humoral factors, such as Ang II, aldosterone, arginine vasopressin, and atrial natriuretic factor, also contribute to the effector limb of the volume reflex.

Neural component

Data obtained primarily from rat experiments indicate that sodium excretion from innervated kidneys is attenuated in rats with CHF compared with sham-operated control rats, whereas the sodium excretion from denervated kidneys of rats with CHF is similar to that from innervated kidneys of sham rats.[50] Furthermore, urine flow and sodium excretion from innervated kidneys, but not from denervated kidneys, were significantly lower in rats with CHF than in sham rats.[50] These results suggest that part of the blunted natriuresis to volume expansion in rats with CHF is from the tonic impact of the renal nerves. The impaired natriuresis to volume expansion in innervated kidneys of rats with CHF may be caused by (1) blunted afferent and central inhibition of RSNA or (2) a hyperactive effect at the neuroeffector junction sites to enhance sodium reabsorption. Recording of RSNA shows that blunted inhibition of RSNA to a given increase in central venous pressure occurs in rats with CHF compared with normal control rats.[50] Because RSNA produces retention of sodium and water, decreased RSNA can contribute to diuresis and natriuresis during volume expansion. The influences of the renal nerves on excretory function are largely mediated by α_1 adrenergic receptors. No studies report the density of adrenergic receptors in the kidneys of rats with CHF. This increased α_1-adrenergic receptor activity in the kidney of rats with CHF may contribute to the increased retention of sodium by the kidney when RSNA is elevated. Despite the accumulating evidence that the neural effector limb of the volume reflex is blunted in CHF, several key questions remain: Is RSNA abnormally elevated before and during acute volume expansion in rats with CHF? Is CHF accompanied by an altered relationship between RSNA and the subsequent release of norepinephrine, which may be affected by various factors, such as turnover of norepinephrine and presynaptic excitation or inhibition? Is the renal excretory response to sympathetic nerve stimulation augmented in rats with CHF? Is renal noradrenergic receptor density increased in CHF? If so, is it specific to a particular tubular segment? Answers to all these questions will identify some of the specific mechanisms through which the renal sympathetic nerves are involved in sodium retention in response to acute volume expansion in CHF.

Humoral component

Several humoral abnormalities have been reported to accompany CHF.[43,60] In light of the direct impact of atrial stretch on the release of ANP, elevated basal ANP levels in CHF are relevant to the renal excretory response to volume expansion. Volume expansion does not increase ANP levels in rats with CHF to the same extent that it does in sham rats.[68] To determine whether renal responses to ANP are altered in the CHF state, the diuretic and natriuretic responses to ANP administration were assessed in innervated and denervated kidneys of anesthetized control rats and those with CHF.[50] Compared with control rats, rats with CHF showed significantly blunted diuretic and natriuretic responses to ANP, and this effect was independent of renal innervation.[50] Glomerular filtration rate measurements indicated that hemodynamic changes did not account for the blunted renal excretory responses in rats with CHF. These results confirm that hemodynamic changes per se are not responsible for the altered volume reflex in rats with CHF, and indicate that renal excretory responses to ANP are blunted in CHF regardless of the presence of renal nerves.

The authors previously showed that renal nerves contribute to the retention of sodium and water in rats with CHF.[50] However, they also showed that although renal denervation normalized the blunted renal diuretic and natriuretic responses to acute volume expansion, these responses were still significantly blunted in rats with CHF compared with control rats. These results suggest that other factors are involved in sodium retention during CHF. The excessive retention of sodium that occurs in CHF may result from a reduced glomerular filtration rate, an enhanced tubular reabsorption, or both.

The key element involved in renal sodium retention is activation of apical epithelial sodium channels (ENaCs) in the collecting tubule by aldosterone and arginine vasopressin. Elevated basal plasma aldosterone and arginine vasopressin levels associated with increased sodium intake have been linked to CHF.[69] However, the roles of various tubular segments and the molecular basis for the inappropriate sodium and water retention remain largely undefined in CHF. In particular, very little, if any, information is available regarding the abundance and functional role of ENaCs in the kidneys of rats with CHF. Chronic administration of aldosterone increases the

α-ENaC subunit and, to a lesser extent, the β and γ subunits[70] at the mRNA and protein levels. In contrast, arginine vasopressin has a different effect from that observed with aldosterone. It primarily increases the expression of the β and γ subunits but not α to any great extent.[71]

Enhanced renal abundance and increased functional activity of ENaC subunits has recently been reported in animals with CHF.[72] This study showed that the mRNA and protein levels of α, β, and γ subunits of ENaC were significantly increased in the cortex and outer medulla of the kidneys in rats with CHF. Immunohistochemistry confirmed the increased α-ENaC, β-ENaC, and γ-ENaC subunits in the collecting duct segments in rats with CHF. These results are consistent with the observations that both aldosterone and arginine vasopressin are increased in rats with CHF.[69] Furthermore, the diuretic and natriuretic responses to the ENaC inhibitor benzamil were increased in rats with CHF. Renal denervation unmasked a greater role for ENaC in CHF.[72] The observed increased expression of ENaC subunits associated with enhanced channel function suggests that dysregulation of renal ENaC subunits could be involved in the retention of sodium chloride and thus contribute to the pathogenesis and development of CHF.

THE CENTRAL RAS AND SYMPATHOEXCITATION IN CHF

The RAS has been implicated in the central processing of sympathetic nerve activity.[73–76] In dogs with CHF, cerebrospinal fluid concentrations of Ang II are markedly elevated[77] and are substantially higher than those in dog plasma.[78] These data raise the important question of the contribution of the central RAS to sympathoexcitation and ABR function in the setting of CHF. Although this is difficult to assess in humans, substantial data strongly implicate activation of the central RAS system in animal models of heart failure.[79]

Much evidence supports the idea that all of the components necessary to synthesize Ang II are located within the central nervous system.[80] Studies in rabbits with pacing-induced heart failure showed that expression of the Ang II type 1 (AT_1) receptor was increased in the rostral ventrolateral medulla (RVLM).[81,82] These data were also confirmed in the rat PVN, RVLM, and NTS.[83–85] Contributing to this central angiotensinergic drive in CHF is the finding that angiotensin-converting enzyme is increased in the brain of animals with CHF.[86] Recently, studies have shown that central Ang II contributes to oxidative stress, which can activate sympathetic neurons.[10,87,88] This effect may be important because reducing central oxidative stress through overexpression of antioxidant enzymes in the setting of CHF not only reduces sympathetic outflow but also improves cardiac function.[11,81]

SYMPATHOEXCITATORY REFLEXES

Although baroreflexes provide a tonic inhibitory influence on sympathetic outflow, several other peripheral autonomic reflexes provide an excitatory influence. These include the cardiac sympathetic (spinal) afferent reflex, the peripheral (carotid body) chemoreflex, and the somatic afferent reflex (or ergoreflex) from exercising skeletal muscle (exercise pressor reflex). These sympathoexcitatory reflexes are enhanced in CHF and thus contribute in a "feed-forward" manner to elevations in sympathetic outflow.

Cardiac Sympathetic Afferent Reflex

The cardiac sympathetic afferent reflex is difficult to study in humans, but the reflex is enhanced in animals with CHF.[89,90] The afferent signal arises from ischemically sensitive endings located mainly in the epicardial regions of the left ventricle. Under normal conditions these afferents have little influence on sympathetic activity, but in CHF they are sensitized to chemical mediators and become tonically active.[91,92] The precise mechanisms through which these endings become sensitized in CHF are not yet understood. These afferent endings are known to be sensitized and activated by a variety of chemical mediators released from ischemic myocardium, including protons, bradykinin, prostaglandins, histamine, reactive oxygen species, ATP, and adenosine.[93] The failing heart enters into a progressive state of functional ischemia because of impaired coronary flow (as seen in patients with myocardial infarctions), increased wall stress secondary to volume overload, and increased myocardial energy expenditure sustained by tonically elevated cardiac sympathetic drive. Studies have confirmed that cardiac sympathetic afferent activity in animals with CHF is enhanced in response to exogenous epicardial bradykinin via a prostaglandin intermediate.[94] The sympathetic reflex in CHF is also enhanced in response to epicardial application of hydrogen peroxide and adenosine.[92] Furthermore, volume expansion of the left ventricle enhances the reflex sympathetic activation in response to chemical stimulation of these afferent endings.[95] Collectively, these studies suggest that the cardiac sympathetic afferent endings are sensitized to a variety of stimuli in CHF associated with cardiac stress.

In addition to an enhancement of the sensory limb of the reflex, it is also well established that the central gain of the cardiac sympathetic afferent reflex is enhanced in CHF.[89,92] This phenomenon was verified through observing an enhanced sympathetic nerve activity in response to electrical stimulation of the cardiac sympathetic afferent nerve, which serves to control the neural input traveling to the central nervous system.[89] Subsequent studies showed that both increased central Ang II with downstream reactive oxygen species activation and reduced central nitric oxide contribute to the increase in central gain of the cardiac reflex in animals with CHF.[96–98] Central Ang II and nitric oxide effects on the reflex have been localized at the levels of the NTS, PVN,[99,100] and RVLM.[101] However, these central mediators are likely acting at multiple autonomic nuclei involved in integration of the reflex. The tonic elevation in cardiac afferent input also impacts the integration of inputs from peripheral reflexes at the level of the NTS through an AT_1 receptor mechanism. Thus, cardiac sympathetic afferents also serve to enhance carotid body chemoreflex activation of sympathetic outflow and to impair baroreflex inhibition of sympathetic outflow in CHF.[84,102]

Carotid Body Chemoreflex

Enhanced activation of sympathetic outflow and ventilation in response to carotid body chemoreflex activation is well documented in CHF. These changes were first shown in humans,[103] but more recent studies in CHF animals have detailed the changes in carotid body chemoreceptor function that contribute to these effects.[104] An enhanced carotid body sensitivity to hypoxia occurs in addition to an elevation in resting afferent chemoreceptor nerve activity under resting normoxic conditions[105] that contributes to a tonic elevation of sympathetic outflow in CHF.[106] The enhanced chemoreceptor nerve activity occurs as a result of synergistic effects within the carotid body involving increased production of reactive oxygen species from elevated Ang II–driven NADPH oxidase activity,[107,108] decreased cytosolic and mitochondrial superoxide dismutase expression,[109,110] and decreased nitric oxide production via down-regulation of nNOS.[105,111]

The neuroexcitatory effect of Ang II superoxide and the neuroinhibitory effect of nitric oxide on carotid body chemoreceptors are consistent with their opposing effects on ion channel function in carotid body glomus cells, the sensory cell of the carotid body. Elevated superoxide derived from Ang II activation of NAPDH oxidase and suppression of superoxide dismutase activity inhibits voltage-gated K^+ currents in these cells in the CHF state.[112] Conversely, nitric oxide, which normally acts on these cells to enhance voltage-gated K^+ currents, is suppressed in CHF.[113,114] The glomus cells also exhibit enhanced voltage-gated Ca^{++} currents in CHF,[114] which is consistent with the known effects of Ang II and nitric oxide on these channels. These changes would facilitate depolarization of glomus cells to hypoxia and may also contribute to the elevation in resting nerve traffic that occurs from the carotid body in CHF.

A recent study has shown that a chronic reduction of carotid body blood flow, similar to that observed in animals with CHF, induces changes in carotid body afferent and reflex function that mimic the CHF state (**Fig. 4**).[115] Thus the impairment in cardiac output and reduced local blood flow associated with CHF are implicated as a primary driving force for altered peripheral chemoreflex function in CHF. This relationship is further supported by evidence that the degree of chemoreflex enhancement correlates with the degree of left ventricular dysfunction[116] and the reduction in carotid blood flow. Further studies are needed to elucidate the mechanisms of flow sensitivity in the carotid body and their impact on carotid body function and autonomic control in CHF.

Exercise Pressor Reflex

A third major reflex input to excitation of sympathetic nerve activity is the exercise pressor reflex or the ergoreflex. The ergoreflex originates from stimulation of mechanically (group III) and metabolically (group IV) sensitive endings in contracting skeletal muscle. Substantial and uniform agreement exists that the ergoreflex is exaggerated in CHF.[117–119] However, the role of the mechanical and metabolic components of the sensory stimulus responsible for this exaggerated reflex in CHF remains controversial. Evidence from human and experimental animal studies suggests that the mechanoreceptor component to the reflex is enhanced, whereas the metabolic component is blunted in CHF.[120–123] In contrast, other studies suggest that the metaboreflex component is enhanced in CHF.[124–126]

Direct recordings from group III and IV afferents from the triceps surae in rats provide some insight into this controversy. These studies have shown that the activation of group III afferents in response to static contraction of the muscle is enhanced in CHF,[127] whereas that of group IV afferents to static

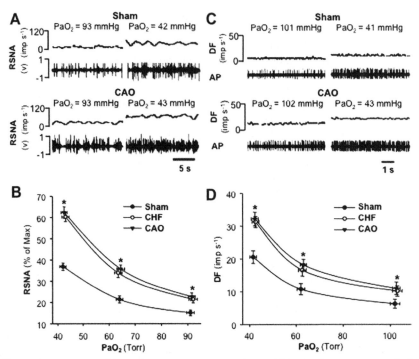

Fig. 4. The effects of normoxic and hypoxic states on RSNA and carotid body chemoreceptor discharge in sham, CHF, and chronic carotid occlusion (CAO) rabbits. (A) Representative recording of RSNA; (B) RSNA response to hypoxia (n = 12); (C) representative recording of carotid body chemoreceptor afferent discharge; (D) carotid body chemoafferent response to hypoxia (n = 6). CAO: bilateral carotid artery flow was decreased chronically (3 wk) to the same extent as that observed in CHF rabbits. Data are mean ± standard error of the mean. *P<.05 CHF and CAO compared with the sham group. AP, action potential; DF, discharge frequency; PaO₂, arterial oxygen partial pressure. (*Reprinted from* Li YL, Schultz HD. Enhanced sensitivity of Kv channels to hypoxia in the rabbit carotid body in heart failure: role of angiotensin II. J Physiol 2006;575:215–27; with permission.)

contraction and to chemical stimulation is blunted in animals with CHF.[127,128] These effects were related to increased purinergic 2X receptor sensitization of group III afferents, and reduced vanilloid receptor (VR1) mediation of group IV activation.[127,128] Other studies have shown that several other chemical mediators also contribute to the enhanced sensitivity of group III mechanosensitive afferents in CHF. These mediators include bradykinin,[129] prostaglandins,[130] and reactive oxygen species.[131]

Studies describing afferent neural responses have used static muscle contraction to activate the afferent sensory endings. In this regard, some of the controversy regarding the role of metabolic muscle afferents in mediating an exaggerated exercise pressor reflex in CHF may be related to the type of muscle work being performed. Important evidence indicates that a significant portion of the elevated muscle sympathetic nerve activation during rhythmic handgrip exercise in patients with CHF can be attributed to metaboreceptors,[125] whereas the metaboreceptor contribution was attenuated during static handgrip

exercise.[123] Metabolic derangements in exercising muscle are likely to be more manifest during rhythmic versus static exercise.[132] Further studies are needed to evaluate the impact of rhythmic versus static exercise on the exercise pressor reflex in CHF.

SUMMARY

Targeting the sympathetic nervous system and hormonal activation has been the focus of treatment of CHF for many years. The control of neurohumoral activation in the setting of CHF is multifactorial but clearly involves abnormalities in both peripheral sensors and the central nervous system. The arterial baroreflex and the volume reflex are major negative feedback systems that contribute to sympathoexcitation in CHF. In addition, excitatory reflexes, such as the carotid body chemoreflex, the ergoreflex, and the cardiac sympathetic afferent reflex, play a role in this sympathoexcitation. Several peripheral and central humoral modulators impact the sensitivity of these reflexes. Ang II, nitric oxide, and reactive oxygen species have been shown to be important regulators of cardiovascular reflex function in CHF. A critical question in this field is the contribution of these mechanisms to early heart failure and the progression of the disease process. This question has been difficult to answer, especially in humans. Most experimental models of CHF are evaluated late in the progression of the disease. The role of the renin-angiotensin system early in CHF is still controversial. Additional human and animal studies are needed to evaluate neurohumoral activation in the earliest phases of CHF.

REFERENCES

1. Esler M. The 2009 Carl Ludwig Lecture: pathophysiology of the human sympathetic nervous system in cardiovascular diseases: the transition from mechanisms to medical management. J Appl Physiol 2010;108:227–37.

2. Ruffolo RR Jr, Feuerstein GZ. Neurohormonal activation, oxygen free radicals, and apoptosis in the pathogenesis of congestive heart failure. J Cardiovasc Pharmacol 1998;32(Suppl 1):S22–30.

3. Cohn JN, Levine TB, Olivari MT, et al. Plasma norepinephrine as a guide to prognosis in patients with chronic congestive heart failure. N Engl J Med 1984;311:819–23.

4. Francis GS, Benedict C, Johnstone DE, et al. Comparison of neuroendocrine activation in patients with left ventricular dysfunction with and without congestive heart failure. A substudy of the Studies of Left Ventricular Dysfunction (SOLVD). Circulation 1990;82:1724–9.

5. Khaper N, Bryan S, Dhingra S, et al. Targeting the vicious inflammation-oxidative stress cycle for the management of heart failure. Antioxid Redox Signal 2010;13:1033–49.

6. Khullar M, Al-Shudiefat AA, Ludke A, et al. Oxidative stress: a key contributor to diabetic cardiomyopathy. Can J Physiol Pharmacol 2010;88:233–40.

7. Robinson T, Smith A, Channer KS. Reversible heart failure: the role of inflammatory activation. Postgrad Med J 2011;87(1024):110–5.

8. Castro PF, Greig D, Pérez O, et al. Relation between oxidative stress, catecholamines, and impaired chronotropic response to exercise in patients with chronic heart failure secondary to ischemic or idiopathic dilated cardiomyopathy. Am J Cardiol 2003;92:215–8.

9. Francis J, Yu L, Guggilam A, et al. Atorvastatin attenuates oxidative stress and improves neuronal nitric oxide synthase in the brain stem of heart failure mice [abstract 814]. Circulation 2007;116: II_157–8.

10. Lindley TE, Infanger DW, Rishniw M, et al. Scavenging superoxide selectively in mouse forebrain is associated with improved cardiac function and survival following myocardial infarction. Am J Physiol Regul Integr Comp Physiol 2009;296:R1–8.

11. Infanger DW, Cao X, Butler SD, et al. Silencing nox4 in the paraventricular nucleus improves myocardial infarction-induced cardiac dysfunction by attenuating sympathoexcitation and periinfarct apoptosis. Circ Res 2010;106:1763–74.

12. Gao L, Wang W, Li YL, et al. Sympathoexcitation by central ANG II: roles for AT1 receptor upregulation and NAD(P)H oxidase in RVLM. Am J Physiol Heart Circ Physiol 2005;288:H2271–9.

13. Ferguson DW, Berg WJ, Sanders JS, et al. Clinical and hemodynamic correlates of sympathetic nerve activity in normal humans and patients with heart failure: evidence from direct microneurographic recordings. J Am Coll Cardiol 1990;16:1125–34.

14. Meredith IT, Eisenhofer G, Lambert GW, et al. Cardiac sympathetic nervous activity in congestive heart failure: evidence for increased neuronal norepinephrine release and preserved neuronal uptake. Circulation 1993;88:136–45.

15. Zucker IH, Schultz HD, Li YF, et al. The origin of sympathetic outflow in heart failure: the roles of angiotensin II and nitric oxide. Prog Biophys Mol Biol 2004;84:217–32.

16. Eckberg DL, Drabinsky M, Braunwald E. Defective cardiac parasympathetic control in patients with heart disease. N Engl J Med 1971;285:877–83.

17. Higgins CB, Vatner SF, Eckberg DL, et al. Alterations in the baroreceptor reflex in conscious dogs with heart failure. J Clin Invest 1972;51:715–24.

18. Chen J-S, Wang W, Bartholet T, et al. Analysis of baroreflex control of heart rate in conscious dogs with pacing-induced heart failure. Circulation 1991;83:260–7.

19. Niebauer MJ, Holmberg MJ, Zucker IH. Aortic baroreceptor characteristics in dogs with chronic high output failure. Basic Res Cardiol 1986;81:111–22.

20. Niebauer MJ, Zucker IH. Static and dynamic responses of carotid sinus baroreceptors in dogs with chronic volume overload. J Physiol (Lond) 1985;369:295–310.

21. Wang W, Chen JS, Zucker IH. Postexcitatory depression of baroreceptors in dogs with experimental heart failure. Am J Physiol Heart Circ Physiol 1991;260:H1160–5.

22. Wang W, Chen J, Zucker IH. Carotid sinus baroreceptor sensitivity in experimental heart failure. Circulation 1990;81:1959–66.

23. Wang W, McClain JM, Zucker IH. Aldosterone reduces baroreceptor discharge in the dog. Hypertension 1992;19:270–7.

24. Wang W, Chen JS, Zucker IH. Carotid sinus baroreceptor reflex in dogs with experimental heart failure. Circ Res 1991;68:1294–301.

25. Grassi G, Seravalle G, Cattaneo BM, et al. Sympathetic activation and loss of reflex sympathetic

control in mild congestive heart failure. Circulation 1995;92:3206–11.

26. Grassi G, Cattaneo BM, Seravalle G, et al. Effects of chronic ACE inhibition on sympathetic nerve traffic and baroreflex control of circulation in heart failure. Circulation 1997;96:1173–9.

27. Brändle M, Patel K, Wang W, et al. Hemodynamic and norepinephrine responses to pacing-induced heart failure in conscious sino-aortic denervated dogs. J Appl Physiol 1996;81:1855–62.

28. Levett JM, Marinelli CC, Lund DD, et al. Effects of beta-blockade on neurohumoral responses and neurochemical markers in pacing-induced heart failure. Am J Physiol Heart Circ Physiol 1994;266: H468–75.

29. Goetz KL, Bond GC, Bloxham DD. Atrial receptors and renal function. Physiol Rev 1975;55:157–205.

30. Schultz HD, Fater DC, Sundet WD, et al. Reflexes elicited by acute stretch of atrial vs. pulmonary receptors in conscious dogs. Am J Physiol Heart Circ Physiol 1982;242:H1065–76.

31. Farrow S, Banta G, Schallhorn S, et al. Vasopressin inhibits diuresis induced by water immersion in humans. J Appl Physiol 1992;73(3):932–6.

32. Gabrielsen A, Sorensen VB, Pump B, et al. Cardio-vascular and neuroendocrine responses to water immersion in compensated heart failure. Am J Physiol Heart Circ Physiol 2000;279:H1931–40.

33. Miki K, Yoshimoto M, Hayashida Y, et al. Role of cardiopulmonary and carotid sinus baroreceptors in regulating renal sympathetic nerve activity during water immersion in conscious dogs. Am J Physiol Regul Integr Comp Physiol 2009;296: R1807–12.

34. Gilmore JP, Zucker IH. Contribution of vagal pathways to the renal responses to head-out immersion in the nonhuman primate. Circ Res 1978;42:263–7.

35. Anjuchovskij EP, Beloshepko GG, Yasinovskuya FP. Characteristics of atrial mechanoreceptor and elastic features following heart failure. Sechenov Physiol J U S S R 1976;62:1210–5.

36. Brändle M, Wang W, Zucker IH. Ventricular mecha-noreflex and chemoreflex alterations in chronic heart failure. Circ Res 1994;74:262–70.

37. Dibner-Dunlap ME, Thames MD. Atrial mechanore-flex control of renal sympathetic nerve activity (RNA) is blunted in heart failure [abstract]. Circula-tion 1989;80:II-393.

38. Dibner-Dunlap ME, Thames MD. Control of sympa-thetic nerve activity by vagal mechanoreflexes is blunted in heart failure. Circulation 1992;86: 1929–34.

39. von Scheidt W, Bohm M, Schneider B, et al. Cholin-ergic baroreflex vasodilatation: defect in heart transplant recipients due to denervation of the ventricular baroreceptor. Am J Cardiol 1992;69: 247–52.

40. Zucker IH, Earle AM, Gilmore JP. Changes in the sensitivity of left atrial receptors following reversal of heart failure. Am J Physiol Heart Circ Physiol 1979;237:H555–9.

41. Zucker IH, Share L, Gilmore JP. Renal effects of left atrial distension in dogs with chronic congestive heart failure. Am J Physiol Heart Circ Physiol 1979;236:H554–60.

42. Zucker IH, Earle AM, Gilmore JP. The mechanism of adaptation of left atrial stretch receptors in dogs with chronic congestive heart failure. J Clin Invest 1977;60:323–31.

43. Mohanty PK, Arrowood JA, Ellenbogen KA, et al. Neurohumoral and hemodynamic effects of lower body negative pressure in patients with congestive heart failure. Am Heart J 1989;118:78–85.

44. Notarius CF, Morris BL, Floras JS. Dissociation between reflex sympathetic and forearm vascular responses to lower body negative pressure in heart failure patients with coronary artery disease. Am J Physiol Heart Circ Physiol 2009;297:H1760–6.

45. Smith ML, Ellenbogen KA, Eckberg DL, et al. Subnormal heart period variability in heart failure: effect of cardiac transplantation. J Am Coll Cardiol 1989;14:106–11.

46. Zehr JE, Hawe A, Tsakiris AG, et al. ADH levels following nonhypotensive hemorrhage in dogs with chronic mitral stenosis. Am J Physiol 1971; 221:312–7.

47. Pliquett RU, Cornish KG, Patel KP, et al. Ameliora-tion of depressed cardiopulmonary reflex control of sympathetic nerve activity by short-term exercise training in male rabbits with heart failure. J Appl Physiol 2003;95:1883–8.

48. DiBona GF, Herman PJ, Sawin LL. Neural control of renal function in edema-forming states. Am J Phys-iol 1988;254:R1017–24.

49. Mizelle HL, Hall JE, Montani JP. Role of renal nerves in control of sodium excretion in chronic congestive heart failure. Am J Physiol Renal Physiol 1989;256(25):F1084–93.

50. Patel KP, Zhang PL, Carmines PK. Neural influ-ences on renal responses to acute volume expan-sion in rats with heart failure. Am J Physiol Heart Circ Physiol 1996;271:H1441–8.

51. Patel KP, Zhang K, Carmines PK. Norepinephrine turnover in peripheral tissues of rats with heart failure. Am J Physiol Regul Integr Comp Physiol 2000;278:R556–62.

52. Feng QP, Carlsson S, Thorén P, et al. Characteris-tics of renal sympathetic nerve activity in experi-mental congestive heart failure in the rat. Acta Physiol Scand 1994;150:259–66.

53. Kidd C. Central neurons activated by cardiac receptors. In: Hainsworth R, Kidd C, Linden RJ, editors. Cardiac receptors. Cambridge (MA): Cam-bridge University Press; 1979. p. 377–403.

54. Swanson LW, Sawchenko PE. Hypothalamic integration: organization of the paraventricular and supraoptic nuclei. Annu Rev Neurosci 1983;6: 269–324.

55. Swanson LW, Sawchenko PE. Paraventricular nucleus: a site for the integration of neuroendocrine and autonomic mechanisms. Neuroendocrinology 1980;31:410–7.

56. Haselton JR, Goering J, Patel KP. Parvocellular neurons of the paraventricular nucleus are involved in the reduction in renal nerve discharge during isotonic volume expansion. J Auton Nerv Syst 1994;50:1–11.

57. Brody MJ, Johnson AK. Role of the anteroventral third ventricle region in fluid and electrolyte balance, arterial pressure regulation and hypertension. In: Martini L, Ganong WF, editors. Frontiers in neuroendocrinology. New York: Raven; 1980. p. 249–92.

58. Patel KP. Neural regulation in experimental heart failure. Baillieres Clin Neurol 1997;6:283–96.

59. Patel KP, Zhang PL, Krukoff TL. Alterations in brain hexokinase activity associated with heart failure in rats. Am J Physiol 1993;265:R923–8.

60. Packer M. Neurohormonal interactions and adaptations in congestive heart failure. Circulation 1988; 77:721–30.

61. Hodsman GP, Kohzuki M, Howes LG, et al. Neurohumoral responses to chronic myocardial infarction in rats. Circulation 1988;78:376–81.

62. Goldsmith SR, Francis GS, Cowley AW Jr, et al. Increased plasma arginine vasopressin levels in patients with congestive heart failure. J Am Coll Cardiol 1983;1:1385–90.

63. Berl T, Quittnat-Pelletier F, Verbalis JG, et al. Oral tolvaptan is safe and effective in chronic hyponatremia. J Am Soc Nephrol 2010;21:705–12.

64. Zheng H, Li YF, Weiss M, et al. Neuronal expression of fos protein in the forebrain of diabetic rats. Brain Res 2002;956:268–75.

65. Li YF, Mayhan WG, Patel KP. Role of the paraventricular nucleus in renal excretory responses to acute volume expansion: role of nitric oxide. Am J Physiol Heart Circ Physiol 2003;285:H1738–46.

66. Li YF, Patel KP. Paraventricular nucleus of the hypothalamus and elevated sympathetic activity in heart failure: the altered inhibitory mechanisms. Acta Physiol Scand 2003;177:17–26.

67. Zhang K, Li YF, Patel KP. Blunted nitric oxide-mediated inhibition of renal nerve discharge within PVN of rats with heart failure. Am J Physiol Heart Circ Physiol 2001;281:H995–1004.

68. Kohzuki M, Hodsman GP, Johnston CI. Attenuated response to atrial natriuretic peptide in rats with myocardial infarction. Am J Physiol 1989;256:H533–8.

69. Pedersen EB, Danielsen H, Jensen T, et al. Angiotensin II, aldosterone and arginine vasopressin in plasma in congestive heart failure. Eur J Clin Invest 1986;16:56–60.

70. Masilamani S, Kim GH, Mitchell C, et al. Aldosterone-mediated regulation of ENaC alpha, beta and gamma subunit proteins in rat kidney. J Clin Invest 1999;104:19–23.

71. Ecelbarger CA, Kim GH, Terris J, et al. Vasopressin-mediated regulation of epithelial sodium channel abundance in rat kidney. Am J Physiol Renal Physiol 2000;270:F46–53.

72. Zheng H, Liu X, Rao US, et al. Increased renal ENaC subunits and sodium retention in rats with chronic heart failure. Am J Physiol Renal Physiol 2011;300:F641–9.

73. Kumagai K, Reid IA. Losartan inhibits sympathetic and cardiovascular responses to carotid occlusion. Hypertension 1994;23:827–31.

74. Quillen EW Jr, Reid IA. Intravertebral ANG II effects on plasma renin and Na excretion in dogs at constant renal artery pressure. Am J Physiol 1995;268:F296–301.

75. Reid IA. Interactions between ANG II, sympathetic nervous system, and baroreceptor reflexes in regulation of blood pressure. Am J Physiol Endocrinol Metab 1992;262:E763–78.

76. Xu L, Brooks VL. ANG II chronically supports renal and lumbar sympathetic activity in sodium-deprived, conscious rats. Am J Physiol Heart Circ Physiol 1996;271:H2591–8.

77. Zucker IH, Wang W, Pliquett RU, et al. The regulation of sympathetic outflow in heart failure. In: Chapleau MW, Abboud FM, editors. Neuro-cardiovascular regulation. New York: New York Academy of Sciences; 2001. p. 431–43.

78. Cardin S, Li D, Thorin-Trescases N, et al. Evolution of the atrial fibrillation substrate in experimental congestive heart failure: angiotensin-dependent and -independent pathways. Cardiovasc Res 2003;60:315–25.

79. Zucker IH, Schultz HD, Patel KP, et al. Regulation of central angiotensin type 1 receptors and sympathetic outflow in heart failure. Am J Physiol Heart Circ Physiol 2009;297:H1557–66.

80. Grobe JL, Xu D, Sigmund CD. An intracellular renin-angiotensin system in neurons: fact, hypothesis, or fantasy. Physiology (Bethesda) 2008;23: 187–93.

81. Gao L, Wang W, Li YL, et al. Superoxide mediates sympathoexcitation in heart failure: roles of angiotensin II and NAD(P)H oxidase. Circ Res 2004;95: 937–44.

82. Liu D, Gao L, Roy SK, et al. Neuronal AT1 receptor upregulation in heart failure: activation of activator protein 1 and Jun N-terminal kinase. Circ Res 2006;99:1004–11.

83. Kang YM, Ma Y, Elks C, et al. Cross-talk between cytokines and renin-angiotensin in hypothalamic

paraventricular nucleus in heart failure: role of nuclear factor-kappaB. Cardiovasc Res 2008;79: 671–8.

84. Wang WZ, Gao L, Wang HJ, et al. Interaction between cardiac sympathetic afferent reflex and chemoreflex is mediated by the NTS AT1 receptors in heart failure. Am J Physiol Heart Circ Physiol 2008;295:H1216–26.

85. Gao L, Wang WZ, Wang W, et al. Imbalance of angiotensin receptor expression and function in the RVLM: Potential mechanism for sympathetic overactivity in heart failure. Hypertension 2008;52: 708–14.

86. Kar S, Gao L, Zucker IH. Exercise training normalizes ACE and ACE2 in the brain of rabbits with pacing induced heart failure. J Appl Physiol 2010; 108:923–34.

87. Zimmerman MC, Dunlay RP, Lazartigues E, et al. Requirement for Rac1-dependent NADPH oxidase in the cardiovascular and dipsogenic actions of angiotensin II in the brain. Circ Res 2004;95:532–9.

88. Zimmerman MC, Lazartigues E, Lang JA, et al. Superoxide mediates the actions of angiotensin II in the central nervous system. Circ Res 2002;91: 1038–45.

89. Ma R, Zucker IH, Wang W. Central gain of the cardiac sympathetic afferent reflex in dogs with heart failure. Am J Physiol Heart Circ Physiol 1997;273:H2664–71.

90. Wang W, Zucker IH. Cardiac sympathetic afferent reflex in dogs with congestive heart failure. Am J Physiol 1996;271:R751–6.

91. Wang W, Schultz HD, Ma R. Cardiac sympathetic afferent sensitivity is enhanced in heart failure. Am J Physiol Heart Circ Physiol 1999;277(46): H812–7.

92. Wang W, Ma R. Cardiac sympathetic afferent reflexes in heart failure. Heart Fail Rev 2000;5:57–71.

93. Fu LW, Longhurst JC. Regulation of cardiac afferent excitability in ischemia. Handb Exp Pharmacol 2009;194:185–225.

94. Wang W. Cardiac sympathetic afferent stimulation by bradykinin in heart failure: role of NO and prostaglandins. Am J Physiol 1998;275:H783–8.

95. Wang W, Schultz HD, Ma R. Volume expansion potentiates cardiac sympathetic afferent reflex in dogs. Am J Physiol Heart Circ Physiol 2001;280: H576–81.

96. Ma R, Zhu GQ, Wang W. Interaction of central Ang II and NO on the cardiac sympathetic afferent reflex in dogs. Auton Neurosci 2005;118:51–60.

97. Ma R, Zucker IH, Wang W. Reduced NO enhances the central gain of cardiac sympathetic afferent reflex in dogs with heart failure. Am J Physiol 1999;276:H19–26.

98. Ma R, Schultz HD, Wang W. Chronic central infusion of ANG II potentiates cardiac sympathetic afferent reflex in dogs. Am J Physiol Heart Circ Physiol 1999;277:H15–22.

99. Zhu GQ, Gao L, Patel KP, et al. ANG II in the paraventricular nucleus potentiates the cardiac sympathetic afferent reflex in rats with heart failure. J Appl Physiol 2004;97:1746–54.

100. Wang WZ, Gao L, Pan YX, et al. Differential effects of cardiac sympathetic afferent stimulation on neurons in the nucleus tractus solitarius. Neurosci Lett 2006;409:146–50.

101. Zhu GQ, Gao XY, Zhang F, et al. Reduced nitric oxide in the rostral ventrolateral medulla enhances cardiac sympathetic afferent reflex in rats with chronic heart failure. Sheng Li Xue Bao 2004;56: 47–53.

102. Gao L, Schultz HD, Patel KP, et al. Augmented input from cardiac sympathetic afferents inhibits baroreflex in rats with heart failure. Hypertension 2005;45:1173–81.

103. Ponikowski P, Chua TP, Pepoli M, et al. Augmented peripheral chemosensitiviy as a potential input to baroreflex impairment and autonomic imbalance in chronic heart failure. Circulation 1997;96:2586–94.

104. Sun SY, Wang W, Zucker IH, et al. Enhanced peripheral chemoreflex function in conscious rabbits with pacing-induced heart failure. J Appl Physiol 1999;86(4):1264–72.

105. Sun SY, Zucker IH, Wang W, et al. Enhanced activity of carotid body chemoreceptors in rabbits with heart failure: role of nitric oxide. J Appl Physiol 1999;86(4):1273–82.

106. Schultz HD, Li YL. Carotid body function in heart failure. Respir Physiol Neurobiol 2007;157:171–85.

107. Li YL, Xia XH, Zheng H, et al. Angiotensin II enhances carotid body chemoreflex control of sympathetic outflow in chronic heart failure rabbits. Cardiovasc Res 2006;71:129–38.

108. Li YL, Gao L, Zucker IH, et al. NADPH oxidase-derived superoxide anion mediates angiotensin II-enhanced carotid body chemoreceptor sensitivity in heart failure rabbits. Cardiovasc Res 2007;75: 546–54.

109. Ding Y, Li YL, Zimmerman MC, et al. Elevated mitochondrial superoxide contributes to enhanced chemoreflex in heart failure rabbits. Am J Physiol Regul Integr Comp Physiol 2010;298:R303–11.

110. Ding Y, Li YL, Zimmerman MC, et al. Role of CuZn superoxide dismutase on carotid body function in heart failure rabbits. Cardiovasc Res 2009;81: 678–85.

111. Li YL, Li YF, Liu D, et al. Gene transfer of neuronal nitric oxide synthase to carotid body reverses enhanced chemoreceptor function in heart failure rabbits. Circ Res 2005;97:260–7.

112. Li YL, Schultz HD. Enhanced sensitivity of Kv channels to hypoxia in the rabbit carotid body in heart failure: role of angiotensin II. J Physiol 2006;575:215–27.

113. Li YL, Sun SY, Overholt JL, et al. Attenuated outward potassium currents in carotid body glomus cells of heart failure rabbit: involvement of nitric oxide. J Physiol 2004;555:219–29.

114. Li YL, Zheng H, Ding Y, et al. Expression of neuronal nitric oxide synthase in rabbit carotid body glomus cells regulates large-conductance Ca2+-activated potassium currents. J Neurophysiol 2010;103:3027–33.

115. Ding Y, Li YL, Schultz HD. Role of blood flow in carotid body chemoreflex function in heart failure. J Physiol 2011;589:245–58.

116. Schmidt H, Francis DP, Rauchhaus M, et al. Chemo- and ergoreflexes in health, disease and ageing. Int J Cardiol 2005;98:369–78.

117. Sinoway LI, Li J. A perspective on the muscle reflex: implications for congestive heart failure. J Appl Physiol 2005;99:5–22.

118. Smith SA, Mitchell JH, Garry MG. The mammalian exercise pressor reflex in health and disease. Exp Physiol 2006;91:89–102.

119. Coats AJ. The "muscle hypothesis" of chronic heart failure. J Mol Cell Cardiol 1996;28:2255–62.

120. Middlekauff HR, Sinoway LI. Increased mechano-receptor/metaboreceptor stimulation explains the exaggerated exercise pressor reflex seen in heart failure. J Appl Physiol 2007;102:492–4.

121. Li J, Sinoway AN, Gao Z, et al. Muscle mechanore-flex and metaboreflex responses after myocardial infarction in rats. Circulation 2004;110:3049–54.

122. Smith SA, Mitchell JH, Naseem RH, et al. Mecha-noreflex mediates the exaggerated exercise pressor reflex in heart failure. Circulation 2005;112:2293–300.

123. Sterns DA, Ettinger SM, Gray KS, et al. Skeletal muscle metaboreceptor exercise responses are attenuated in heart failure. Circulation 1991;84:2034–9.

124. Piepoli MF, Coats AJ. Increased metaboreceptor stimulation explains the exaggerated exercise pressor reflex seen in heart failure. J Appl Physiol 2007;102:494–6.

125. Silber DH, Sutliff G, Yang QX, et al. Altered mech-anisms of sympathetic activation during rhythmic forearm exercise in heart failure. J Appl Physiol 1998;84:1551–9.

126. Scott AC, Davies LC, Coats AJ, et al. Relationship of skeletal muscle metaboreceptors in the upper and lower limbs with the respiratory control in patients with heart failure. Clin Sci (Lond) 2002;102:23–30.

127. Wang HJ, Li YL, Gao L, et al. Alteration in skeletal muscle afferents in rats with chronic heart failure. J Physiol 2010;588:5033–47.

128. Smith SA, Williams MA, Mitchell JH, et al. The capsaicin-sensitive afferent neuron in skeletal muscle is abnormal in heart failure. Circulation 2005;111:2056–65.

129. Koba S, Xing J, Sinoway LI, et al. Bradykinin receptor blockade reduces sympathetic nerve response to muscle contraction in rats with ischemic heart failure. Am J Physiol Heart Circ Physiol 2010;298:H1438–44.

130. Middlekauff HR, Chiu J, Hamilton MA, et al. Cyclo-oxygenase products sensitize muscle mechanore-ceptors in humans with heart failure. Am J Physiol Heart Circ Physiol 2008;294:H1956–62.

131. Koba S, Gao Z, Sinoway LI. Oxidative stress and the muscle reflex in heart failure. J Physiol 2009;587:5227–37.

132. Schunk K, Kersjes W, Schadmand-Fischer S, et al. [Dynamic 31phosphorus magnetic resonance spectroscopy of the quadriceps muscle: metabolic changes under 2 different forms of loading]. Rofo 1997;166:317–23 [in German].

Role of Oxidative Stress in Disease Progression in Stage B, a Pre-cursor of Heart Failure

Arvind Bhimaraj, MD, MPH[a], W.H. Wilson Tang, MD[b],*

KEYWORDS

- Oxidative stress • Progression of heart failure
- Stage B heart failure

Oxidative stress represents a persistent imbalance between the production and the compensation of reactive oxygen species (ROS). Multiple animal studies have shown the critical role of ROS (and hence redox balance) in maintaining cellular homeostasis and their role as second-messenger systems in various physiologic and adaptive mechanisms.[1–3] However, excessive ROS can lead to the accumulation of peroxides and free radicals that damage proteins, lipids, and genes. The balance between reactive cellular species and natural antioxidant systems is therefore key to minimizing adverse cellular consequences of ROS, while maintaining their physiologic functions. Hence, oxidative stress has been implicated in many disease states, including senescence, malignant diseases,[4] diabetes,[5,6] ischemia/reperfusion injury, neurodegenerative diseases, certain infectious processes, rheumatoid arthritis, atherosclerosis, and hypertension.[7–10] When considering oxidative stress as a contributor of chronic heart failure disease progression, it can be broadly divided into two categories: exogenous (mediated by inflammatory cells) and endogenous (mediated by dysfunctional myocardial tissues). However, these processes are difficult to identify and quantify, and challenging to separate from related processes such as inflammation and neurohormonal upregulation in humans.

Oxidative stress has been linked to heart failure over the past decades, with most studies focused on patient populations with symptomatic or advanced heart failure. Study focus has ranged from cytokine-targeted therapy,[11,12] to inhibitors of xanthine oxidase,[13] and to various nonspecific immunomodulatory therapy.[12] Clearly the main objective to include these "relatively ill" patient populations was to allow adequate event rates to demonstrate statistically significant differences. However, most studies identify eligible patients with clinical characteristics because there is a lack of reliable in vivo tools that can aid the identification and quantification of ongoing oxidative stress.

Markers of inflammation and/or oxidative stress have been associated with incident heart failure[14,15] even after controlling for coronary artery disease, suggesting that inflammation has a direct effect (possibly through exogenous oxidative stress) on the myocardium. However, these studies also assumed that oxidative stress was generated as the primary mediator of heart failure disease progression. In reality, such an assumption has never been validated in humans, in part because our contemporary understanding of the

Dr Bhimaraj has nothing to disclose. Dr Tang is a consultant for Medtronic and St. Jude Medical, Inc, and has research support from Abbott Laboratories and the National Institutes of Health (1R01HL103931-01).

[a] Methodist DeBakey Cardiology Associates, Smith Tower, 6550 Fannin, Suite 1901, Houston, TX 77030, USA
[b] Section of Heart Failure and Cardiac Transplantation Medicine, Heart and Vascular Institute, Cleveland Clinic, 9500 Euclid Avenue, Desk J3-4, Cleveland, OH 44195, USA
* Corresponding author.
E-mail address: tangw@ccf.org

role of ROS (particularly in an individual patient) is limited. Nevertheless, it is important to recognize that even if oxidative stress may not directly cause cardiac dysfunction, appropriate modulation of such potential secondary pathologic processes may still yield favorable therapeutic interventions (as in the case of neurohormonal antagonism). This article summarizes the current understanding of the role of oxidative stress leading to the development of heart failure in at-risk individuals, and highlights the current diagnostic and therapeutic options under active investigation.

ROLE OF OXIDATIVE STRESS IN DISEASE PROGRESSION OF HEART FAILURE
Ischemic Heart Disease

Involvement of oxidative stress in disease progression has been best described in the setting of ischemic heart disease, one of the most common causes of heart failure secondary to structural heart disease (Stage B heart failure). Direct myocardial damage mediated by downstream oxidative stress

processes can lead to progressive enlargement and contractile impairment known as "cardiac re-modeling." Adverse myocardial remodeling is the likely basis of unrelenting myocardial dysfunction in ischemic heart disease, with progression of initial myocardial damage from both adaptive and maladaptive changes leading to overt heart failure.[16] Production of ROS occurs during ischemia/reperfusion injury[17] while ongoing chronic ischemia can lead to high and sustained levels of ROS caused by dysfunctional electron transport chain systems in the mitochondria. The accumulation of ROS can lead to diverse downstream negative consequences, including cardioinhibition, hypertrophy, and matrix metalloproteinase stimulation. These intentionally compensatory processes can directly lead to progression of negative myocardial remodeling (**Fig. 1**). The precise mechanisms are complex, but can be in part explained by their role as intracellular second messengers that mediate the remodeling effects of the renin-angiotensin and adrenergic systems.[18,19] Furthermore, heightened oxidative stress can lead to unwanted

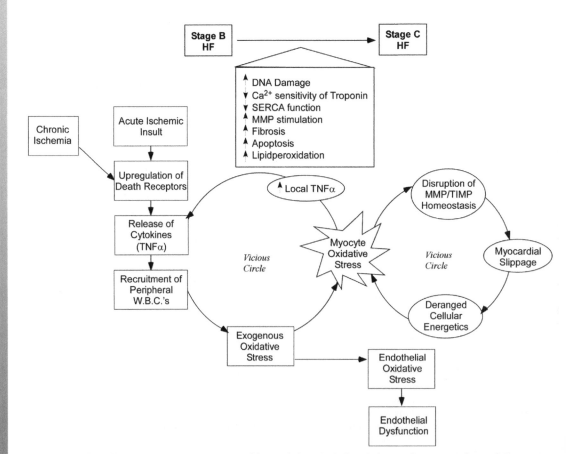

Fig. 1. Role of oxidative stress in progression of heart failure in ischemic heart disease. HF, heart failure; MMP, matrix metalloprotein; SERCA, sarco/endoplasmic reticulum Ca^{2+} adenosine triphosphatase; TIMP, tissue inhibitor of MMP; TNF, tumor necrosis factor; W.B.C, white blood cells.

modulation of lipids and proteins (eg, low-density lipoprotein [LDL] cholesterol) and deposition of such oxidized LDL in atherosclerotic plaque, leading to further inflammation and progression of atherosclerotic coronary artery disease,[20,21] and further ischemic insult.

Antioxidant systems are known to be upregulated in the setting of ischemia, with overexpression of superoxide dismutase (SOD) being associated with reduced infarct size.[21,22] Whereas such data may imply the harmful effect of ROS, other molecular studies paradoxically show that ROS mediate adaptive mechanisms vital for cell survival, such as angiogenesis, upregulation of glucose transport proteins, erythropoiesis, apoptosis, and inflammation during hypoxic episodes.[23,24] Apart from identification of increased levels of ROS in the peri-infarct area,[25] upregulation of these molecules in the remote myocardium suggests more diffuse remodeling and cardioinhibitory effects of ROS being operational.[26] Therefore, it is unclear whether complete suppression of potential adaptive mechanisms can promote or prevent disease progression. Endothelial dysfunction in the noninfarct-related artery has also been noted,[27,28] but the exact mechanisms of this phenomenon have not been elucidated and despite decades of research, treatment to improve endothelial function remains a theoretical rather than a practical clinical application.

Hypertensive Heart Disease

Epidemiologic studies have shown that hypertension increases the risk of developing heart failure by twofold in men and threefold in women.[29] Hypertension is also one of the most common risk factors for coronary artery disease, and hence indirectly contributes to heart failure incidence. Hypertension in the absence of coronary artery disease is best known to cause adaptive left ventricular hypertrophy in response to increased pressure load. Treatment of blood pressure with diuretics, β-blockers, and angiotensin-converting enzyme (ACE) inhibitors may decrease the incident development of heart failure, and such effects can in part be due to reducing progression of such hypertrophic processes.[30–32] The role of ROS in progression of direct myocardial changes from hypertrophy to clinical heart failure was first suggested based on experiments in guinea pigs. Vitamin E–treated aortic-banded hearts showed more adaptive left ventricular hypertrophy and fewer clinical signs of heart failure compared with sham animals with no supplementation.[33]

Emerging evidence from animal (and now human) studies has implicated a role for neuronal, renal, and vascular endothelial ROS for initiation and perpetuation of hypertension.[34–38] As systemic endothelial oxidative stress can contribute to vascular stiffness, coronary endothelial dysfunction[39] may augment myocardial oxidative stress, leading to further ischemic insult. Furthermore, poorly controlled blood pressure can also cause increased generation of ROS in the cardiomyocytes that can activate a wide array of intracellular hypertrophic signaling redox-sensitive kinases, with or without interactions with neurohormonal systems.[40–42] In fact, both sympathetically mediated and renin-mediated hypertension can cause myocardial negative remodeling using oxidative stress as an intermediate. In addition, ROS have also been shown to mediate myocyte hypertrophy secondary to mechanical stress and stimulate mitochondrial permeability protein.[43] Such promoters of cell necrosis can create a vicious circle of recruitment of exogenous oxidative stress in the form of inflammation, which in turn worsens endogenous oxidative stress. Hence, hypertension can culminate through multiple pathways to create an oxidative stress load in the myocardium that mediates negative remodeling and ultimately maladaptive changes, leading to heart failure.[44]

Insulin Resistance: Type 2 Diabetes Mellitus, Metabolic Syndrome, and Obesity

Diabetes and insulin resistance is a significant risk factor for atherosclerotic heart disease and contributes to incident heart failure in the form of macrovascular and microvascular atherosclerosis, leading to ischemia. Apart from accelerating atherogenesis, diabetes mellitus can contribute to derangement of myocardial metabolism via intracellular accumulation of fatty acids and triglycerides, leading to cellular lipotoxicity. Such derangement can lead to cellular apoptosis, contractile dysfunction, and relaxation abnormalities.[45–48] Although altered cardiac metabolism in diabetes mellitus has not been consistently reproduced in humans,[49–51] epidemiologic data show an 8% increased risk of heart failure for every 1% increase in hemoglobin A_{1c} (even after correcting for underlying coronary artery disease).[52]

There is accumulating evidence to suggest that diastolic dysfunction may predate the onset of systolic dysfunction in diabetic mellitus.[53,54] The prevalence of preclinical diastolic dysfunction varies from 20% to 60% based on the criteria used. Epidemiologic data from Olmstead County suggested that the presence of preclinical diastolic dysfunction predicts future onset of heart failure independent of age, body mass index, coronary artery disease, hypertension, and echocardiographic cardiac structural and functional abnormalities.[55] This finding recognizes the importance of identifying patients with underlying diastolic dysfunction as "Stage B heart failure" in the setting of diabetes mellitus.

Metabolic syndrome has been associated with future development of heart failure,[56] but more recent data have identified the presence of hyperglycemia, abdominal adiposity, and coronary artery disease as confounding factors rather than the syndrome itself.[57,58] In other patients, metabolic derangements secondary to hyperglycemia and insulin resistance may play a role in what is called diabetic or insulin-resistance cardiomyopathy, but the nebulousness of these ill-defined clinical phenotypes have precluded more rigorous clinical investigations.[59]

Specific mechanism(s) of oxidative stress that are pertinent in patients with diabetes mellitus are complex but may be worthy of some discussion. Oxidative stress in diabetes mellitus can mediate direct downstream consequences such as apoptosis, mediated through apoptosis-stimulating kinase 1, and increased ceramide accumulation, as well as direct cellular, genetic, and mitochondrial damage.[60–63] Inflammatory markers such as tumor necrosis factor α are elevated in patients with insulin resistance, probably contributing to exogenous oxidative stress.[64,65] Hyperglycemia-induced overproduction of SOD by the mitochondrial electron transport chain is suggested to be the first and important event that cascades further cellular derangements.[66] One mouse transgenic model showed protection from developing diabetic cardiomyopathy when the antioxidant protein metallothionein was overexpressed.[67] Nitroso-oxidative stress has also been implicated with the finding of increased inducible nitric oxide synthase in streptozotocin-induced diabetic rats.[68] Novel adipokines (proteins secreted from adipocytes) have been associated with the pathophysiology of insulin resistance and obesity. These adipokines can possess primary anti-inflammatory (such as adiponectin) and/or proinflammatory properties (such as resistin), and have been shown to correlate with concentrations of plasma cytokines or cardiac-specific markers of dysfunction.[69,70] The latter may potentially be perpetuating its deleterious effects through intracellular ROS. Epidemiologic studies have demonstrated that high levels of resistin are associated with increased incident heart failure during long-term follow-up,[71,72] even after adjusting for risk score for heart failure.[73]

Valvular Heart Diseases

Geometric changes and physical stretch in volume overload conditions as a result of valvular regurgitation can increase stretch-mediated upregulation of intracellular ROS, contributing to oxidative stress in a heart that already is overusing the available substrates. Studies using myocardial strips from patients with mitral regurgitation have shown derangement of calcium-handling proteins and increased cytokines, which could be attributed to oxidative stress.[74–76] In patients with severe mitral regurgitation and normal ejection fraction, the total serum oxidant stress was significantly higher when compared with that of normal controls.[77] Also, the serum oxidant stress was higher in those with atrial fibrillation than in individuals in sinus rhythm, while the oxidant stress index correlated with atrial size. Using lateral endocardial biopsy specimens from patients undergoing mitral valve surgery, protein content of tissue xanthine dehydrogenase and transiently modified xanthine oxidase was increased more than fivefold in density in patients with mitral regurgitation when compared with that of control subjects.[78]

BIOMARKERS OF OXIDATIVE STRESS

The ability to measure markers of oxidative stress in various disease states has been challenging, due to the nonspecific nature of many of the markers. Myeloperoxidase, biopyrrins, F-2 isoprostanes, malondialdehyde and thiobarbituric acid–reactive substances (TBARS), oxidized LDL, and uric acid have been studied, while newer markers such as allantoin and S-nitrosohemoglobin are emerging as evidence of nitrosoreactive species.

The contribution of systemic oxidative stress in the development of heart failure following acute coronary syndromes can be demonstrated by detectable circulating markers of inflammation and oxidative stress. One of the most widely studied of such markers is myeloperoxidase (MPO), a hemoprotein released from neutrophils and monocytes that has been implicated in progression and destabilization of atherosclerotic plaque.[79] In vivo magnetic resonance studies[80] have identified local expression of MPO in areas of plaque rupture in humans. In patients presenting with acute coronary syndrome (ACS), high levels of MPO (as a marker of inflammation and probably as a source of exogenous oxidative stress) have been associated with future development of cardiovascular death and ischemic events.[81,82] Biomarker data from large clinical trials have confirmed the incremental value of MPO in short-term[83] as well as long-term risk prediction.[82] Recent data also identified an MPO level greater than 670 pmol/L on admission, in the setting of non-ST elevation myocardial infarction, has a 1.6-fold increased risk of subsequent development of heart failure over 1 year of follow-up.[84] These findings indicate the long-term impact of the acute oxidative stress elicited as a response to an acute ischemic event.

Epidemiologic and clinical trial data from hypertensive individuals have shown mixed results of association with increased levels of TBARS, 8-isoprostanes, and biomarkers of lipid peroxidation in comparison to normotensive individuals.[85,86]

Uric acid has been used as a biomarker of oxidative stress because of its generation from xanthine oxidase (during production of ROS in the xanthine oxidase system). Hyperuricemia has been associated with worse clinical outcomes, and animal studies have suggested a cardioprotective role of xanthine oxidase inhibitors. However, clinical trials have not reproduced the same results in established heart failure.[13] In a propensity-matched control study using data from the Cardiovascular Health Study in 5461 community-dwelling adults older than 65 years, the presence of hyperuricemia was associated with incident heart failure, particularly in the subgroups with normal kidney function (hazard ratio [HR] 1.23, 95% confidence interval [CI] 1.02–1.49, P = .031), those not receiving thiazide diuretics (HR 1.2, 95% CI 1.01–1.42, P = .044), and without hyperinsulinemia (HR 1.35, 95% CI 1.06–1.72, P = .013).[87] The true incidence of structural abnormality in these studies is difficult to assess, but the prevalence of risk factors makes it highly likely that most of them would qualify as Stage B heart failure. For example, in the Cardiovascular Health Study, only 7% had left ventricular hypertrophy by electrocardiographic criteria despite a high percentage with a diagnosis of hypertension.

THERAPEUTIC CONSIDERATIONS

As the extent of ROS might cause direct myocardial damage, antioxidant therapy seems to be a logical strategy to limit the amount of jeopardized tissue and lower the risk of subsequent development of heart failure in patients experiencing insults to the myocardium. In animal myocardial infarction models, allopurinol has been shown to reduce infarct size[88] and limit left ventricular cavity dilatation and dysfunction, along with a markedly reduced myocardial hypertrophy and interstitial fibrosis.[26] Similar findings were noted in an MPO knock-out mouse model.[89] Clinical studies of antioxidant supplementation during acute ischemia are lacking in the contemporary era. In fact, small human clinical studies in the setting of coronary artery bypass surgery and myocardial infarction have shown contradictory findings, and there have been no large-scale randomized studies of xanthine oxidase inhibitors in the ACS or post–myocardial infarction settings.[90–92]

Statins, with their "antioxidant" properties, have been suggested to have a role in reducing reperfusion injury in the setting of an acute myocardial infarction in the short term.[93] By reducing recurrent ischemic events, statins should result in reduction of heart failure. There are limited clinical trial data in this regard. Moreover, markers of oxidative stress often have not been analyzed, and their benefits have focused on those before overt heart failure ensues.[94] A randomized controlled study done at the University of Michigan in 774 ACS patients older than 65 years found that statin initiation less than 24 hours from admission reduced the incidence of in-hospital heart failure.[95] In another Japanese study comprising mostly ST-elevation myocardial infarction patients, a similar hypothesis was studied, with a 96-hour window showing benefit of statin therapy in the composite end point that was driven primarily by heart failure hospitalization and revascularizations.[96] Statins have been time tested in many trials to improve mortality and adverse clinical outcomes in patients with coronary artery disease and post–myocardial infarction. The pleiotropic effects of statins broadly encompass all beneficial non–cholesterol-lowering effects. Statins have been shown to reduce inflammation and oxidative stress through their effects on reducing isoprenylation. Nicotinamide adenine dinucleotide phosphate (NADPH) oxidase (NOX) is an important source of oxidative radical synthesis in the cells (more so in endothelial cells). Rac-1 protein acts as a second messenger immediately after NOX stimulation in the ROS pathway, and statins inhibit Rac-1 as isoprenylated proteins are needed for the latter's activation.[97] On the contrary, statins are postulated to bind and decrease levels of coenzyme Q and hence possibly increase oxidative stress. Although in patients with established heart failure statins have shown inconsistent benefits (even in ischemic cardiomyopathy), they have at least not led to worsening heart failure.[98] One explanation for the inconsistent benefit is reflected by the variable effects and lipid-soluble properties of different statins. In the context of patients with coronary artery disease and post–myocardial infarction patients, data from the Pravastatin or Atorvastatin Evaluation and Infection Therapy—Thrombolysis in Myocardial Infarction 22 (PROVE IT TIMI-22) study showed that 80 mg/d of atorvastatin significantly reduced the rate of hospitalization for heart failure (1.6% vs 3.1%; HR, 0.55; 95% CI, 0.35–0.85; P = .008) compared with pravastatin independent of recurrent myocardial infarction or prior heart failure.[99] In the Incremental Decrease in Events through Aggressive Lipid Lowering (IDEAL) study, 80 mg/d of atorvastatin was associated with a 26% decrease in new heart failure events compared with 20–40 mg/d of simvastatin. Atorvastatin was associated with fewer heart failure events even in patients without a history of myocardial infarction. However, none of these studies specifically analyzed markers of oxidative stress.[100]

Omega-3 polyunsaturated fatty acids have antioxidant properties and have been extensively studied for both primary and secondary prevention of ischemic events. Supplementation in post–myocardial infarction patients has been shown to improve survival and reduce sudden cardiac death.[101–103] Other studies did not show any benefit in reducing adverse cardiovascular events.[104,105]

Although many trials have not used heart failure as an outcome, data from HOPE (Heart Outcomes Prevention Evaluation) and HOPE TOO (Heart Outcomes Prevention Evaluation–The Ongoing Outcomes) trials, which studied the impact of Vitamin E supplementation in a population at high risk for cardiovascular disease, showed a paradoxic increase in heart failure incidence (relative risk [RR] 1.13, 95% CI 1.01–1.26; P = .03) and heart failure hospitalizations (RR 1.21, 95% CI 1.00–1.47).[106] Approximately 80% of trial participants had coronary artery disease and up to 50% had a previous myocardial infarction. Such controversial data make it difficult to interpret the role of oxidative stress but do emphasize that oxidative stress might have an adaptive role.

There are no clinical trials data suggesting beneficial effects of antioxidants in hypertensive patients in preventing heart failure. Of note, 47% of the study population in the HOPE TOO trial, which showed an increased heart failure incidence, had hypertension. Hypertension was also prevalent in the statin trials, but incident heart failure as an outcome was never analyzed.

Multiple cardiovascular medications such as ACE inhibitors, statins, and angiotensin receptor blockers are postulated to have antioxidant properties and hence to be beneficial in diabetics. Yet, there are no data from studies on incident heart failure in at-risk individuals. The potent antioxidant vitamin E has been shown in a diabetic rat model to improve ventricular function and attenuate myocardial accumulation of markers of oxidative stress (8-iso-prostaglandin $F_{2\alpha}$ and oxidized glutathione).[63] In a similar rat model, Vitamin E supplementation showed a significant reduction in lipid peroxidation and protein oxidation, and an increase in the antioxidant defense systems and apoptosis in the myocardium.[107] The adverse finding from the HOPE TOO study as detailed here remains puzzling and concerning. Approximately 40% were diabetic in this study.

Thiazolidinediones (TZDs) are insulin sensitizers that have come under recent scrutiny for adverse cardiac events. However, animal studies have shown that this class of drugs, through its action on peroxisome proliferator–activated receptor, improves cardiac function in parallel with reduction of oxidative stress.[108] In a small human clinical trial, Von Bibra and colleagues[109] studied the effect of rosiglitazone in comparison with a sulfanylurea on a background of metformin therapy. Although both groups had similar hemoglobin A_{1c} reductions, the glitazone group of patients at the end of 16 weeks had significantly lower levels of malondialdehyde and C-reactive protein. Improvement of echocardiographic tissue velocity from baseline was also shown. The future use of glitazones to reduce incident heart failure in diabetic patients might be limited, due to their effects on fluid retention.

SUMMARY

There is a common theme in our contemporary understanding of the contribution of oxidative stress to the progression of Stage B heart failure. First, most of our understanding of this topic is based on experimental findings from animal heart failure models, many of which are crude and simplistic. In humans the process of oxidative stress is complex, and largely dependent on the nature and extent of the insult, the underlying substrate vulnerability (ie, host defenses in the form of "antioxidant" systems), and the contribution of coexisting conditions. In other words, what we learn from experimental models may not directly translate into human pathophysiology. Second, alterations in the overall "nitroso-redox system" can be appreciated as a disruption of the fine balance between oxidative and antioxidative processes at various stages of disease process, but our ability to identify and target the precise pathways is lacking (in part because many of these processes are subcellular and localized). In fact, even the best markers may only provide a snap-shot of oxidative destruction rather than an appreciation or identification of the underlying process of oxidative damage that is targetable for intervention. For example, whether lowering MPO or uric acid can lead to reduction in the future development of heart failure is still unproved. Third, our understanding of the impact of different therapeutic interventions can affect various pathways of oxidative stress is seriously lacking, as they are rarely translatable from animal studies. Such disconnect can be best illustrated by the example of α-tocopherol, which despite being an "antioxidant" may attenuate the anti-inflammatory effects of statins[110] while being a pro-oxidant in the setting of an oxidative milieu.[111] The doses of α-tocopherol used as supplements are often far lower than those tested in animal studies. Newer agents that selectively block NADPH oxidase enzymes NOX2 and NOX4 are being developed. As we unravel the specifics and identify the molecular pathways of maladaptive versus adaptive effects of ROS, the future holds promise in our making breakthroughs in manipulating oxidative stress in the heart.

REFERENCES

1. Sawyer DB, Siwik DA, Xiao L, et al. Role of oxidative stress in myocardial hypertrophy and failure. J Mol Cell Cardiol 2002;34(4):379–88.

2. Thannickal VJ, Fanburg BL. Reactive oxygen species in cell signaling. Am J Physiol Lung Cell Mol Physiol 2000;279(6):L1005–28.

3. Griendling KK, FitzGerald GA. Oxidative stress and cardiovascular injury: part I: basic mechanisms and in vivo monitoring of ROS. Circulation 2003; 108(16):1912–6.

4. Dreher D, Junod AF. Role of oxygen free radicals in cancer development. Eur J Cancer 1996;32A(1): 30–8.

5. Baynes JW. Role of oxidative stress in development of complications in diabetes. Diabetes 1991;40(4): 405–12.

6. Wolff SP. Diabetes mellitus and free radicals. Free radicals, transition metals and oxidative stress in the aetiology of diabetes mellitus and complications. Br Med Bull 1993;49(3):642–52.

7. Cathcart MK, McNally AK, Morel DW, et al. Superoxide anion participation in human monocyte-mediated oxidation of low-density lipoprotein and conversion of low-density lipoprotein to a cytotoxin. J Immunol 1989;142(6):1963–9.

8. Cathcart MK, Chisolm GM 3rd, McNally AK, et al. Oxidative modification of low density lipoprotein (LDL) by activated human monocytes and the cell lines U937 and HL60. In Vitro Cell Dev Biol 1988; 24(10):1001–8.

9. Griendling KK, Minieri CA, Ollerenshaw JD, et al. Angiotensin II stimulates NADH and NADPH oxidase activity in cultured vascular smooth muscle cells. Circ Res 1994;74(6):1141–8.

10. Halliwell B. Free radicals, reactive oxygen species and human disease: a critical evaluation with special reference to atherosclerosis. Br J Exp Pathol 1989;70(6):737–57.

11. Mann DL, McMurray JJ, Packer M, et al. Targeted anticytokine therapy in patients with chronic heart failure: results of the Randomized Etanercept Worldwide Evaluation (RENEWAL). Circulation 2004;109(13):1594–602.

12. Chung ES, Packer M, Lo KH, et al. Randomized, double-blind, placebo-controlled, pilot trial of infliximab, a chimeric monoclonal antibody to tumor necrosis factor-alpha, in patients with moderate-to-severe heart failure: results of the anti-TNF Therapy Against Congestive Heart Failure (ATTACH) trial. Circulation 2003;107(25):3133–40.

13. Hare JM, Mangal B, Brown J, et al. Impact of oxypurinol in patients with symptomatic heart failure. Results of the OPT-CHF study. J Am Coll Cardiol 2008;51(24):2301–9.

14. Vasan RS, Sullivan LM, Roubenoff R, et al. Inflammatory markers and risk of heart failure in elderly subjects without prior myocardial infarction: the Framingham Heart Study. Circulation 2003; 107(11):1486–91.

15. Cesari M, Penninx BW, Newman AB, et al. Inflammatory markers and onset of cardiovascular events: results from the Health ABC study. Circulation 2003;108(19):2317–22.

16. Pfeffer MA, Braunwald E. Ventricular remodeling after myocardial infarction. Experimental observations and clinical implications. Circulation 1990; 81(4):1161–72.

17. Kukielka GL, Smith CW, LaRosa GJ, et al. Interleukin-8 gene induction in the myocardium after ischemia and reperfusion in vivo. J Clin Invest 1995;95(1):89–103.

18. Nakamura K, Fushimi K, Kouchi H, et al. Inhibitory effects of antioxidants on neonatal rat cardiac myocyte hypertrophy induced by tumor necrosis factor-alpha and angiotensin II. Circulation 1998; 98(8):794–9.

19. Remondino A, Kwon SH, Communal C, et al. Beta-adrenergic receptor-stimulated apoptosis in cardiac myocytes is mediated by reactive oxygen species/c-Jun NH$_2$-terminal kinase-dependent activation of the mitochondrial pathway. Circ Res 2003;92(2):136–8.

20. Steinberg D, Parthasarathy S, Carew TE, et al. Beyond cholesterol. Modifications of low-density lipoprotein that increase its atherogenicity. N Engl J Med 1989;320(14):915–24.

21. Chen EP, Bittner HB, Davis RD, et al. Extracellular superoxide dismutase transgene overexpression preserves postischemic myocardial function in isolated murine hearts. Circulation 1996;94(Suppl 9): II412–7.

22. Wang P, Chen H, Qin H, et al. Overexpression of human copper, zinc-superoxide dismutase (SOD1) prevents postischemic injury. Proc Natl Acad Sci U S A 1998;95(8):4556–60.

23. Giordano FJ, Johnson RS. Angiogenesis: the role of the microenvironment in flipping the switch. Curr Opin Genet Dev 2001;11(1):35–40.

24. Iyer NV, Kotch LE, Agani F, et al. Cellular and developmental control of O$_2$ homeostasis by hypoxia-inducible factor 1 alpha. Genes Dev 1998;12(2):149–62.

25. Irwin MW, Mak S, Mann DL, et al. Tissue expression and immunolocalization of tumor necrosis factor-alpha in postinfarction dysfunctional myocardium. Circulation 1999;99(11):1492–8.

26. Engberding N, Spiekermann S, Schaefer A, et al. Allopurinol attenuates left ventricular remodeling and dysfunction after experimental myocardial infarction: a new action for an old drug? Circulation 2004;110(15):2175–9.

27. Heras M, Sanz G, Roig E, et al. Endothelial dysfunction of the non-infarct related, angiographically normal, coronary artery in patients with an acute myocardial infarction. Eur Heart J 1996; 17(5):715–20.

28. Werns SW, Walton JA, Hsia HH, et al. Evidence of endothelial dysfunction in angiographically normal coronary arteries of patients with coronary artery disease. Circulation 1989;79(2):287–91.

29. Levy D, Larson MG, Vasan RS, et al. The progression from hypertension to congestive heart failure. JAMA 1996;275(20):1557–62.

30. Moser M, Hebert PR. Prevention of disease progression, left ventricular hypertrophy and congestive heart failure in hypertension treatment trials. J Am Coll Cardiol 1996;27(5):1214–8.

31. Kostis JB, Davis BR, Cutler J, et al. Prevention of heart failure by antihypertensive drug treatment in older persons with isolated systolic hypertension. SHEP Cooperative Research Group. JAMA 1997; 278(3):212–6.

32. Psaty BM, Smith NL, Siscovick DS, et al. Health outcomes associated with antihypertensive therapies used as first-line agents. A systematic review and meta-analysis. JAMA 1997;277(9): 739–45.

33. Dhalla AK, Hill MF, Singal PK. Role of oxidative stress in transition of hypertrophy to heart failure. J Am Coll Cardiol 1996;28(2):506–14.

34. Lob HE, Marvar PJ, Guzik TJ, et al. Induction of hypertension and peripheral inflammation by reduction of extracellular superoxide dismutase in the central nervous system. Hypertension 2010; 55(2):277–83, 276p following 283.

35. Peterson JR, Burmeister MA, Tian X, et al. Genetic silencing of Nox2 and Nox4 reveals differential roles of these NADPH oxidase homologues in the vasopressor and dipsogenic effects of brain angiotensin II. Hypertension 2009;54(5): 1106–14.

36. Jackson EK, Gillespie DG, Zhu C, et al. Alpha2-adrenoceptors enhance angiotensin II-induced renal vasoconstriction: role for NADPH oxidase and RhoA. Hypertension 2008;51(3):719–26.

37. Carlstrom M, Persson AE. Important role of NAD(P)H oxidase 2 in the regulation of the tubuloglomerular feedback. Hypertension 2009;53(3): 456–7.

38. Gongora MC, Qin Z, Laude K, et al. Role of extracellular superoxide dismutase in hypertension. Hypertension 2006;48(3):473–81.

39. Lavi S, Yang EH, Prasad A, et al. The interaction between coronary endothelial dysfunction, local oxidative stress, and endogenous nitric oxide in humans. Hypertension 2008;51(1):127–33.

40. Sabri A, Hughie HH, Lucchesi PA. Regulation of hypertrophic and apoptotic signaling pathways by reactive oxygen species in cardiac myocytes. Antioxid Redox Signal 2003;5(6):731–40.

41. Wei S, Rothstein EC, Fliegel L, et al. Differential MAP kinase activation and Na(+)/H(+) exchanger phosphorylation by H(2)O(2) in rat cardiac myocytes. Am J Physiol Cell Physiol 2001;281(5):C1542–50.

42. Tanaka K, Honda M, Takabatake T. Redox regulation of MAPK pathways and cardiac hypertrophy in adult rat cardiac myocyte. J Am Coll Cardiol 2001;37(2):676–85.

43. Shahbaz AU, Kamalov G, Zhao W, et al. Mitochondria-targeted cardioprotection in aldosteronism. J Cardiovasc Pharmacol 2011;57(1):37–43.

44. Mohammed SF, Ohtani T, Korinek J, et al. Mineralocorticoid accelerates transition to heart failure with preserved ejection fraction via "nongenomic effects". Circulation 2010;122(4):370–8.

45. Cai L, Li W, Wang G, et al. Hyperglycemia-induced apoptosis in mouse myocardium: mitochondrial cytochrome C-mediated caspase-3 activation pathway. Diabetes 2002;51(6):1938–48.

46. Carroll R, Carley AN, Dyck JR, et al. Metabolic effects of insulin on cardiomyocytes from control and diabetic db/db mouse hearts. Am J Physiol Endocrinol Metab 2005;288(5):E900–6.

47. Young ME, Guthrie PH, Razeghi P, et al. Impaired long-chain fatty acid oxidation and contractile dysfunction in the obese Zucker rat heart. Diabetes 2002;51(8):2587–95.

48. Buchanan J, Mazumder PK, Hu P, et al. Reduced cardiac efficiency and altered substrate metabolism precedes the onset of hyperglycemia and contractile dysfunction in two mouse models of insulin resistance and obesity. Endocrinology 2005;146(12):5341–9.

49. Avogaro A, Nosadini R, Doria A, et al. Myocardial metabolism in insulin-deficient diabetic humans without coronary artery disease. Am J Physiol 1990;258(4 Pt 1):E606–18.

50. Jagasia D, Whiting JM, Concato J, et al. Effect of non-insulin-dependent diabetes mellitus on myocardial insulin responsiveness in patients with ischemic heart disease. Circulation 2001;103(13): 1734–9.

51. Utriainen T, Takala T, Luotolahti M, et al. Insulin resistance characterizes glucose uptake in skeletal muscle but not in the heart in NIDDM. Diabetologia 1998;41(5):555–9.

52. Iribarren C, Karter AJ, Go AS, et al. Glycemic control and heart failure among adult patients with diabetes. Circulation 2001;103(22):2668–73.

53. From AM, Scott CG, Chen HH. Changes in diastolic dysfunction in diabetes mellitus over time. Am J Cardiol 2009;103(10):1463–6.

54. Poirier P, Bogaty P, Garneau C, et al. Diastolic dysfunction in normotensive men with well-controlled type 2 diabetes: importance of maneuvers in echocardiographic screening for preclinical diabetic cardiomyopathy. Diabetes Care 2001;24(1):5–10.

55. From AM, Scott CG, Chen HH. The development of heart failure in patients with diabetes mellitus and pre-clinical diastolic dysfunction a population-based study. J Am Coll Cardiol 2010;55(4):300–5.

56. Ingelsson E, Arnlov J, Lind L, et al. Metabolic syndrome and risk for heart failure in middle-aged men. Heart 2006;92(10):1409–13.

57. Bahrami H, Bluemke DA, Kronmal R, et al. Novel metabolic risk factors for incident heart failure and their relationship with obesity: the MESA (Multi-Ethnic Study of Atherosclerosis) study. J Am Coll Cardiol 2008;51(18):1775–83.

58. Butler J, Rodondi N, Zhu Y, et al. Metabolic syndrome and the risk of cardiovascular disease in older adults. J Am Coll Cardiol 2006;47(8): 1595–602.

59. Witteles RM, Fowler MB. Insulin-resistant cardiomyopathy clinical evidence, mechanisms, and treatment options. J Am Coll Cardiol 2008;51(2):93–102.

60. Hayat SA, Patel B, Khattar RS, et al. Diabetic cardiomyopathy: mechanisms, diagnosis and treatment. Clin Sci (Lond) 2004;107(6):539–57.

61. Barouch LA, Berkowitz DE, Harrison RW, et al. Disruption of leptin signaling contributes to cardiac hypertrophy independently of body weight in mice. Circulation 2003;108(6):754–9.

62. Thandavarayan RA, Watanabe K, Ma M, et al. 14-3-3 protein regulates Ask1 signaling and protects against diabetic cardiomyopathy. Biochem Pharmacol 2008;75(9):1797–806.

63. Hamblin M, Friedman DB, Hill S, et al. Alterations in the diabetic myocardial proteome coupled with increased myocardial oxidative stress underlies diabetic cardiomyopathy. J Mol Cell Cardiol 2007; 42(4):884–95.

64. Itoh H, Doi K, Tanaka T, et al. Hypertension and insulin resistance: role of peroxisome proliferator-activated receptor gamma. Clin Exp Pharmacol Physiol 1999;26(7):558–60.

65. Winkler G, Lakatos P, Salamon F, et al. Elevated serum TNF-alpha level as a link between endothelial dysfunction and insulin resistance in normotensive obese patients. Diabet Med 1999;16(3):207–11.

66. Rolo AP, Palmeira CM. Diabetes and mitochondrial function: role of hyperglycemia and oxidative stress. Toxicol Appl Pharmacol 2006;212(2):167–78.

67. Wang J, Song Y, Elsherif L, et al. Cardiac metallothionein induction plays the major role in the prevention of diabetic cardiomyopathy by zinc supplementation. Circulation 2006;113(4):544–54.

68. El-Omar MM, Lord R, Draper NJ, et al. Role of nitric oxide in posthypoxic contractile dysfunction of diabetic cardiomyopathy. Eur J Heart Fail 2003;5(3): 229–39.

69. Reilly MP, Lehrke M, Wolfe ML, et al. Resistin is an inflammatory marker of atherosclerosis in humans. Circulation 2005;111(7):932–9.

70. Ouchi N, Kihara S, Funahashi T, et al. Reciprocal association of C-reactive protein with adiponectin in blood stream and adipose tissue. Circulation 2003;107(5):671–4.

71. Frankel DS, Vasan RS, D'Agostino RB Sr, et al. Resistin, adiponectin, and risk of heart failure the Framingham offspring study. J Am Coll Cardiol 2009;53(9):754–62.

72. Butler J, Kalogeropoulos A, Georgiopoulou V, et al. Serum resistin concentrations and risk of new onset heart failure in older persons: the health, aging, and body composition (Health ABC) study. Arterioscler Thromb Vasc Biol 2009;29(7):1144–9.

73. Butler J, Kalogeropoulos A, Georgiopoulou V, et al. Incident heart failure prediction in the elderly: the health ABC heart failure score. Circ Heart Fail 2008;1(2):125–33.

74. Leszek P, Korewicki J, Klisiewicz A, et al. Reduced myocardial expression of calcium handling protein in patients with severe chronic mitral regurgitation. Eur J Cardiothorac Surg 2006;30(5):737–43.

75. Mulieri LA, Leavitt BJ, Martin BJ, et al. Myocardial force-frequency defect in mitral regurgitation heart failure is reversed by forskolin. Circulation 1993; 88(6):2700–4.

76. Oral H, Sivasubramanian N, Dyke DB, et al. Myocardial proinflammatory cytokine expression and left ventricular remodeling in patients with chronic mitral regurgitation. Circulation 2003;107(6):831–7.

77. Chen MC, Chang JP, Liu WH, et al. Increased serum oxidative stress in patients with severe mitral regurgitation: a new finding and potential mechanism for atrial enlargement. Clin Biochem 2009; 42(10–11):943–8.

78. Ahmed MI, Gladden JD, Litovsky SH, et al. Increased oxidative stress and cardiomyocyte myofibrillar degeneration in patients with chronic isolated mitral regurgitation and ejection fraction >60%. J Am Coll Cardiol 2010;55(7):671–9.

79. Sugiyama S, Okada Y, Sukhova GK, et al. Macrophage myeloperoxidase regulation by granulocyte macrophage colony-stimulating factor in human atherosclerosis and implications in acute coronary syndromes. Am J Pathol 2001;158(3):879–91.

80. Ronald JA, Chen JW, Chen Y, et al. Enzyme-sensitive magnetic resonance imaging targeting

myeloperoxidase identifies active inflammation in experimental rabbit atherosclerotic plaques. Circulation 2009;120(7):592–9.

81. Baldus S, Heeschen C, Meinertz T, et al. Myeloperoxidase serum levels predict risk in patients with acute coronary syndromes. Circulation 2003; 108(12):1440–5.

82. Mocatta TJ, Pilbrow AP, Cameron VA, et al. Plasma concentrations of myeloperoxidase predict mortality after myocardial infarction. J Am Coll Cardiol 2007; 49(20):1993–2000.

83. Morrow DA, Sabatine MS, Brennan ML, et al. Concurrent evaluation of novel cardiac biomarkers in acute coronary syndrome: myeloperoxidase and soluble CD40 ligand and the risk of recurrent ischaemic events in TACTICS-TIMI 18. Eur Heart J 2008;29(9):1096–102.

84. Scirica BM, Sabatine MS, Jarolim P, et al. Assessment of multiple cardiac biomarkers in non-ST-segment elevation acute coronary syndromes: observations from the MERLIN-TIMI 36 Trial. Eur Heart J 2011;32(6):697–705.

85. Ward NC, Hodgson JM, Puddey IB, et al. Oxidative stress in human hypertension: association with antihypertensive treatment, gender, nutrition, and lifestyle. Free Radic Biol Med 2004;36(2):226–32.

86. Redon J, Oliva MR, Tormos C, et al. Antioxidant activities and oxidative stress byproducts in human hypertension. Hypertension 2003;41(5):1096–101.

87. Desai RV, Ahmed MI, Fonarow GC, et al. Effect of serum insulin on the association between hyperuricemia and incident heart failure. Am J Cardiol 2010;106(8):1134–8.

88. Werns SW, Shea MJ, Mitsos SE, et al. Reduction of the size of infarction by allopurinol in the ischemic-reperfused canine heart. Circulation 1986;73(3): 518–24.

89. Askari AT, Brennan ML, Zhou X, et al. Myeloperoxidase and plasminogen activator inhibitor 1 play a central role in ventricular remodeling after myocardial infarction. J Exp Med 2003;197(5):615–24.

90. Coghlan JG, Flitter WD, Clutton SM, et al. Allopurinol pretreatment improves postoperative recovery and reduces lipid peroxidation in patients undergoing coronary artery bypass grafting. J Thorac Cardiovasc Surg 1994;107(1):248–56.

91. Coetzee A, Roussouw G, Macgregor L. Failure of allopurinol to improve left ventricular stroke work after cardiopulmonary bypass surgery. J Cardiothorac Vasc Anesth 1996;10(5):627–33.

92. Taggart DP, Young V, Hooper J, et al. Lack of cardioprotective efficacy of allopurinol in coronary artery surgery. Br Heart J 1994;71(2):177–81.

93. Fonarow GC, Wright RS, Spencer FA, et al. Effect of statin use within the first 24 hours of admission for acute myocardial infarction on early morbidity and mortality. Am J Cardiol 2005;96(5):611–6.

94. Tang WH, Francis GS. Statin treatment for patients with heart failure. Nat Rev Cardiol 2010;7(5): 249–55.

95. Saab FA, Petrina M, Kline-Rogers E, et al. Early statin therapy in elderly patients presenting with acute coronary syndrome causing less heart failure. Indian Heart J 2006;58(4):321–4.

96. Sakamoto T, Kojima S, Ogawa H, et al. Effects of early statin treatment on symptomatic heart failure and ischemic events after acute myocardial infarction in Japanese. Am J Cardiol 2006;97(8): 1165–71.

97. Brown JH, Del Re DP, Sussman MA. The Rac and Rho hall of fame: a decade of hypertrophic signaling hits. Circ Res 2006;98(6):730–42.

98. Lipinski MJ, Cauthen CA, Biondi-Zoccai GG, et al. Meta-analysis of randomized controlled trials of statins versus placebo in patients with heart failure. Am J Cardiol 2009;104(12):1708–16.

99. Scirica BM, Morrow DA, Cannon CP, et al. Intensive statin therapy and the risk of hospitalization for heart failure after an acute coronary syndrome in the PROVE IT-TIMI 22 study. J Am Coll Cardiol 2006;47(11):2326–31.

100. Strandberg TE, Holme I, Faergeman O, et al. Comparative effect of atorvastatin (80 mg) versus simvastatin (20 to 40 mg) in preventing hospitalizations for heart failure in patients with previous myocardial infarction. Am J Cardiol 2009;103(10): 1381–5.

101. Stephens NG, Parsons A, Schofield PM, et al. Randomised controlled trial of vitamin E in patients with coronary disease: Cambridge Heart Antioxidant Study (CHAOS). Lancet 1996;347(9004): 781–6.

102. Rapola JM, Virtamo J, Ripatti S, et al. Randomised trial of alpha-tocopherol and beta-carotene supplements on incidence of major coronary events in men with previous myocardial infarction. Lancet 1997;349(9067):1715–20.

103. Boaz M, Smetana S, Weinstein T, et al. Secondary prevention with antioxidants of cardiovascular disease in endstage renal disease (SPACE): randomised placebo-controlled trial. Lancet 2000; 356(9237):1213–8.

104. Dietary supplementation with n-3 polyunsaturated fatty acids and vitamin E after myocardial infarction: results of the GISSI-Prevenzione trial. Gruppo Italiano per lo Studio della Sopravvivenza nell'Infarto miocardico. Lancet 1999;354(9177):447–55.

105. Yusuf S, Dagenais G, Pogue J, et al. Vitamin E supplementation and cardiovascular events in high-risk patients. The Heart Outcomes Prevention Evaluation Study Investigators. N Engl J Med 2000; 342(3):154–60.

106. Lonn E, Bosch J, Yusuf S, et al. Effects of long-term vitamin E supplementation on cardiovascular

events and cancer: a randomized controlled trial. JAMA 2005;293(11):1338–47.

107. Shirpoor A, Salami S, Khadem-Ansari MH, et al. Cardioprotective effect of vitamin E: rescues of diabetes-induced cardiac malfunction, oxidative stress, and apoptosis in rat. J Diabetes Complications 2009;23(5):310–6.

108. Ren J, Dominguez LJ, Sowers JR, et al. Troglitazone attenuates high-glucose-induced abnormalities in relaxation and intracellular calcium in rat ventricular myocytes. Diabetes 1996;45(12):1822–5.

109. Von Bibra H, Diamant M, Scheffer PG, et al. Rosiglitazone, but not glimepiride, improves myocardial diastolic function in association with reduction in oxidative stress in type 2 diabetic patients without overt heart disease. Diab Vasc Dis Res 2008;5(4):310–8.

110. Tousoulis D, Antoniades C, Vassiliadou C, et al. Effects of combined administration of low dose atorvastatin and vitamin E on inflammatory markers and endothelial function in patients with heart failure. Eur J Heart Fail 2005;7(7):1126–32.

111. Bowry VW, Ingold KU, Stocker R. Vitamin E in human low-density lipoprotein. When and how this antioxidant becomes a pro-oxidant. Biochem J 1992;288(Pt 2):341–4.

From Risk Factors to Structural Heart Disease: The Role of Inflammation

Andreas P. Kalogeropoulos, MD[a],
Vasiliki V. Georgiopoulou, MD[b], Javed Butler, MD, MPH[c],*

KEYWORDS

- Heart failure • Inflammation
- Left ventricular dysfunction • Cytokines

Inflammation, an integral component of homeostasis, is a complex tissue response to stressors that attempts to mitigate their effect and initiate the healing process.[1] Inflammatory responses in the cardiovascular system are regulated by, and interact with, the immune response system,[2] the renin-angiotensin-aldosterone system (RAAS),[3,4] the sympathetic nervous system,[5] nitroso-redox homeostasis,[6] calcium homeostasis,[7] and the heme-oxygenase system,[8] among others. Therefore, depending on the balance between these complex regulating processes and the timing of inflammatory response in relation to the inciting event, inflammation can exert both beneficial and detrimental effects to the cardiovascular system.

Pathophysiological inflammatory responses can cause alterations in myocardial function during both acute (either cardiac-specific, eg, acute myocardial infarction, viral myocarditis, or systemic, eg, sepsis, shock) and chronic inflammatory states. The latter can be broadly categorized into either manifest chronic inflammatory conditions or subclinical, low-grade inflammation. In manifest inflammatory conditions, cardiac and vascular involvement is part of a systemic disorder with distinct clinical characteristics and involvement of specific systems (eg, chronic infections, connective tissue disorders, psoriatic arthritis, lupus). The overall impact of these conditions on the prevalence of structural heart disease at the population level is probably limited.[9] By contrast, low-grade, nonspecific, subclinical inflammatory activity, which can be detected as elevated levels of circulating proinflammatory cytokines in the blood, is highly prevalent in the population.[9] Thus, any effect of low-grade inflammation on structural heart disease progression is of major interest from an epidemiologic and public health perspective.

Elevated levels of circulating proinflammatory cytokines, mostly C-reactive protein (CRP), interleukin (IL)-6, and tumor necrosis factor (TNF)-α, have been repeatedly associated with increased risk for clinically manifest heart failure (HF), that is, Stage C HF, in multiple large cohort studies (**Table 1**).[10–17] However, the role of inflammation in the transition from risk factors (Stage A HF) to structural heart disease (Stage B HF) is less well understood; it is only recently that basic and translational research has started shedding light on

Financial disclosures: The authors have nothing to disclose.
Funding Support: None.
[a] Emory Clinical Cardiovascular Research Institute, 1462 Clifton Road Northeast, Suite 535B, Atlanta, GA 30322, USA
[b] Emory Clinical Cardiovascular Research Institute, 1462 Clifton Road Northeast, Suite 535A, Atlanta, GA 30322, USA
[c] Emory Clinical Cardiovascular Research Institute, 1462 Clifton Road Northeast, Suite 504, Atlanta, GA 30322, USA
* Corresponding author.
E-mail address: javed.butler@emory.edu

Table 1
Major cohort studies demonstrating association between baseline levels of circulating proinflammatory cytokines and risk for heart failure

Study	Population	Markers
Health, Aging, and Body Composition Study[10]	n = 2610, ≥65 y	CRP, IL-6, TNF-α
Health, Aging, and Body Composition Study[11]	n = 2902, ≥65 y	Resistin
Framingham Offspring Study[12]	n = 2739, mean age 61 y	Resistin
Malmö Diet and Cancer (MDC) Study[13]	n = 4691, >40 y, no MI or stroke	CRP
Cardiovascular Health Study[14]	n = 4017, ≥65 y, no diabetes	CRP, IL-6
Multi-Ethnic Study of Atherosclerosis (MESA)[15]	n = 6814, ≥45 y, no CVD	CRP, IL-6
Suleiman et al[16]	n = 1044, acute MI	CRP
Framingham Heart Study[17]	n = 732, mean age 78 y, no MI	CRP, IL-6, TNF-α

Abbreviations: CRP, C-reactive protein; CVD, cardiovascular disease; IL, interleukin; MI, myocardial infarction; TNF, tumor necrosis factor.

the mechanistic links between inflammatory processes, circulating proinflammatory cytokines, and structural heart disease progression. This review focuses on the evidence that links low-grade inflammatory activity with progression of structural heart disease and transition to Stage B HF.

RISK FACTORS ASSOCIATED WITH LOW-GRADE INFLAMMATORY ACTIVITY

As outlined in **Fig. 1**, low-grade inflammatory activity characterizes atherosclerotic disease and various noncardiovascular conditions, including chronic kidney disease and chronic obstructive pulmonary disease (COPD) among others, all known to increase HF risk. However, elevated levels of inflammatory biomarkers have been also associated with modifiable risk factors; these

include smoking, dietary elements, sedentary lifestyle, and obesity. In fact, an inflammatory component underlies all adiposity-related disorders, including metabolic syndrome, type 2 diabetes, and obstructive sleep apnea.[18] The role of inflammation in atherosclerosis,[19] chronic kidney disease,[20] and COPD[21] has been extensively reviewed. The authors describe here briefly the evidence regarding modifiable risk factors and the modulatory effects of aging.

Obesity and Adiposity-Related Disorders

Obesity is characterized by a state of chronic low-grade inflammation, initiated by excess nutrients in metabolic cells (thus the term "metaflammation"), primarily adipocytes.[22] Adipocytes are capable of secreting both nonspecific proinflammatory

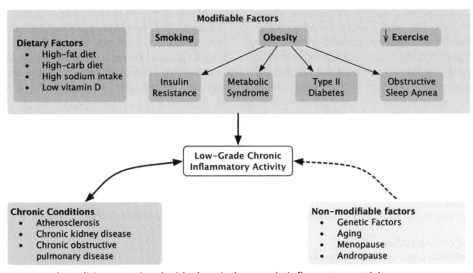

Fig. 1. Factors and conditions associated with chronic, low-grade inflammatory activity.

cytokines, including TNF-α, IL-6, and IL-1β, and also adipose tissue–specific proteins with pleiotropic regulatory properties ("adipokines").[18] Among the latter, leptin and resistin possess proinflammatory properties, whereas adiponectin has anti-inflammatory effects.[18] In obese states, the hypertrophied adipocytes demonstrate a proinflammatory secretory profile, with increased expression of TNF-α, IL-6, and leptin, and decreased expression of adiponectin.[18,23] Preliminary data suggest that weight loss is capable of reversing this unfavorable inflammatory profile.[23] Proinflammatory cytokines and adipokines may play a causative role and can also exacerbate insulin resistance, metabolic syndrome, and type 2 diabetes.[18,24] TNF-α and IL-6 interfere with insulin signaling and regulation of peroxisomal proliferator-activated receptor γ (PPAR-γ) receptors, whereas IL-6 exerts inhibitory effects on gene transcription of PPAR-γ, accompanied by a marked reduction in insulin-stimulated tyrosine phosphorylation and reduced insulin-stimulated glucose transport.[18] Of note, production of proinflammatory cytokines appears to be greater in visceral adipose tissue than in subcutaneous adipose tissue.[18]

Obstructive sleep apnea exacerbates low-grade inflammation in obese states, as a result of repeated episodes of hypoxia; circulating levels of proinflammatory cytokines and adipokines (CRP, TNF-α, IL-6, IL-1β, leptin, resistin) are elevated in patients with obstructive sleep apnea relative to controls matched for body mass index.[18,25] In addition, obstructive sleep apnea is accompanied by increased oxidative stress, as evident by increased production of reactive oxygen species, which further triggers activation of inflammatory pathways.[18,25]

Sedentary Lifestyle and Exercise

Acutely, physical exercise causes a short-term inflammatory response; however, regular physical activity has been associated with lower levels of circulating inflammatory markers both in cross-sectional and prospective exercise intervention studies.[26] In randomized studies, increases in daily physical activity resulted in reductions in CRP and IL-6 levels both in healthy individuals and in patients with adiposity-related disease burden.[27]

Smoking

Chronic smoking induces release of proinflammatory markers, including CRP, IL-6, IL-1, and TNF-α, and decreases production of anti-inflammatory cytokines.[28] In a large cohort of elderly men, IL-6 levels were elevated in both current and former smokers in comparison with nonsmokers.[29] There is a dose-response relation between years of smoking and levels of proinflammatory cytokines in past smokers.[30] Although the inflammatory profile reverts toward normal after smoking cessation over the years, a long time (up to 20 years) is required for levels of proinflammatory cytokines to normalize, especially in heavier smokers.[30]

Dietary Factors

In epidemiologic studies, higher fat intake has been consistently associated with increased levels of proinflammatory cytokines, whereas a more favorable inflammatory profile has been observed with higher intake of dietary fiber, vegetables, fruit, and fish.[27] Data on dietary sodium intake are limited. In a recent report from a large United Kingdom community cohort, CRP levels were only modestly associated with 24-hour urine sodium.[31] Dietary sodium restriction has yielded mixed results on inflammatory profile. In two small trials in patients with asthma, sodium restriction yielded small or no reduction in circulating inflammatory markers,[32,33] whereas a low-sodium diet (<1500 mg/d) caused increases in circulating inflammatory markers in untreated patients with hypertension.[34] Finally, vitamin D deficiency, which is highly prevalent in the general population, is associated with increased inflammatory activity, cardiometabolic burden, and cardiovascular risk; these effects are thought to be mediated by increases in parathyroid hormone, which in turn induces insulin resistance.[7]

Aging

Aging is associated not only with increase in body fat but also with redistribution of fat from the periphery to central (abdominal and visceral) locations. Age-related changes in adiposity play a central role in the proinflammatory profile shift observed with aging.[35] Other mechanisms include declining levels of sex hormones after menopause and andropause, and cumulative oxidative damage.[35] In vitro studies suggest that IL-6 gene transcription is repressed by estrogen and androgen and that these hormones inhibit secretion of IL-6.[36] Several studies describe an increase in IL-6 levels after the onset of menopause, and preliminary data suggest development of a proinflammatory state with declining levels of testosterone.[37,38] However, exogenous hormone therapy does not appear to reverse these changes.[37]

INFLAMMATION AND PROGRESSION OF STRUCTURAL HEART DISEASE: OVERVIEW

The transition from Stage A to Stage B HF in the absence of direct myocardial damage (eg, ischemic injury) remains incompletely understood. Data from basic and translational research studies suggest that, among other mechanisms, inflammation plays a key role in this transition, through direct and indirect effects on the myocardium (**Fig. 2**). Also, inflammation-mediated changes in the vascular bed contribute to progression of structural heart disease, precipitation of symptoms, and transition to Stage C HF.

DIRECT EFFECTS OF PROINFLAMMATORY CYTOKINES ON MYOCARDIAL CONTRACTILITY

Proinflammatory cytokines exert cardiodepressant effects that lead to decreased myocardial contractility and left ventricular (LV) performance.[39] The ultimate goal of this adaptive response is to decrease energy demands and protect the myocardium during stress[39]; however, protracted exposure to inflammatory stimuli has adverse consequences on LV function.[40] TNF-α and interleukins have been extensively studied in this aspect, and exemplify the double-edged nature of inflammatory responses. In isolated hamster papillary muscles, TNF-α, IL-6, and IL-2 inhibit contractility in a concentration-dependent, reversible manner; removal of the endocardial endothelium does not alter these responses, suggesting a direct negative inotropic effect of cytokines.[41] Cardiac-specific overexpression of TNF-α in transgenic mice results in a dilated cardiomyopathy phenotype.[42] Both TNF-α and IL-6 can reduce myocardial contractility directly through cytosolic Ca^{2+} reduction during systole; this effect is mediated by alterations in the sarcoplasmic reticulum function, and is fully reversible when the cytokine exposure is removed.[43] Also, TNF-α decreases myocyte contractility indirectly through nitric oxide (NO)-dependent attenuation of myofilament Ca^{2+} sensitivity.[44] Myocytes have TNF-α receptors on their surfaces; the adult human heart expresses both mRNA and receptor proteins for TNF receptors 1 and 2 (TNF-R1 and TNF-R2, respectively). The negative inotropic effects of TNF-α in cardiac myocytes appear to be initiated by activation of TNF-R1.[45]

Resistin, a proinflammatory adipokine now known to be produced also by nonadipose cells, has demonstrated several direct myocardial effects as well.[46] In neonatal rats, adenovirus-mediated overexpression of resistin results in increased sarcomere organization, cell size, and protein synthesis in cardiomyocytes, and expression of atrial natriuretic factor and β-myosin heavy chain.[46] Overexpression of resistin in adult rat cardiomyocytes alters mechanics by depressing cell contractility as well as contraction and relaxation velocities.[46]

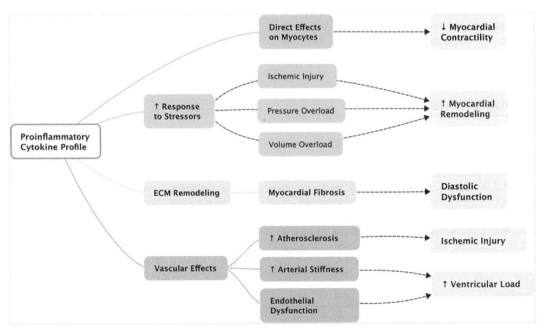

Fig. 2. Potential mechanisms linking a proinflammatory cytokine profile with transition to Stage B heart failure. ECM, extracellular matrix.

INFLAMMATION AND LEFT VENTRICULAR REMODELING

In contrast to static tissues, the process of stress response and damage repair is significantly more challenging in a continuously beating organ.[47] First, the proliferative capacity of cardiac myocytes is limited. Second, the heart needs to maintain adequate function to meet the body needs throughout stress adaptation processes, such as those observed in mechanical overload, or tissue repair processes, for example, after a myocardial infarction. Finally, necrotic cells need to be replaced immediately for cardiac chambers to maintain mechanical integrity.[47] Thus, although the ultimate goal of inflammatory responses is to protect against stress induced by mechanical stressors and to repair damaged tissue, this process can result in extensive remodeling of the myocardium at the molecular and structural level. This situation is clinically evident by alterations in the size and geometry of the affected chambers, most frequently the left ventricle.

Remodeling After Ischemic Injury

The role of inflammation in myocardial healing has been extensively studied after ischemic or ischemia-reperfusion injury.[48] During this process, fibrotic tissue (scar) replaces damaged cells whereas remote, intact myocardial cells respond with hypertrophy.[49] Remodeling continues over the weeks and months after the initial inciting event, mediated by active inflammation, fibrosis, and cardiomyocyte loss.[50] Initially, products of tissue injury, including reactive oxygen species and intracellular proteins released from necrotic cells, activate several nonantigen-specific mechanisms that initiate the inflammatory response; these include pattern recognition receptors such as Toll-like receptors, the transcription nuclear factor κB (NF-κB), and the complement.[48] These mechanisms converge to an activation of the immune system resembling that observed after infection. This activation leads to release of several inflammatory mediators, which in turn recruit inflammatory cells to the site of injury.[48] Of note, proinflammatory cytokines, such as TNF-α, IL-1β, and IL-6, are not constitutively expressed in the normal heart, but robust upregulation of cytokine mRNA expression takes place in the infarct area as well as in the noninfarcted myocardium within the first hours after infarction.[39] This proinflammatory response induces progressive myocyte apoptosis and hypertrophy, defects in contractility, and inflammatory signal transduction.[39] Proinflammatory cytokine levels normally decrease 1 week after myocardial injury. However, depending on the degree of injury and the presence of ongoing myocardial stress factors (oxidative, mechanical, and neurohormonal stress), chronic cytokine upregulation may persist, particularly in remote myocardial sites. This upregulation initiates a vicious circle between chronic inflammatory activity and myocardial remodeling.[39]

In human studies, levels of proinflammatory cytokines after acute myocardial infarction strongly correlate with LV remodeling and clinical outcomes. In patients with acute myocardial infarction, serum CRP measured within 12 to 24 h of symptom onset predicts 30-day mortality and HF development,[51] whereas IL-6 levels remain elevated even 12 weeks after infarction, and predischarge IL-6 levels are associated with HF and depressed LV function.[52] In patients with acute myocardial infarction receiving contemporary treatment, increases in circulating CRP and IL-6 levels parallel infarct size, microvascular obstruction, and parameters of LV remodeling up to 2 months after percutaneous coronary intervention.[53] Also, serial assessment of TNF-α and IL-10, a cytokine with anti-inflammatory properties, revealed that an unfavorable inflammatory profile persists for up to 6 months in patients demonstrating extensive LV remodeling after percutaneous coronary intervention.[54] These data support the hypothesis that a proinflammatory cytokine profile contributes to the progression of LV remodeling.

Response to Pressure Overload

Beyond the well-recognized role of inflammation in cardiac remodeling after acute myocardial events, recent experimental evidence suggests a distinct role for inflammatory cytokines in cardiac remodeling induced by pressure and volume overload. Transverse aortic constriction (a procedure used to create an experimental model of pressure overload) leads to exaggerated decline in circumferential fiber shortening, more prominent cardiac hypertrophy and fibrosis, and enhanced inflammation, oxidative stress, and RAAS activation in transgenic mice overexpressing CRP, in comparison with nontransgenic mice.[55] These effects of CRP overexpression are preceded by augmented macrophage infiltration, presence of activated NF-κB in cardiomyocytes, myocardial expression of inflammatory cytokines, oxidative stress, and p38 mitogen-activated protein kinase signaling (which is reported to play an important role in the development of myocardial hypertrophy in models of chronic pressure overload); in addition, NO production is attenuated.[55]

Although circulating and cardiac TNF-α levels were long known to be elevated in human and experimental pressure overload conditions, it is only recently that studies in animal models have shed light on the role of TNF-α in cardiac remodeling and dysfunction in pressure overload states. In an experimental model of pressure overload caused by banding of the descending aorta, TNF-knockout mice showed attenuated cardiac apoptosis, hypertrophy, inflammatory response, cardiac matrix metalloproteinase (MMP)-9 activity, and reparative fibrosis compared with their wild-type counterparts[56]; this attenuated response was accompanied by relatively preserved cardiac function.[56] These findings suggest that inflammation plays an important role in pressure overload–induced ventricular hypertrophy, remodeling, and dysfunction.

Response to Volume Overload

In an experimental model of volume overload induced by aortocaval fistula in rats, activation of MMPs and degradation of interstitial collagen are preceded by inflammation and increased oxidative stress.[57] These extracellular myocardial events are thought to be central in adverse eccentric LV remodeling and progression to HF through a process of myocyte and myofiber slippage along with cardiomyocyte elongation.[58] The response to stretch is initiated, partially at least, by TNF-α, as shown by elevated TNF-α expression in the left ventricle early after induction of volume overload.[57] TNF-α is known to induce activation of MMPs and collagen degradation, and is also a potent chemoattractant for mast cells; conversely, TNF-α is a major component of mast cells. Mast cell degranulation mediates extracellular matrix (ECM) remodeling through secretion of cytokines and proteases (eg, tryptase, chymase). Of note, pharmacologic inhibition of mast cell degranulation prevents LV remodeling induced by volume overload, whereas mast cell–deficient rats do not demonstrate the upregulation in TNF-α and MMP activity and increase in collagen degradation after initiation of aortocaval fistula observed in wild-type rats.[59] In volume-overloaded mice, TNF-α inhibition preserves LV function and limits cardiac dilation.[60,61] Of note, circulating levels of TNF-α and TNF receptors are elevated in patients with mitral regurgitation.[62]

ROLE OF INFLAMMATION IN FIBROSIS AND DIASTOLIC DYSFUNCTION

Although abnormalities not directly related to LV diastolic function have been described in patients with HF and preserved LV ejection fraction,[63] abnormalities in active relaxation and passive stiffness of the myocardium are considered the key pathophysiological features in these patients.[64] The molecular mechanisms of diastolic dysfunction are still under active investigation. Current evidence suggests that the elastic properties of the heart are largely determined by the dynamic regulation of the giant muscle protein titin[65] and the composition and mass of ECM.[66] Pathologic ECM remodeling, often referred to as myocardial fibrosis, is therefore a major contributor to increased myocardial stiffness. In fact, impaired diastolic function is related to fibrosis rather than to myocardial hypertrophy in renovascular hypertensive rats.[67] Although the fibrotic process most extensively studied is ischemic scar,[68] there is accumulating evidence that diffuse myocardial fibrosis is present in a variety of conditions in the absence of ischemia.[66] Activation of inflammatory pathways appears to play a central role in myocardial fibrosis, a role that seems to be augmented by aging, estrogen deficiency, and glucose metabolism disorders among others, all associated with clinical diastolic dysfunction.

Recent evidence suggests that inflammatory cells play a key role in myocardial fibrosis via release of profibrogenic cytokines. In a pressure overload model created by suprarenal abdominal aorta constriction in rats (a model of cardiac hypertrophy associated with preserved systolic but impaired diastolic function without overt HF), transforming growth factor (TGF)-β activates fibroblasts, leading to marked reactive myocardial fibrosis accompanied by diastolic dysfunction.[69] Blocking TGF-β activity prevents fibrosis and ameliorates diastolic dysfunction.[69] Perivascular accumulation of macrophages, mainly recruited by the monocyte chemoattractant protein (MCP)-1,[70] is central in this process because perivascular fibrosis is followed by interstitial fibrosis. Treatment with an anti–MCP-1 antibody inhibits macrophage accumulation, TGF-β induction, and fibroblast proliferation in rats, attenuating thus myocardial fibrosis (but not myocyte hypertrophy), and ameliorating diastolic dysfunction without affecting blood pressure and systolic function.[71] In endomyocardial biopsies from humans with HF and preserved ejection fraction, there is evidence of cardiac collagen accumulation accompanied by decreased MMP-1 and presence of inflammatory cells expressing TGF-β.[72] The amount of cardiac collagen and inflammatory cells correlate with the degree of diastolic dysfunction, suggesting a direct role of inflammation and fibrosis in diastolic dysfunction.[72] Activation of RAAS in conditions of pressure overload appears to play a central role in triggering myocardial inflammation and perivascular myocardial fibrosis; notably, angiotensin II directly stimulates secretion of TGF-β.[4]

Circulating inflammatory cytokines have also been implicated in diastolic dysfunction. In spontaneously hypertensive rats, cardiac hypertrophy and diastolic dysfunction with increased expression of B-type natriuretic peptide and downregulation of β-adrenergic receptors parallels upregulation of IL-6, indicating an active proinflammatory process during early stages of cardiac hypertrophy and diastolic dysfunction.[73] In humans, levels of TNF-α and IL-6 correlate with degree of diastolic dysfunction in patients with acute myocardial infarction or stable coronary heart disease, and in those with glucose metabolism disorders.[74–77] In 2610 participants of the Health, Aging, and Body Composition Study (Health ABC Study) (≥65 years old) without prevalent HF, baseline levels of IL-6 and TNF-α were strongly predictive of incident HF over the next 10 years in models controlling for clinical characteristics, ankle-arm index, and incident coronary heart disease; this strong association persisted after accounting for competing mortality.[10] Of note, inflammatory markers had a stronger association with HF with preserved ejection fraction in this elderly cohort.[10] In the younger cohort of the Multi-Ethnic Study of Atherosclerosis (MESA), where 65% of incident HF cases had preserved LV systolic function, serum IL-6 and CRP predicted HF independent of obesity and other established risk factors.[15]

Aging, estrogen deficiency, and glucose metabolism appear to modulate the effects of inflammation on interstitial myocardial fibrosis. In an experimental model of progressive diastolic dysfunction in rats, fibroblast infiltration and collagen expression in the heart was a function of age, paralleling progressive diastolic dysfunction over 30 months.[2] These cellular and functional changes were associated with progressive increases in mRNA for MCP-1 and IL-13, which correlated temporally and quantitatively with fibrosis and cellular procollagen levels, suggesting a causative relationship between age-dependent immunoinflammatory dysfunction, fibrosis, and diastolic dysfunction.[2] In a recent experimental study, estrogen deficiency has been shown to augment cardiac inflammation and oxidative stress in hypertensive female rats, thus aggravating myocardial fibrosis and diastolic dysfunction.[78] Finally, glucose metabolism disorders appear to play an important role in inflammatory signaling via increased oxidative stress, protein kinase C activation, and advanced glycosylation end products.[79]

VASCULAR EFFECTS OF INFLAMMATION AND VENTRICULAR DYSFUNCTION

Chronic inflammation is involved in vascular pathophysiology at 3 levels, all contributing to structural heart disease (see **Fig. 2**). First, inflammation has an established, pivotal role in the progression of atherosclerosis. Second, inflammation is involved in vascular remodeling and increased arterial stiffness. The resulting decreased distensibility of large arteries reduces their capacity to accommodate pulsatile pressure and amplifies pressure waves reflected from the periphery; this increases LV end-systolic pressure and LV work.[80] Increased arterial stiffness is considered a major pathophysiologic determinant of HF with preserved ejection fraction.[81] Third, recent data suggest that inflammation is an important pathway for endothelial dysfunction, which is present early in HF[82] and may contribute to progression of ventricular dysfunction through various pathways, including impaired nitroso-redox balance in the periphery, which results in vasoconstriction and enhanced afterload, and myocardial perfusion abnormalities.[83] The role of inflammation in atherosclerosis has been extensively reviewed elsewhere.[19] The authors focus here briefly on the role of inflammation in endothelial dysfunction and arterial stiffness.

Arterial Stiffness

In healthy individuals, higher CRP levels are associated with increased arterial stiffness, as measured by the carotid-femoral pulse-wave velocity (PWV),[84] and in patients with untreated essential hypertension, PWV correlates with circulating levels of high-sensitivity CRP, TNF-α, and IL-6.[85] In a large prospective cohort study in Italy encompassing individuals from a wide age spectrum, higher circulating CRP and leptin levels were associated with increased PWV independent of age, sex, metabolic syndrome, and other cardiovascular risk factors.[86]

Endothelial Dysfunction

In a recent experimental study, the relaxation response of aortic tissue to acetylcholine, but not to sodium nitroprusside, was significantly decreased after 16 weeks of high-fat diet in female mice.[87] This impaired relaxation response was accompanied by decreased expression of endothelial NO synthase and increased expression of TNF-α in the aorta; notably, inhibition of NF-κB corrected the relaxation response abnormalities.[87] In a recent human study, vitamin D–deficient individuals, who are known to have elevated levels of proinflammatory cytokines, demonstrated impaired brachial artery flow-mediated dilation (FMD), a measure of endothelium-dependent dilation[88]; this was accompanied by higher endothelial cell expression of NF-κB and IL-6 compared with sufficient individuals.[88] Of importance, inhibition of NF-κB improved FMD in vitamin D–deficient individuals.[88] Taken together, these data suggest a distinct role of inflammation via the NF-κB pathway in endothelial dysfunction.

SUMMARY AND FUTURE DIRECTIONS

Low-grade inflammatory activity is involved in most mechanisms that underlie progression of structural heart disease, including ventricular remodeling, response to pressure and volume overload, and myocardial fibrosis. Inflammation also contributes to progression of peripheral vascular changes that eventually impose an increased load on ventricular function. However, how to translate this knowledge into clinical practice is still unclear. One potential application would be to use circulating levels of proinflammatory cytokines as markers of subclinical disease with the aim of improving risk prediction for HF and identifying individuals at higher risk. For example, addition of IL-6 significantly improved the predictive properties of a clinical HF risk prediction model,[10] the Health ABC HF Score.[89,90] Similarly, CRP and IL-6 substantially reclassified HF risk assessment over clinical risk factors in the Cardiovascular Health Study.[14] However, attempts to directly manipulate inflammatory responses with the goal of preventing progression of structural heart disease are still at a very early experimental stage. Despite encouraging results from animal models,[91,92] the disappointing results of anti-inflammatory therapy in patients with Stage C HF[93] temper enthusiasm for inflammation as a therapeutic target. On the other hand, a wealth of evidence suggests that the inflammatory profile in humans can be favorably manipulated by non-pharmacologic means, including weight loss, healthier dietary habits, smoking cessation, and regular exercise. Considering the collateral benefits of these interventions, this may be an avenue worth exploring further, especially among individuals at higher risk for Stage C HF.

REFERENCES

1. Khaper N, Bryan S, Dhingra S, et al. Targeting the vicious inflammation-oxidative stress cycle for the management of heart failure. Antioxid Redox Signal 2010;13:1033–49.

2. Cieslik KA, Taffet GE, Carlson S, et al. Immune-inflammatory dysregulation modulates the incidence of progressive fibrosis and diastolic stiffness in the aging heart. J Mol Cell Cardiol 2011;50:248–56.

3. Sekiguchi K, Li X, Coker M, et al. Cross-regulation between the renin-angiotensin system and inflammatory mediators in cardiac hypertrophy and failure. Cardiovasc Res 2004;63:433–42.

4. Sciarretta S, Paneni F, Palano F, et al. Role of the renin-angiotensin-aldosterone system and inflammatory processes in the development and progression of diastolic dysfunction. Clin Sci (Lond) 2009;116:467–77.

5. Felder RB. Mineralocorticoid receptors, inflammation and sympathetic drive in a rat model of systolic heart failure. Exp Physiol 2010;95:19–25.

6. Hori M, Nishida K. Oxidative stress and left ventricular remodelling after myocardial infarction. Cardiovasc Res 2009;81:457–64.

7. Lee JH, O'Keefe JH, Bell D, et al. Vitamin D deficiency an important, common, and easily treatable cardiovascular risk factor? J Am Coll Cardiol 2008;52:1949–56.

8. Ndisang JF. Role of heme oxygenase in inflammation, insulin-signalling, diabetes and obesity. Mediators Inflamm 2010;2010:359732.

9. Dhingra R, Gona P, Nam BH, et al. C-reactive protein, inflammatory conditions, and cardiovascular disease risk. Am J Med 2007;120:1054–62.

10. Kalogeropoulos A, Georgiopoulou V, Psaty BM, et al. Inflammatory markers and incident heart failure risk in older adults: the Health ABC (Health, Aging, and Body Composition) study. J Am Coll Cardiol 2010;55:2129–37.

11. Butler J, Kalogeropoulos A, Georgiopoulou V, et al. Serum resistin concentrations and risk of new onset heart failure in older persons: the Health, Aging, and Body Composition (Health ABC) study. Arterioscler Thromb Vasc Biol 2009;29:1144–9.

12. Frankel DS, Vasan RS, D'Agostino RBS, et al. Resistin, adiponectin, and risk of heart failure the Framingham offspring study. J Am Coll Cardiol 2009;53:754–62.

13. Engstrom G, Melander O, Hedblad B. Carotid intima-media thickness, systemic inflammation, and incidence of heart failure hospitalizations. Arterioscler Thromb Vasc Biol 2009;29:1691–5.

14. Suzuki T, Katz R, Jenny NS, et al. Metabolic syndrome, inflammation, and incident heart failure in the elderly: the cardiovascular health study. Circ Heart Fail 2008;1:242–8.

15. Bahrami H, Bluemke DA, Kronmal R, et al. Novel metabolic risk factors for incident heart failure and their relationship with obesity: the MESA (Multi-Ethnic Study of Atherosclerosis) study. J Am Coll Cardiol 2008;51:1775–83.

16. Suleiman M, Khatib R, Agmon Y, et al. Early inflammation and risk of long-term development of heart

failure and mortality in survivors of acute myocardial infarction predictive role of C-reactive protein. J Am Coll Cardiol 2006;47:962–8.

17. Vasan RS, Sullivan LM, Roubenoff R, et al. Inflammatory markers and risk of heart failure in elderly subjects without prior myocardial infarction: the Framingham Heart Study. Circulation 2003;107: 1486–91.

18. Alam I, Lewis K, Stephens JW, et al. Obesity, metabolic syndrome and sleep apnoea: all pro-inflammatory states. Obes Rev 2007;8:119–27.

19. Libby P, Ridker PM, Hansson GK. Inflammation in atherosclerosis: from pathophysiology to practice. J Am Coll Cardiol 2009;54:2129–38.

20. Vidt DG. Inflammation in renal disease. Am J Cardiol 2006;97:20A–7A.

21. Maestrelli P, Saetta M, Mapp CE, et al. Remodeling in response to infection and injury. Airway inflammation and hypersecretion of mucus in smoking subjects with chronic obstructive pulmonary disease. Am J Respir Crit Care Med 2001;164:S76–80.

22. Gregor MF, Hotamisligil GS. Inflammatory mechanisms in obesity. Annu Rev Immunol 2010;29: 415–45.

23. Forsythe LK, Wallace JM, Livingstone MB. Obesity and inflammation: the effects of weight loss. Nutr Res Rev 2008;21:117–33.

24. Shoelson SE, Herrero L, Naaz A. Obesity, inflammation, and insulin resistance. Gastroenterology 2007; 132:2169–80.

25. Kasai T, Bradley TD. Obstructive sleep apnea and heart failure: pathophysiologic and therapeutic implications. J Am Coll Cardiol 2011;57:119–27.

26. Kasapis C, Thompson PD. The effects of physical activity on serum C-reactive protein and inflammatory markers: a systematic review. J Am Coll Cardiol 2005;45:1563–9.

27. O'Connor MF, Irwin MR. Links between behavioral factors and inflammation. Clin Pharmacol Ther 2010;87:479–82.

28. Arnson Y, Shoenfeld Y, Amital H. Effects of tobacco smoke on immunity, inflammation and autoimmunity. J Autoimmun 2010;34:J258–65.

29. Helmersson J, Larsson A, Vessby B, et al. Active smoking and a history of smoking are associated with enhanced prostaglandin F(2alpha), interleukin-6 and F2-isoprostane formation in elderly men. Atherosclerosis 2005;181:201–7.

30. Wannamethee SG, Lowe GD, Shaper AG, et al. Associations between cigarette smoking, pipe/cigar smoking, and smoking cessation, and haemostatic and inflammatory markers for cardiovascular disease. Eur Heart J 2005;26:1765–73.

31. Fogarty AW, Lewis SA, McKeever TM, et al. Is higher sodium intake associated with elevated systemic inflammation? A population-based study. Am J Clin Nutr 2009;89:1901–4.

32. Mickleborough TD, Lindley MR, Ray S. Dietary salt, airway inflammation, and diffusion capacity in exercise-induced asthma. Med Sci Sports Exerc 2005;37:904–14.

33. Forrester DL, Britton J, Lewis SA, et al. Impact of adopting low sodium diet on biomarkers of inflammation and coagulation: a randomised controlled trial. J Nephrol 2010;23:49–54.

34. Nakandakare ER, Charf AM, Santos FC, et al. Dietary salt restriction increases plasma lipoprotein and inflammatory marker concentrations in hypertensive patients. Atherosclerosis 2008;200: 410–6.

35. Singh T, Newman AB. Inflammatory markers in population studies of aging. Ageing Res Rev 2011; 10(3):319–29.

36. Papanicolaou DA, Wilder RL, Manolagas SC, et al. The pathophysiologic roles of interleukin-6 in human disease. Ann Intern Med 1998;128:127–37.

37. Davison S, Davis SR. New markers for cardiovascular disease risk in women: impact of endogenous estrogen status and exogenous postmenopausal hormone therapy. J Clin Endocrinol Metab 2003; 88:2470–8.

38. Maggio M, Basaria S, Ceda GP, et al. The relationship between testosterone and molecular markers of inflammation in older men. J Endocrinol Invest 2005;28:116–9.

39. Nian M, Lee P, Khaper N, et al. Inflammatory cytokines and postmyocardial infarction remodeling. Circ Res 2004;94:1543–53.

40. Hedayat M, Mahmoudi MJ, Rose NR, et al. Proinflammatory cytokines in heart failure: double-edged swords. Heart Fail Rev 2010;15:543–62.

41. Finkel MS, Oddis CV, Jacob TD, et al. Negative inotropic effects of cytokines on the heart mediated by nitric oxide. Science 1992;257:387–9.

42. Kubota T, McTiernan CF, Frye CS, et al. Dilated cardiomyopathy in transgenic mice with cardiac-specific overexpression of tumor necrosis factor-alpha. Circ Res 1997;81:627–35.

43. Yokoyama T, Vaca L, Rossen RD, et al. Cellular basis for the negative inotropic effects of tumor necrosis factor-alpha in the adult mammalian heart. J Clin Invest 1993;92:2303–12.

44. Jozefowicz E, Brisson H, Rozenberg S, et al. Activation of peroxisome proliferator-activated receptor-alpha by fenofibrate prevents myocardial dysfunction during endotoxemia in rats. Crit Care Med 2007;35: 856–63.

45. Torre-Amione G, Kapadia S, Lee J, et al. Expression and functional significance of tumor necrosis factor receptors in human myocardium. Circulation 1995; 92:1487–93.

46. Kim M, Oh JK, Sakata S, et al. Role of resistin in cardiac contractility and hypertrophy. J Mol Cell Cardiol 2008;45:270–80.

47. Jiang B, Liao R. The paradoxical role of inflammation in cardiac repair and regeneration. J Cardiovasc Transl Res 2010;3:410–6.

48. Frantz S, Bauersachs J, Ertl G. Post-infarct remodelling: contribution of wound healing and inflammation. Cardiovasc Res 2009;81:474–81.

49. Sam F, Sawyer DB, Chang DL, et al. Progressive left ventricular remodeling and apoptosis late after myocardial infarction in mouse heart. Am J Physiol Heart Circ Physiol 2000;279:H422–8.

50. Dorn GW 2nd. Novel pharmacotherapies to abrogate postinfarction ventricular remodeling. Nat Rev Cardiol 2009;6:283–91.

51. Suleiman M, Aronson D, Reisner SA, et al. Admission C-reactive protein levels and 30-day mortality in patients with acute myocardial infarction. Am J Med 2003;115:695–701.

52. Gabriel AS, Martinsson A, Wretlind B, et al. IL-6 levels in acute and post myocardial infarction: their relation to CRP levels, infarction size, left ventricular systolic function, and heart failure. Eur J Intern Med 2004;15:523–8.

53. Orn S, Manhenke C, Ueland T, et al. C-reactive protein, infarct size, microvascular obstruction, and left-ventricular remodelling following acute myocardial infarction. Eur Heart J 2009;30:1180–6.

54. Laura PA, Michela DR, Silvia M, et al. Pro/anti-inflammatory cytokine imbalance in postischemic left ventricular remodeling. Mediators Inflamm 2010; 2010:974694.

55. Nagai T, Anzai T, Kaneko H, et al. C-reactive protein overexpression exacerbates pressure overload-induced cardiac remodeling through enhanced inflammatory response. Hypertension 2011;57: 208–15.

56. Sun M, Chen M, Dawood F, et al. Tumor necrosis factor-alpha mediates cardiac remodeling and ventricular dysfunction after pressure overload state. Circulation 2007;115:1398–407.

57. Chen Y, Pat B, Zheng J, et al. Tumor necrosis factor-alpha produced in cardiomyocytes mediates a predominant myocardial inflammatory response to stretch in early volume overload. J Mol Cell Cardiol 2010;49:70–8.

58. Ulasova E, Gladden JD, Chen Y, et al. Loss of interstitial collagen causes structural and functional alterations of cardiomyocyte subsarcolemmal mitochondria in acute volume overload. J Mol Cell Cardiol 2011;50:147–56.

59. Levick SP, Gardner JD, Holland M, et al. Protection from adverse myocardial remodeling secondary to chronic volume overload in mast cell deficient rats. J Mol Cell Cardiol 2008;45:56–61.

60. Kadokami T, Frye C, Lemster B, et al. Anti-tumor necrosis factor-alpha antibody limits heart failure in a transgenic model. Circulation 2001;104: 1094–7.

61. Jobe LJ, Melendez GC, Levick SP, et al. TNF-alpha inhibition attenuates adverse myocardial remodeling in a rat model of volume overload. Am J Physiol Heart Circ Physiol 2009;297:H1462–8.

62. Kapadia SR, Yakoob K, Nader S, et al. Elevated circulating levels of serum tumor necrosis factor-alpha in patients with hemodynamically significant pressure and volume overload. J Am Coll Cardiol 2000;36:208–12.

63. Tschope C, Westermann D. Heart failure with normal ejection fraction. Pathophysiology, diagnosis, and treatment. Herz 2009;34:89–96.

64. Zile MR, Baicu CF, Gaasch WH. Diastolic heart failure–abnormalities in active relaxation and passive stiffness of the left ventricle. N Engl J Med 2004;350:1953–9.

65. Kruger M, Linke WA. Titin-based mechanical signalling in normal and failing myocardium. J Mol Cell Cardiol 2009;46:490–8.

66. Jellis C, Martin J, Narula J, et al. Assessment of nonischemic myocardial fibrosis. J Am Coll Cardiol 2010;56:89–97.

67. Matsubara LS, Matsubara BB, Okoshi MP, et al. Myocardial fibrosis rather than hypertrophy induces diastolic dysfunction in renovascular hypertensive rats. Can J Physiol Pharmacol 1997;75:1328–34.

68. Cleutjens JP, Creemers EE. Integration of concepts: cardiac extracellular matrix remodeling after myocardial infarction. J Card Fail 2002;8:S344–8.

69. Kuwahara F, Kai H, Tokuda K, et al. Transforming growth factor-beta function blocking prevents myocardial fibrosis and diastolic dysfunction in pressure-overloaded rats. Circulation 2002;106: 130–5.

70. Reape TJ, Groot PH. Chemokines and atherosclerosis. Atherosclerosis 1999;147:213–25.

71. Kuwahara F, Kai H, Tokuda K, et al. Hypertensive myocardial fibrosis and diastolic dysfunction: another model of inflammation? Hypertension 2004;43:739–45.

72. Westermann D, Lindner D, Kasner M, et al. Cardiac inflammation contributes to changes in the extracellular matrix in patients with heart failure and normal ejection fraction. Circ Heart Fail 2011;4:44–52.

73. Haugen E, Chen J, Wikstrom J, et al. Parallel gene expressions of IL-6 and BNP during cardiac hypertrophy complicated with diastolic dysfunction in spontaneously hypertensive rats. Int J Cardiol 2007;115:24–8.

74. Dinh W, Futh R, Nickl W, et al. Elevated plasma levels of TNF-alpha and interleukin-6 in patients with diastolic dysfunction and glucose metabolism disorders. Cardiovasc Diabetol 2009;8:58.

75. Kosmala W, Derzhko R, Przewlocka-Kosmala M, et al. Plasma levels of TNF-alpha, IL-6, and IL-10 and their relationship with left ventricular diastolic function in patients with stable angina pectoris and

preserved left ventricular systolic performance. Coron Artery Dis 2008;19:375–82.

76. Williams ES, Shah SJ, Ali S, et al. C-reactive protein, diastolic dysfunction, and risk of heart failure in patients with coronary disease: Heart and Soul Study. Eur J Heart Fail 2008;10:63–9.

77. Arruda-Olson AM, Enriquez-Sarano M, Bursi F, et al. Left ventricular function and C-reactive protein levels in acute myocardial infarction. Am J Cardiol 2010;105:917–21.

78. Mori T, Kai H, Kajimoto H, et al. Enhanced cardiac inflammation and fibrosis in ovariectomized hypertensive rats: a possible mechanism of diastolic dysfunction in postmenopausal women. Hypertens Res 2011;34(4):496–502.

79. Watts GF, Marwick TH. Ventricular dysfunction in early diabetic heart disease: detection, mechanisms and significance. Clin Sci (Lond) 2003;105:537–40.

80. Ooi H, Chung W, Biolo A. Arterial stiffness and vascular load in heart failure. Congest Heart Fail 2008;14:31–6.

81. Kang S, Fan HM, Li J, et al. Relationship of arterial stiffness and early mild diastolic heart failure in general middle and aged population. Eur Heart J 2010;31:2799–807.

82. Heitzer T, Baldus S, von Kodolitsch Y, et al. Systemic endothelial dysfunction as an early predictor of adverse outcome in heart failure. Arterioscler Thromb Vasc Biol 2005;25:1174–9.

83. Lapu-Bula R, Ofili E. From hypertension to heart failure: role of nitric oxide-mediated endothelial dysfunction and emerging insights from myocardial contrast echocardiography. Am J Cardiol 2007;99: 7D–14D.

84. Yasmin McEniery CM, Wallace S, Mackenzie IS, et al. C-reactive protein is associated with arterial stiffness in apparently healthy individuals. Arterioscler Thromb Vasc Biol 2004;24:969–74.

85. Mahmud A, Feely J. Arterial stiffness is related to systemic inflammation in essential hypertension. Hypertension 2005;46:1118–22.

86. Scuteri A, Orru M, Morrell C, et al. Independent and additive effects of cytokine patterns and the metabolic syndrome on arterial aging in the SardiNIA Study. Atherosclerosis 2010;215(2):459–64.

87. Kobayasi R, Akamine EH, Davel AP, et al. Oxidative stress and inflammatory mediators contribute to endothelial dysfunction in high-fat diet-induced obesity in mice. J Hypertens 2010;28:2111–9.

88. Jablonski KL, Chonchol M, Pierce GL, et al. 25-Hydroxyvitamin D deficiency is associated with inflammation-linked vascular endothelial dysfunction in middle-aged and older adults. Hypertension 2011;57:63–9.

89. Butler J, Kalogeropoulos A, Georgiopoulou V, et al. Incident heart failure prediction in the elderly: the health ABC heart failure score. Circ Heart Fail 2008;1:125–33.

90. Kalogeropoulos A, Psaty BM, Vasan RS, et al. Validation of the health ABC heart failure model for incident heart failure risk prediction: the Cardiovascular Health Study. Circ Heart Fail 2010;3:495–502.

91. Li J, Leschka S, Rutschow S, et al. Immunomodulation by interleukin-4 suppresses matrix metalloproteinases and improves cardiac function in murine myocarditis. Eur J Pharmacol 2007;554:60–8.

92. Li S, Zhong S, Zeng K, et al. Blockade of NF-kappaB by pyrrolidine dithiocarbamate attenuates myocardial inflammatory response and ventricular dysfunction following coronary microembolization induced by homologous microthrombi in rats. Basic Res Cardiol 2010;105:139–50.

93. Gullestad L, Aukrust P. Review of trials in chronic heart failure showing broad-spectrum anti-inflammatory approaches. Am J Cardiol 2005;95:17C–23C [discussion: 38C–40C].

Diabetes and the Risk of Heart Failure

Ravi Dhingra, MD, MPH[a],
Ramachandran S. Vasan, MD, DM[b],*

KEYWORDS

- Diabetes mellitus • Heart failure • Prediabetic state
- Ventricular remodeling

The current American Heart Association heart failure classification schema designates the presence of diabetes mellitus as stage A heart failure, which raises the risk of developing stage B heart failure or asymptomatic left ventricular (LV) dysfunction. The present body of scientific evidence suggests that individuals with diabetes have a much higher risk for heart failure than those without diabetes.[1] Several clinical and experimental studies have shown that diabetes mellitus leads to functional, biochemical, and morphologic abnormalities of the heart, independent of promoting myocardial ischemia, and some of these changes happen earlier in the natural history of diabetes. In this review, the authors summarize some of the epidemiologic evidence that supports that diabetes is an independent risk factor for heart failure and promotes myocardial remodeling (a precursor of heart failure). The authors also provide a brief overview of the mechanisms (beyond ischemia) that lead to the development of heart failure in individuals with varying degrees of impaired glucose homeostasis (diabetes itself representing the most overt form of the spectrum of dysglycemic disorders).

INCIDENCE AND PREVALENCE OF DIABETES AND HEART FAILURE: 2 CONDITIONS INCREASING IN MAGNITUDE WORLDWIDE

Heart failure remains a major medical illness in individuals aged 65 years or more, with an estimated annual incidence of 10 per 1000.[2] At age 40 years, the lifetime risk of developing heart failure is about 1 in 5 for both men and women.[3] Similarly, prevalence and incidence of diabetes is increasing at an exponential rate, with an observed age-adjusted increase in incidence of 90% in the last decade.[4] Current estimated prevalence of diagnosed diabetes in the United States is approximately 7.8% for individuals older than 20 years, another 14.6% have undiagnosed diabetes, and nearly 37% have prediabetes. Each year, about 1.6 million cases of diabetes are newly diagnosed in the United States.[2] In addition, an estimated 23.1% of individuals aged 60 years or more have diabetes as assessed in the year 2007 by the National Health Interview Survey.[5] The estimated lifetime risk of developing diabetes ranges from 33% (men) to 39% (women), rivaling and exceeding that of heart failure.[6] Thus, diabetes and heart failure represent twin epidemics that pose a substantial population burden.

DIABETES AS AN INDEPENDENT RISK FACTOR FOR HEART FAILURE

More than a century ago, heart failure was noted to be a complication of diabetes.[7] In 1974, Kannel and colleagues[8] reported diabetes to be "another discrete cause of congestive heart failure" and postulated the mechanism as caused by small vessel disease or associated metabolic disturbances. These observations have been confirmed

This work was supported by contract NO1 25195 from the National Health Institute.

[a] Section of Cardiology, Heart and Vascular Center, Dartmouth Hitchcock Medical Center, One Medical Center Drive, Lebanon, NH 03756, USA

[b] Section of Preventive Medicine and Epidemiology, Department of Medicine, The Framingham Heart Study, Boston University School of Medicine, 73 Mount Wayte Avenue, Suite 2, Framingham, MA 01702-5803, USA

* Corresponding author.
E-mail address: vasan@bu.edu

Heart Failure Clin 8 (2012) 125–133
doi:10.1016/j.hfc.2011.08.008
1551-7136/12/$ – see front matter © 2012 Elsevier Inc. All rights reserved.

by several recent epidemiologic studies.[9] Data also support the hypothesis that individuals with diabetes who have poor blood glucose control are at much higher risk for heart failure.[10] In addition, other studies indicate that individuals without overt diabetes but who have insulin resistance[11] or have higher hemoglobin A1C values[12] (5.5%–6.0%) also incur greater risk for heart failure on follow-up.

Framingham researchers had estimated a 2-fold increase in risk of heart failure in men and about a 5-fold increase in risk in women with diabetes.[13] In fact, even in a cohort of postmenopausal women with prior history of coronary disease, diabetes was recognized to be the strongest predictor of heart failure.[14] Prevalence and incidence of diabetes among patients with heart failure is observed to be growing,[15,16] whereas mortality among those with heart failure with diabetes is also noted to be alarmingly high.[15,17]

DIABETES, IMPAIRED FASTING GLUCOSE, AND LV REMODELING

Individuals with diabetes frequently have echocardiographic evidence of LV remodeling; both increased LV mass and dilatation have been reported,[18] and these phenotypes are well-known predictors of heart failure in community studies.[19,20] Subclinical LV remodeling in diabetes is more prevalent in women.[21] These sex-related differences, with greater impact of dysglycemia in women, are also consistently seen among studies that observed that LV mass increases with worsening glucose tolerance and with greater insulin resistance.[22,23] More recently, longitudinal data from the Framingham cohort indicate that individuals with diabetes mellitus experienced greater age-associated increases in LV wall thickness and a lesser decrease in LV diastolic dimensions with increasing age.[24] In the Multi Ethnic Study of Atherosclerosis, researchers observed ethnicity-related variability in the prevalence of greater LV mass (in Hispanics and blacks), smaller LV end-diastolic volume, and reduced stroke volume (in whites, blacks and Chinese) in diabetic patients independent of the presence of subclinical atherosclerosis.[25] In addition, insulin levels and insulinlike growth factor 1 (IGF-1) are also associated with greater LV mass, although insulin resistance assessed by hemostasis model is related to LV remodeling in some[26–29] but not all studies.[23,30,31]

SYSTOLIC AND DIASTOLIC DYSFUNCTION IN DIABETES

Several studies have observed that individuals with diabetes have a greater risk of developing LV diastolic dysfunction.[32–35] Prior epidemiologic studies have observed higher prevalence and increased incidence of clinical heart failure among individuals with diabetes after controlling for other traditional risk factors.[15,36,37] Subclinical diastolic and systolic dysfunction progress to clinical heart failure[38] and are associated with greater cardiovascular mortality.[39] Researchers have also observed that factors associated with insulin resistance syndrome predate the development of LV systolic dysfunction by 2 decades, adjusting for ischemic heart disease and other risk factors.[40]

DIABETES AND VASCULAR STIFFNESS

Pulse wave velocity is a well-known indicator of target organ damage in patients with diabetes.[41] Higher peripheral pulse pressure is associated with a greater risk of subsequent cardiovascular disease events in the general population[42,43] and in high-risk patients with LV dysfunction.[44] In a recent meta-analysis, greater stiffness in large arteries was associated with higher cardiovascular events and all-cause mortality.[45] Vascular stiffness coupled with ventricular systolic stiffness is positively related with increase in age.[46] Furthermore, it is also evident that large artery compliance is reduced with age in patients with diastolic heart failure.[47] Aortic stiffness as measured by carotid-femoral pulse wave velocity increases in the presence of diabetes and also with age and obesity.[48] Researchers have observed that individuals with diabetes and diastolic dysfunction are prone to have ventricular and arterial stiffening beyond that expected because of aging or hypertension.[49] Although several studies have shown positive associations between diabetes, impaired fasting glucose, and lower large artery compliance,[50–52] a recent study suggested that only frank diabetes but not impaired fasting glucose increased aortic stiffness.[53] Some investigators have suggested that the impact of diabetes on vascular stiffness attenuates beyond age 65 years.[54] Of note, despite the lack of unanimous consensus regarding effect modification by age, most investigators agree that the evolution of the "diabetic heart" is mediated in part by altered ventriculovascular coupling.[52,55]

ASSOCIATION OF DIABETES WITH OTHER CLINICAL RISK FACTORS

Most established risk factors for atherosclerosis also increase the risk of heart failure.[56] As previously known, coronary disease is the most common cause of heart failure. In the presence of coronary disease, the risk of heart failure is increased several fold among individuals with diabetes. It is conceivable that individuals with diabetes may have a decreased awareness of chest discomfort due to acute ischemia that could result in delay in seeking medical attention, and consequently they may accrue greater myocardial damage. After myocardial infarction, ventricular remodeling may occur at a faster pace among those with diabetes, which greatly elevates the risk for development of overt heart failure.[57]

Diabetes and Dyslipidemia

In general, individuals with diabetes who have insulin resistance also have higher circulating levels of triglycerides and lower high-density lipoprotein (HDL)-cholesterol concentrations and commonly manifest the metabolic syndrome.[58] The metabolic syndrome is a predictor of future risk of cardiovascular disease.[59] Specifically, it is widely recognized that higher levels of small dense low-density lipoprotein particles are a major contributor of increased risk for cardiovascular disease in insulin-resistant patients.[60] The association of different lipid fractions (especially the total cholesterol to HDL-cholesterol ratio) with incident heart failure is not the same as that for incident atherosclerotic cardiovascular events.[61] Evidence supports that higher triglyceride levels[62] or higher non-HDL–cholesterol levels[63] increase the risk of developing heart failure, perhaps because of the presence of insulin resistance that predisposes to metabolic changes characterized by impaired myocardial fatty acid oxidation and greater uncoupling of mitochondrial proteins in the heart.[64] Thus, in an insulin-resistant patient, myocardial glucose uptake is decreased.[65] Indeed, patients with non-ischemic cardiomyopathy may still exhibit relatively preserved myocardial glucose uptake in the presence of insulin sensitivity.[66] Another possible lipid fraction that could be associated in raising the risk for heart failure in those with diabetes is higher levels of lipoprotein (a).[67] Underexpression of peroxisome proliferator-activated receptor α (PPAR-α) increases glucose metabolism and prevents cardiac dilatation, whereas its overexpression leads to severe cardiomyopathy. The multiple mechanistic steps implicating PPAR-α in the development of heart failure and the use of fibrates that act as agonists to PPAR-α in heart failure have been reviewed recently.[68]

Diabetes and Hypertension

Individuals with hypertension are prone to develop clinical heart failure.[69] A study from human autopsies showed that the alterations in myocardial cells and capillaries in diabetic patients leading to ventricular systolic and diastolic dysfunction are more pronounced in individuals with a history of hypertension.[70] Hypertensive patients with type 2 diabetes are observed to have higher LV mass and LV hypertrophy compared with their normotensive counterparts with diabetes.[26,71] Although intensive blood pressure control (systolic blood pressure <120 mm Hg) with medications in patients with diabetes has not shown reduction in fatal or nonfatal cardiovascular events consistently in recent trials,[72–74] prior observational data demonstrate that lower blood pressure in diabetes is generally associated with lesser risk of cardiovascular disease.[75–77] Recommendations from JNC 7 (The Seventh Report of the Joint National Committee on Prevention, Detection, Evaluation, and Treatment of High Blood Pressure) guidelines suggest treating patients with diabetes with a systolic blood pressure goal of less than 130 mm Hg.[78]

Diabetes and Obesity

The Framingham Heart Study data have shown a significant positive association of obesity with incident heart failure independent of diabetes status.[79] In the presence of insulin resistance, obesity is known to increase free fatty acid use that further leads to decreased cardiac bioenergetic efficiency (cardiac work/myocardial oxygen consumption).[80] Among obese individuals with insulin resistance[81] and those with frank diabetes, LV mass increase is potentiated,[82] although some reports are inconsistent.[30]

MECHANISMS FOR DIABETES-ASSOCIATED HEART FAILURE RISK

Insulin resistance and diabetes have a considerable effect on myocardium.[83,84] It is beyond the scope of this review to describe all molecular pathways that may act as a mediator for raising the risk of heart failure. There are several postulated mechanisms that may be responsible for causing diastolic and systolic dysfunction of heart in an insulin-resistant patient or in overt diabetes. The authors describe briefly some mechanisms that have been the focus of considerable research.

Metabolic Derangements in Diabetes

The basic metabolic defects in patients with diabetes include hyperglycemia, insulin resistance, and increased circulating levels of free fatty acids. The inability of the myocardial cells to metabolize pyruvate in diabetes results in lipid accumulation in the myocardium and decrease in glucose uptake by the myocardial cells, a long-postulated mechanism for the impact of diabetes on the heart.[85] Glucose uptake by myocardial cells is primarily determined by local concentrations of insulin and the intensity of cardiac contraction.[83] However, the mechanisms by which free fatty acid metabolism and glucose oxidation are interrelated are quite complex.[86] Increased activation of different isomers of protein kinase C has been noted to play a role in inhibition of insulin secretion by free fatty acids.[87] On the other hand, hyperinsulinemia in diabetic patients is also associated with increased free fatty acid levels, elevated heart rate, and increased activation of sympathetic nervous system; all these factors subsequently lead to cardiac hypertrophy and intracellular accumulation of triglycerides. In the presence of hyperinsulinemia and insulin resistance, the human heart has also been shown to reduce protein degradation, which may then promote myocardial hypertrophy.[88] In addition, dyslipidemia and production of free radicals result in alteration of genetic transcription factors and coding, which subsequently alters the translation of nucleoprotein genes such as those in the renin-angiotensin system (RAS) and IGF-1. Increased expression of RAS genes promotes insulin resistance, whereas greater expression of the IGF-1 gene increases sensitivity of cardiac myocytes to calcium concentrations and increases myocardial contractility. IGF-1 also acts synergistically with angiotensin II in promoting cellular and myocardial hypertrophy.[89]

In experimental models of diabetes[90] and glucose intolerance,[91] increased collagen-bound advanced glycation end products (AGEs) are recognized to promote ventricular hypertrophy by increasing myocardial collagen deposition and fibrosis. In clinical studies, serum levels of AGEs are associated with greater diastolic dysfunction or ventricular stiffness.[92] AGEs and their potential role in increasing vascular stiffness in diabetic patients has also been postulated,[93] and the existence of higher levels of AGEs in diabetes has been known for several decades.[94] In addition, besides the collagen binding effect, AGEs also bind to the endothelial cells and promote oxidative stress.[93] Furthermore, upregulation of soluble AGE receptor is also postulated to promote vascular stiffness and increases risk of incident cardiovascular disease and mortality in diabetes.[95] Of note, an AGE "breaker" does attenuate diabetes-induced myocardial damage.[96]

Oxidative Stress in Diabetes

Hyperglycemia increases the production of reactive nitrogen and oxygen species, leading to increased glucose auto-oxidation and cardiac lipid peroxidation that in turn promotes abnormal gene expression and alters the signal transduction leading to myocardial cell death.[97] In experiment studies, treatment with antioxidant protein (metallothionein) has been shown to reverse myocardial effects of diabetes in mice.[98] Furthermore, depressed expression of sarcoendoplasmic reticulum Ca^{2+}–adenosine triphosphatase (SERCA2) protein (resulting in decreased sodium-calcium exchange leading to intracellular calcium overload) is another postulated mechanism that has been demonstrated in diabetic rats.[99] Several other mechanisms have also been proposed in addition to depressed SERCA2 expression in relation to impaired calcium metabolism in diabetes; these include reduced activity of adenosine triphosphatases, decreased activity of sacroplasmic reticulum to take up Ca^{2+}, and reduced activity of other exchangers such as Na^{2+}-Ca^{2+} pump.[100]

Mitochondrial Dysfunction in Diabetes

Studies over the last 3 decades have reported structural and functional mitochondrial alterations in diabetes.[101–104] Most experimental studies have shown that these mitochondrial alterations eventually cause a reduction in adenosine triphosphate (ATP) production by lower creatine phosphate activity,[105,106] lower ATP synthase activity,[102] and lower creatine-stimulated respiration,[107] which then promotes cardiac dysfunction. These results are supported by similar findings in human heart.[108] In addition, reactive oxygen species–mediated mitochondrial uncoupling may also play a role in the development of myocardial dysfunction in diabetes.[86]

Autonomic Neuropathy in Diabetes

Abnormal myocardial contractile response to exercise suggestive of impaired sympathetic innervation has been observed in type 1 diabetes.[109] This observation is further supported by the observed higher incidence of abnormal LV diastolic function by myocardial radionuclide imaging studies[110] and echocardiography[111] in diabetic patients with impaired autonomic responses. Presence of autonomic neuropathy in patients with diabetes also increases the likelihood of having abnormal radionuclide perfusion imaging results[112] and manifesting LV diastolic dysfunction.[113]

In addition, there are several other postulated mechanisms by which diabetes may cause cardiac dysfunction; these include increased activation of protein kinase C or upregulation of RAS, angiotensin II–induced or aldosterone-induced fibrosis, coronary vasomotor abnormalities,[114] endothelial dysfunction,[115] impaired angiogenesis with upregulation of microRNA,[116] and vascular endothelial growth factor expression.[117] A detailed discussion of these mechanisms is beyond the scope of the present review.

SUMMARY

There is substantial and consistent evidence in the literature to indicate that diabetes is a premier risk factor for heart failure, independent of its association with ischemic disease. The most common abnormality observed in asymptomatic diabetics is LV diastolic dysfunction, likely resulting from greater LV myocardial and vascular stiffness. There is also growing evidence that some, if not all, of these structural and biochemical myocardial abnormalities start at the prediabetic stage. Further research is needed to identify more sensitive markers of early myocardial abnormalities in asymptomatic individuals with diabetes and to formulate strategies for reversing these subclinical abnormalities to lower the risk of heart failure on long-term follow-up.

REFERENCES

1. Schocken DD, Benjamin EJ, Fonarow GC, et al. Prevention of heart failure: a scientific statement from the American Heart Association Councils on Epidemiology and Prevention, Clinical Cardiology, Cardiovascular Nursing, and High Blood Pressure Research; Quality of Care and Outcomes Research Interdisciplinary Working Group; and Functional Genomics and Translational Biology Interdisciplinary Working Group. Circulation 2008;117: 2544–65.
2. Roger VL, Go AS, Lloyd-Jones DM, et al. Heart disease and stroke statistics—2011 update: a report from the American Heart Association. Circulation 2011;123(4):e18–209.
3. Lloyd-Jones DM, Larson MG, Leip EP, et al. Lifetime risk for developing congestive heart failure: the Framingham Heart Study. Circulation 2002; 106:3068–72.
4. Available at: http://www.cdc.gov/mmwr/preview/ mmwrhtml/mm5743a2.htm. Accessed September 21, 2011.
5. Available at: http://www.cdc.gov/diabetes/pubs/ pdf/ndfs_2007.pdf. Accessed September 21, 2011.
6. Narayan KM, Boyle JP, Thompson TJ, et al. Lifetime risk for diabetes mellitus in the United States. JAMA 2003;290:1884–90.
7. Leyden D. Asthma und diabetes mellitus. Zeitschr Klin Med 1881;3:358–64.
8. Kannel WB, Hjortland M, Castelli WP. Role of diabetes in congestive heart failure: the Framingham study. Am J Cardiol 1974;34:29–34.
9. de Simone G, Devereux RB, Chinali M, et al. Diabetes and incident heart failure in hypertensive and normotensive participants of the Strong Heart Study. J Hypertens 2010;28:353–60.
10. Iribarren C, Karter AJ, Go AS, et al. Glycemic control and heart failure among adult patients with diabetes. Circulation 2001;103:2668–73.
11. Ingelsson E, Sundström J, Arnlöv J, et al. Insulin resistance and risk of congestive heart failure. JAMA 2005;294:334–41.
12. Matsushita K, Blecker S, Pazin-Filho A, et al. The association of hemoglobin A1c with incident heart failure among people without diabetes: the Atherosclerosis Risk in Communities Study. Diabetes 2010;59:2020–6.
13. Kannel WB, McGee DL. Diabetes and cardiovascular disease. The Framingham study. JAMA 1979;241:2035–8.
14. Bibbins-Domingo K, Lin F, Vittinghoff E, et al. Predictors of heart failure among women with coronary disease. Circulation 2004;110:1424–30.
15. Bertoni AG, Hundley WG, Massing MW, et al. Heart failure prevalence, incidence, and mortality in the elderly with diabetes. Diabetes Care 2004;27: 699–703.
16. Owan TE, Hodge DO, Herges RM, et al. Trends in prevalence and outcome of heart failure with preserved ejection fraction. N Engl J Med 2006; 355:251–9.
17. Murcia AM, Hennekens CH, Lamas GA, et al. Impact of diabetes on mortality in patients with myocardial infarction and left ventricular dysfunction. Arch Intern Med 2004;164:2273–9.
18. Lindman BR, Arnold SV, Madrazo JA, et al. The adverse impact of diabetes mellitus on left ventricular remodeling and function in patients with severe aortic stenosis. Circ Heart Fail 2011;4(3): 286–92.
19. Levy D, Garrison RJ, Savage DD, et al. Prognostic implications of echocardiographically determined left ventricular mass in the Framingham Heart Study. N Engl J Med 1990;322:1561–6.
20. Vasan RS, Larson MG, Benjamin EJ, et al. Left ventricular dilatation and the risk of congestive heart failure in people without myocardial infarction. N Engl J Med 1997;336:1350–5.
21. Galderisi M, Anderson KM, Wilson PW, et al. Echocardiographic evidence for the existence of a distinct diabetic cardiomyopathy (the Framingham Heart Study). Am J Cardiol 1991;68:85–9.
22. Henry RM, Kamp O, Kostense PJ, et al. Left ventricular mass increases with deteriorating glucose tolerance, especially in women: independence of increased arterial stiffness or decreased flow-mediated dilation. Diabetes Care 2004;27:522–9.
23. Rutter MK, Parise H, Benjamin EJ, et al. Impact of glucose intolerance and insulin resistance on

cardiac structure and function: sex-related differences in the Framingham Heart Study. Circulation 2003;107:448–54.

24. Cheng S, Xanthakis V, Sullivan LM, et al. Correlates of echocardiographic indices of cardiac remodeling over the adult life course: longitudinal observations from the Framingham Heart Study. Circulation 2010;122:570–8.

25. Bertoni AG, Goff DC, D Agostino RB, et al. Diabetic cardiomyopathy and subclinical cardiovascular disease. Diabetes Care 2006;29:588–94.

26. Palmieri V, Bella JN, Arnett DK, et al. Effect of type 2 diabetes mellitus on left ventricular geometry and systolic function in hypertensive subjects: Hypertension Genetic Epidemiology Network (HyperGEN) study. Circulation 2001;103:102–7.

27. Sundstrom J, Lind L, Nystrom N, et al. Left ventricular concentric remodeling rather than left ventricular hypertrophy is related to the insulin resistance syndrome in elderly men. Circulation 2000;101:2595–600.

28. Uusitupa M, Siitonen O, Pyorala K, et al. Relationship of blood pressure and left ventricular mass to serum insulin levels in newly diagnosed non-insulin-dependent (type 2) diabetic patients and in non-diabetic subjects. Diabetes Res 1987;4: 19–25.

29. Witteles RM, Tang WH, Jamali AH, et al. Insulin resistance in idiopathic dilated cardiomyopathy: a possible etiologic link. J Am Coll Cardiol 2004; 44:78–81.

30. Galvan AQ, Galetta F, Natali A, et al. Insulin resistance and hyperinsulinemia: no independent relation to left ventricular mass in humans. Circulation 2000;102:2233–8.

31. Verdecchia P, Reboldi G, Schillaci G, et al. Circulating insulin and insulin growth factor-1 are independent determinants of left ventricular mass and geometry in essential hypertension. Circulation 1999;100:1802–7.

32. Raev DC. Which left ventricular function is impaired earlier in the evolution of diabetic cardiomyopathy? An echocardiographic study of young type I diabetic patients. Diabetes Care 1994;17:633–9.

33. Poirier P, Bogaty P, Garneau C, et al. Diastolic dysfunction in normotensive men with well-controlled type 2 diabetes. Diabetes Care 2001; 24:5–10.

34. Rijzewijk LJ, van der Meer RW, Lamb HJ, et al. Altered myocardial substrate metabolism and decreased diastolic function in nonischemic human diabetic cardiomyopathy: studies with cardiac positron emission tomography and magnetic resonance imaging. J Am Coll Cardiol 2009;54:1524–32.

35. Schannwell CM, Schneppenheim M, Perings S, et al. Left ventricular diastolic dysfunction as an early manifestation of diabetic cardiomyopathy. Cardiology 2002;98:33–9.

36. Aronow WS, Ahn C. Incidence of heart failure in 2,737 older persons with and without diabetes mellitus. Chest 1999;115:867–8.

37. Nichols GA, Gullion CM, Koro CE, et al. The incidence of congestive heart failure in type 2 diabetes. Diabetes Care 2004;27:1879–84.

38. Aurigemma GP, Gottdiener JS, Shemanski L, et al. Predictive value of systolic and diastolic function for incident congestive heart failure in the elderly: the Cardiovascular Health Study. J Am Coll Cardiol 2001;37:1042–8.

39. Vasan RS, Larson MG, Benjamin EJ, et al. Congestive heart failure in subjects with normal versus reduced left ventricular ejection fraction: prevalence and mortality in a population-based cohort. J Am Coll Cardiol 1999;33:1948–55.

40. Arnlov J, Lind L, Zethelius BR, et al. Several factors associated with the insulin resistance syndrome are predictors of left ventricular systolic dysfunction in a male population after 20 years of follow-up. Am Heart J 2001;142:720–4.

41. Woolam GL, Schnur PL, Vallbona C, et al. The pulse wave velocity as an early indicator of atherosclerosis in diabetic subjects. Circulation 1962;25: 533–9.

42. Franklin SS, Khan SA, Wong ND, et al. Is pulse pressure useful in predicting risk for coronary heart disease? The Framingham Heart Study. Circulation 1999;100:354–60.

43. Haider AW, Larson MG, Franklin SS, et al. Systolic blood pressure, diastolic blood pressure, and pulse pressure as predictors of risk for congestive heart failure in the Framingham Heart Study. Ann Intern Med 2003;138:10–6.

44. Mitchell GF, Moye LA, Braunwald E, et al. Sphygmomanometrically determined pulse pressure is a powerful independent predictor of recurrent events after myocardial infarction in patients with impaired left ventricular function. Circulation 1997;96:4254–60.

45. Vlachopoulos C, Aznaouridis K, Stefanadis C. Prediction of cardiovascular events and all-cause mortality with arterial stiffness: a systematic review and meta-analysis. J Am Coll Cardiol 2010;55:1318–27.

46. Chen CH, Nakayama M, Nevo E, et al. Coupled systolic-ventricular and vascular stiffening with age: Implications for pressure regulation and cardiac reserve in the elderly. J Am Coll Cardiol 1998;32:1221–7.

47. Hundley WG, Kitzman DW, Morgan TM, et al. Cardiac cycle-dependent changes in aortic area and distensibility are reduced in older patients with isolated diastolic heart failure and correlate with exercise intolerance. J Am Coll Cardiol 2001; 38:796–802.

48. Mitchell GF, Guo CY, Benjamin EJ, et al. Cross-sectional correlates of increased aortic stiffness in the community: the Framingham Heart Study. Circulation 2007;115:2628–36.

49. Kawaguchi M, Hay I, Fetics B, et al. Combined ventricular systolic and arterial stiffening in patients with heart failure and preserved ejection fraction: implications for systolic and diastolic reserve limitations. Circulation 2003;107:714–20.

50. Henry RM, Kostense PJ, Spijkerman AM, et al. Arterial stiffness increases with deteriorating glucose tolerance status: the Hoorn Study. Circulation 2003;107:2089–95.

51. Schram MT, Henry RM, van Dijk RA, et al. Increased central artery stiffness in impaired glucose metabolism and type 2 diabetes: the Hoorn Study. Hypertension 2004;43:176–81.

52. van Heerebeek L, Hamdani N, Handoko ML, et al. Diastolic stiffness of the failing diabetic heart: importance of fibrosis, advanced glycation end products, and myocyte resting tension. Circulation 2008;117:43–51.

53. Rerkpattanapipat P, D'Agostino RB, Link KM, et al. Location of arterial stiffening differs in those with impaired fasting glucose versus diabetes. Diabetes 2009;58:946–53.

54. Stacey RB, Bertoni AG, Eng J, et al. Modification of the effect of glycemic status on aortic distensibility by age in the multi-ethnic study of atherosclerosis. Hypertension 2010;55:26–32.

55. Antonini-Canterin F, Carerj S, Di Bello V, et al. Arterial stiffness and ventricular stiffness: a couple of diseases or a coupling disease? A review from the cardiologist's point of view. Eur J Echocardiogr 2009;10:36–43.

56. Kenchaiah S, Narula J, Vasan RS. Risk factors for heart failure. Med Clin North Am 2004;88:1145–72.

57. Lewis EF, Moye LA, Rouleau JL, et al. Predictors of late development of heart failure in stable survivors of myocardial infarction: the CARE study. J Am Coll Cardiol 2003;42:1446–53.

58. Grundy SM, Cleeman JI, Daniels SR, et al. Diagnosis and management of the metabolic syndrome. an American Heart Association/National Heart, Lung, and Blood Institute Scientific statement. Circulation 2005;112(17):2735–52.

59. Wilson PW, D'Agostino RB, Parise H, et al. Metabolic syndrome as a precursor of cardiovascular disease and type 2 diabetes mellitus. Circulation 2005;112:3066–72.

60. Kathiresan S, Otvos JD, Sullivan LM, et al. Increased small low-density lipoprotein particle number: a prominent feature of the metabolic syndrome in the Framingham Heart Study. Circulation 2006;113:20–9.

61. Dhingra R, Sesso HD, Kenchaiah S, et al. Differential effects of lipids on the risk of heart failure and coronary heart disease: the Physicians' Health Study. Am Heart J 2008;155:869–75.

62. Pillutla P, Hwang YC, Augustus A, et al. Perfusion of hearts with triglyceride-rich particles reproduces the metabolic abnormalities in lipotoxic cardiomyopathy. Am J Physiol Endocrinol Metab 2005;288: E1229–35.

63. Velagaleti RS, Massaro J, Vasan RS, et al. Relations of lipid concentrations to heart failure incidence: the Framingham Heart Study. Circulation 2009; 120:2345–51.

64. Murray AJ, Anderson RE, Watson GC, et al. Uncoupling proteins in human heart. Lancet 2004;364: 1786–8.

65. Dutka DP, Pitt M, Pagano D, et al. Myocardial glucose transport and utilization in patients with type 2 diabetes mellitus, left ventricular dysfunction, and coronary artery disease. J Am Coll Cardiol 2006;48:2225–31.

66. Dávila-Román VG, Vedala G, Herrero P, et al. Altered myocardial fatty acid and glucose metabolism in idiopathic dilated cardiomyopathy. J Am Coll Cardiol 2002;40:271–7.

67. The Emerging Risk Factors Collaboration. Lipoprotein(a) concentration and the risk of coronary heart disease, stroke, and nonvascular mortality. JAMA 2009;302:412–23.

68. Sarma S, Ardehali H, Gheorghiade M. Enhancing the metabolic substrate: PPAR-alpha agonists in heart failure. Heart Fail Rev 2010. [Epub ahead of print].

69. Levy D, Larson MG, Vasan RS, et al. The progression from hypertension to congestive heart failure. JAMA 1996;275:1557–62.

70. Kawaguchi M, Techigawara M, Ishihata T, et al. A comparison of ultrastructural changes on endomyocardial biopsy specimens obtained from patients with diabetes mellitus with and without hypertension. Heart Vessels 1997;12:267–74.

71. Grossman E, Shemesh J, Shamiss A, et al. Left ventricular mass in diabetes-hypertension. Arch Intern Med 1992;152:1001–4.

72. ACCORD Study Group, Cushman WC, Evans GW, et al. Effects of intensive blood-pressure control in type 2 diabetes mellitus. N Engl J Med 2010;362: 1575–85.

73. Patel A. Effects of a fixed combination of perindopril and indapamide on macrovascular and microvascular outcomes in patients with type 2 diabetes mellitus (the ADVANCE trial): a randomised controlled trial. Lancet 2007;370:829–40.

74. Wing LMH, Reid CM, Ryan P, et al. A comparison of outcomes with angiotensin-converting–enzyme inhibitors and diuretics for hypertension in the elderly. N Engl J Med 2003;348:583–92.

75. Adler AI, Stratton IM, Neil HA, et al. Association of systolic blood pressure with macrovascular and

microvascular complications of type 2 diabetes (UKPDS 36): prospective observational study. BMJ 2000;321:412–9.

76. Tight blood pressure control and risk of macrovascular and microvascular complications in type 2 diabetes: UKPDS 38. BMJ 1998;317:703–13.

77. Turnbull F, Blood Pressure Lowering Treatment Trialists' Collaboration. Effects of different blood-pressure-lowering regimens on major cardiovascular events: results of prospectively-designed overviews of randomised trials. Lancet 2003;362: 1527–35.

78. Chobanian AV, Bakris GL, Black HR, et al. The seventh report of the joint national committee on prevention, detection, evaluation, and treatment of high blood pressure. JAMA 2003;289:2560–71.

79. Kenchaiah S, Evans JC, Levy D, et al. Obesity and the risk of heart failure. N Engl J Med 2002;347: 305–13.

80. Peterson LR, Herrero P, Schechtman KB, et al. Effect of obesity and insulin resistance on myocardial substrate metabolism and efficiency in young women. Circulation 2004;109:2191–6.

81. Sasson Z, Rasooly Y, Bhesania T, et al. Insulin resistance is an important determinant of left ventricular mass in the obese. Circulation 1993; 88:1431–6.

82. Kuperstein R, Hanly P, Niroumand M, et al. The importance of age and obesity on the relation between diabetes and left ventricular mass. J Am Coll Cardiol 2001;37:1957–62.

83. Taegtmeyer H, McNulty P, Young ME. Adaptation and maladaptation of the heart in diabetes: part I: general concepts. Circulation 2002;105:1727–33.

84. Young ME, McNulty P, Taegtmeyer H. Adaptation and maladaptation of the heart in diabetes: part II: potential mechanisms. Circulation 2002;105:1861–70.

85. Ungar I, Gilbert M, Siegel A, et al. Studies on myocardial metabolism. IV. Myocardial metabolism in diabetes. Am J Med 1955;18:385–96.

86. Boudina S, Abel ED. Diabetic cardiomyopathy revisited. Circulation 2007;115:3213–23.

87. Itani SI, Zhou Q, Pories WJ, et al. Involvement of protein kinase C in human skeletal muscle insulin resistance and obesity. Diabetes 2000;49: 1353–8.

88. McNulty PH, Louard RJ, Deckelbaum LI, et al. Hyperinsulinemiainhibits myocardial protein degradation in patients with cardiovascular disease and insulin resistance. Circulation 1995;92:2151–6.

89. Ren J, Samson WK, Sowers JR. Insulin-like growth factor I as a cardiac hormone: physiological and pathophysiological implications in heart disease. J Mol Cell Cardiol 1999;31:2049–61.

90. Bhimji S, Godin DV, McNeill JH. Biochemical and functional changes in hearts from rabbits with diabetes. Diabetologia 1985;28:452–7.

91. Avendano GF, Agarwal RK, Bashey RI, et al. Effects of glucose intolerance on myocardial function and collagen-linked glycation. Diabetes 1999; 48:1443–7.

92. Berg TJ, Snorgaard O, Faber J, et al. Serum levels of advanced glycation end products are associated with left ventricular diastolic function in patients with type 1 diabetes. Diabetes Care 1999;22:1186–90.

93. Wautier JL, Wautier MP, Schmidt AM, et al. Advanced glycation end products (AGEs) on the surface of diabetic erythrocytes bind to the vessel wall via a specific receptor inducing oxidant stress in the vasculature: a link between surface-associated AGEs and diabetic complications. Proc Natl Acad Sci U S A 1994;91:7742–6.

94. Brownlee M, Cerami A, Vlassara H. Advanced glycosylation end products in tissue and the biochemical basis of diabetic complications. N Engl J Med 1988;318:1315–21.

95. Nin JW, Jorsal A, Ferreira I, et al. Higher plasma soluble receptor for advanced glycation end products (sRAGE) levels are associated with incident cardiovascular disease and all-cause mortality in type 1 diabetes. Diabetes 2010;59:2027–32.

96. Candido R, Forbes JM, Thomas MC, et al. A breaker of advanced glycation end products attenuates diabetes-induced myocardial structural changes. Circ Res 2003;92:785–92.

97. Singal PK, Bello-Klein A, Farahmand F, et al. Oxidative stress and functional deficit in diabetic cardiomyopathy. Adv Exp Med Biol 2001;498:213–20.

98. Liang Q, Carlson EC, Donthi RV, et al. Overexpression of metallothionein reduces diabetic cardiomyopathy. Diabetes 2002;51:174–81.

99. Abe T, Ohga Y, Tabayashi N, et al. Left ventricular diastolic dysfunction in type 2 diabetes mellitus model rats. Am J Physiol Heart Circ Physiol 2002; 282:H138–48.

100. Cesario DA, Brar R, Shivkumar K. Alterations in ion channel physiology in diabetic cardiomyopathy. Endocrinol Metab Clin North Am 2006;35: 601–10.

101. Kuo TH, Moore KH, Giacomelli F, et al. Defective oxidative metabolism of heart mitochondria from genetically diabetic mice. Diabetes 1983;32:781–7.

102. Pierce GN, Dhalla NS. Heart mitochondrial function in chronic experimental diabetes in rats. Can J Cardiol 1985;1:48–54.

103. Tanaka Y, Konno N, Kako KJ. Mitochondrial dysfunction observed in situ in cardiomyocytes of rats in experimental diabetes. Cardiovasc Res 1992;26:409–14.

104. Shen X, Zheng S, Thongboonkerd V, et al. Cardiac mitochondrial damage and biogenesis in a chronic model of type 1 diabetes. Am J Physiol Endocrinol Metab 2004;287:E896–905.

105. Savabi F. Mitochondrial creatine phosphokinase deficiency in diabetic rat heart. Biochem Biophys Res Commun 1988;154:469–75.

106. Awaji Y, Hashimoto H, Matsui Y, et al. Isoenzyme profiles of creatine kinase, lactate dehydrogenase, and aspartate aminotransferase in the diabetic heart: comparison with hereditary and catecholamine cardiomyopathies. Cardiovasc Res 1990; 24:547–54.

107. Veksler VI, Murat I, Ventura-Clapier R. Creatine kinase and mechanical and mitochondrial functions in hereditary and diabetic cardiomyopathies. Can J Physiol Pharmacol 1991;69: 852–8.

108. Scheuermann-Freestone M, Madsen PL, Manners D, et al. Abnormal cardiac and skeletal muscle energy metabolism in patients with type 2 diabetes. Circulation 2003;107:3040–6.

109. Scognamiglio R, Avogaro A, Casara D, et al. Myocardial dysfunction and adrenergic cardiac innervation in patients with insulin-dependent diabetes mellitus. J Am Coll Cardiol 1998;31: 404–12.

110. Kahn JK, Zola B, Juni JE, et al. Radionuclide assessment of left ventricular diastolic filling in diabetes mellitus with and without cardiac autonomic neuropathy. J Am Coll Cardiol 1986;7: 1303–9.

111. Monteagudo PT, Moisés VA, Kohlmann O Jr, et al. Influence of autonomic neuropathy upon left ventricular dysfunction in insulin-dependent diabetic patients. Clin Cardiol 2000;23:371–5.

112. Young LH, Wackers FJT, Chyun DA, et al. Cardiac outcomes after screening for asymptomatic coronary artery disease in patients with type 2 diabetes. JAMA 2009;301:1547–55.

113. Sacre JW, Franjic B, Jellis CL, et al. Association of cardiac autonomic neuropathy with subclinical myocardial dysfunction in type 2 diabetes. JACC Cardiovasc Imaging 2010;3:1207–15.

114. Ones MJ, Hemandez-Pampaloni M, Schelbert H, et al. Coronary vasomotor abnormalities in insulin-resistant individuals. Ann Intern Med 2004;140: 700–8.

115. Taylor PD, Graves JE, Poston L. Selective impairment of acetylcholine-mediated endothelium-dependent relaxation in isolated resistance arteries of the streptozotocin-induced diabetic rat. Clin Sci (Lond) 1995;88:519–24.

116. Caporali A, Meloni M, Vollenkle C, et al. Deregulation of microRNA-503 contributes to diabetes mellitus-induced impairment of endothelial function and reparative angiogenesis after limb ischemia. Circulation 2011;123:282–91.

117. Chou E, Suzuma I, Way KJ, et al. Decreased cardiac expression of vascular endothelial growth factor and its receptors in insulin-resistant and diabetic states: a possible explanation for impaired collateral formation in cardiac tissue. Circulation 2002;105:373–9.

Arterial Stiffness/ Elasticity in the Contribution to Progression of Heart Failure

Daniel A. Duprez, MD, PhD

KEYWORDS

- Arterial stiffness • Arterial elasticity • Augmentation index
- Large artery elasticity • Pulse-wave velocity
- Small artery elasticity

Early identification of those at risk for heart failure can help prevent clinical overt heart failure or at least to delay the progression to heart failure. Individuals at risk for heart failure events are currently identified by screening for risk factors such as elevated blood pressure.[1,2] By identifying individuals on a trajectory of development for the development of heart failure, prior to the occurrence of symptoms or morbid events, a subpopulation may be identified that is likely to progress to clinical events, beyond prediction possible from classic risk factors for heart failure alone.

Systolic and diastolic blood pressure provides information only about the two extreme points of the arterial pressure waveform.[3] Arterial stiffness (which increases as arterial elasticity decreases) is a functional vascular marker that likely can capture an earlier phase of progression to heart failure. This article reviews the concepts of arterial stiffness/elasticity, the different measurement techniques, its predictive value for heart failure, and the effect of cardiovascular therapy on preventing heart failure or delaying its progression.

CONCEPT OF ARTERIAL STIFFNESS/ ELASTICITY
Physiologic Role of Arteries

A current approach consists of considering the blood pressure curve as the summation of a steady component, mean arterial blood pressure, and a pulsatile component, pulse pressure. Mean arterial blood pressure, the product of cardiac output multiplied by total peripheral resistance, is the pressure for the average flow of blood and oxygen to peripheral tissues and organs. The pulse pressure is linked to clinical events. The pulse pressure is influenced by several cardiac and vascular factors, but it is the role of large conduit arteries, mainly the aorta, to minimize pulsatility. In addition to the pattern of left ventricular ejection, the determinants of pulse pressure and systolic blood pressure include the cushioning capacity of arteries and the timing and intensity of wave reflections.[4] The former is influenced by arterial stiffness, usually expressed in the quantitative terms of compliance and distensibility. The latter results from the summation of a forward wave coming

Financial Disclosures: Dr Daniel Duprez received grant support from NIH, Roche, Genetech, Novartis, Merck; has been on advisory board of Novartis, Genetech, Abbott, Pfizer; received honorarium from Novartis, Pfizer, Forest Laboratories.
Cardiovascular Division, University of Minnesota, Minneapolis, 420 Delaware Street South East, MMC 508, Minneapolis, MN 55455, USA
E-mail address: dupre007@umn.edu

Heart Failure Clin 8 (2012) 135–141
doi:10.1016/j.hfc.2011.08.001
1551-7136/12/$ – see front matter © 2012 Elsevier Inc. All rights reserved.

from the heart and propagating at a given speed (pulse-wave velocity [PWV]) toward the origin of resistance vessels and a backward wave returning toward the heart from particular sites characterized by specific reflection indices.[5,6] Information about the interaction between the left ventricle and the physical properties of the arterial circulation can be derived by the descriptive and quantitative analysis of the arterial pressure pulse waveform.

Ejection of blood into the aorta generates a pressure wave that is propagated to other arteries throughout the body. As in elastic conduits, this forward-traveling pressure wave may be reflected at all points of structural and/or functional discontinuity of the arterial tree. From these different points of discontinuity, mainly located in the distal arteries at the branching origins of arterioles, a reflected wave is generated that travels backward toward the ascending aorta. Thus, incident and reflected pressure waves are in constant interaction along the arterial circuit and are summed up into the actual pressure wave. The final amplitude and shape of the measured aortic blood pressure wave are determined by the phase relationship (timing) between these two component waves. The timing of incident and reflected pressure waves depends on PWV, the traveling distance of pressure waves, and the duration of ventricular ejection. In young subjects, under physiologic conditions the backward pressure wave returns from the distal arterial compartment during diastole, making pulse pressure higher in peripheral than in central arteries. This physiologic phenomenon is called pulse pressure amplification. With heightened PWV, the reflecting sites of the distal compartment appear closer to the ascending aorta and the reflected waves occur earlier, being more closely in phase with incident waves in this region. Such an earlier return of wave reflections means that the reflected wave affects the central arteries during systole and not during diastole. This disturbed signal results in an augmentation of aortic and ventricular pressures during systole, and reduces aortic pressure during diastole. Altered mechanical properties of the aortic wall influence the level of aortic systolic blood pressure, which is increased, and diastolic blood pressure, which is decreased, as a consequence of early wave reflections. Both animal and human studies have demonstrated that a loading sequence characterized by prominent late systolic load adversely affects the left ventricular structure and function.[7,8,9] Finally, all these findings taken together indicate that a disturbed pressure signal arising from the distal arteries through disturbed wave reflections may alter the ventricular-

vascular coupling and lead to an increased risk for heart failure.[10]

Wave reflections alter the ventricular-vascular coupling not only through increased arterial stiffness and changed timing but also through modifications in their amplitude.[11] Such possibilities depend on the arterial wave reflection properties arising from the distal part of the arterial tree. These wave reflections are influenced by the geometry, number, structure, and function of smaller muscular arteries and arterioles. Arterial and arteriolar constriction results in earlier wave reflections at the aortic level and consequently an increased pulse pressure. It appears that elastic arteries buffer the pulsations, muscular arteries actively alter propagation velocity, and arterioles serve as major reflection sites. Each of these alterations (or their combination) enables a cross-talk between the proximal and distal compartments of the arterial tree, which leads to the predominant or selective increases of systolic blood pressure and pulse pressure. In the presence of decreased ventricular ejection, these frequency-dependent factors disturb the ventricular-vascular coupling, increase the load of the heart, and favor cardiac hypertrophy, heart failure and, ultimately, cardiovascular death.

Physiologic Effects of Vascular Wall Alterations

All arteries have certain characteristics of compliance that can be defined as the increase in caliber for a given increase in pressure (dV/dP, where dV is the change in artery volume over a linear length and dP is the increase in pressure during the cardiac cycle). The smaller arteries and arterioles only provide resistance to flow, which is sensitive to changes in the caliber of these vessels. Conduit artery compliance is a critical determinant of their storage capacity during systole. Much of the stroke volume delivered by the ventricle is accommodated in the pressure-dependent increase in arterial caliber, and this volume is released during diastole to help maintain diastolic pressure. With reduced conduit artery compliance there is decreased storage of stroke volume, leading to a greater increase in systolic pressure to distend the noncompliant arterial bed. This process results in an increased workload on the left ventricle and a decrease in aortic diastolic pressure.

The stiffness/elasticity of the more distal arterial system serves to dampen the arterial pulse wave during its transmission through the arterial bed. A decrease in cushioning effect results in a greater magnitude and frequency of oscillations, which have their origin at these sites in the vascular bed.[4] The pressure response to these oscillations results from a complex interaction of the storage volume of these cushioning vessels, the compliance of the more proximal arterial system, and the PWV that influences the rate at which these reflections are transmitted back to the root of the aorta. Compliance of the arterioles also will influence pulsatile vascular resistance. To the extent that pulsatile pressure is transmitted to the arterioles, the caliber of these vessels, and thus the resistance, will vary throughout the cardiac cycle, depending on the compliance of these vessels.

It is well known that arterial wave reflections affect the left ventricular afterload.[12–14] Due to the finite wave transit time from the heart to reflection sites and back to the proximal aorta, wave reflections typically increase left ventricular afterload in mid-to-late systole. For any given level of systolic blood pressure, a pattern characterized by prominent late-systolic load has been unequivocally demonstrated to exert deleterious effects on left ventricular structure and function. Wave reflections are thought to occur predominantly in muscular (medium-sized) and smaller arterial segments, and can be modified by pharmacologic agents.

MEASUREMENT OF ARTERIAL STIFFNESS

The arterial pressure wave has two principal components: the wave generated by the heart, which travels away from the heart, and the reflected wave, which returns to the heart from peripheral sites, predominantly in the lower part of the body. In considering arterial stiffness it is important to recognize that stiffness of the aorta, the muscular conduit arteries, the more peripheral branch points, and microvascular components all differ in mechanism and significance.[3] Aging affects all segments of the vasculature because of structural alterations in collagen, elastin, and interstitium, but functional changes in vascular smooth muscle predominantly the microcirculation.[4] Pulse pressure, the difference between the systolic and diastolic blood pressure, has been considered in the past to be one of the simplest measures of arterial stiffness.[3] However, pulse pressure alone is inadequate to assess arterial stiffness accurately. Problems include the "normal" amplification of the pressure wave as it travels from the aorta to the periphery.

Noninvasive measurement of arterial stiffness entails measurement of surrogate parameters that are intrinsically associated with stiffness. This evaluation involves 3 main methodologies: (1) pulse transit time or PWV; (2) analysis of the arterial pressure pulse and its wave contour; and

(3) direct stiffness estimation using measurements of diameter and distending pressure.[4,15] These surrogate parameters are related to the functional effects of arterial stiffness, and as such can be used to quantify changes. Several computerized devices are now available that enable quantification of global indices of stiffness, as well as regional and local abnormalities.

The velocity of propagation of the pulse wave through the arterial tree is directly related to the stiffness of the arterial system between the sensors detecting the waveform. PWV is limited to the assessment of conduit artery structural changes. The most frequent assessment is between the carotid artery, as equivalent to the root of the aorta, and more distal accessible sites such as the femoral artery. This relationship has served as the basis for measuring PWV as a guide to arterial health. Many studies have demonstrated its correlation in a variety of clinical conditions with future atherosclerotic morbid events.[16–21]

Another approach to estimate arterial stiffness is the systolic pulse contour analysis.[15,22] The systolic arterial pressure wave is composed of an initial incident wave generated by the left ventricle and reflected waves from oscillations induced by interaction of the incident wave at branch points in the circulation. The magnitude of these wave reflections is dependent in part on the elasticity characteristics of the small arteries, and the timing of this reflection to be superimposed on the incident wave. A second systolic peak or plateau can usually be detected in peripheral artery waveforms, and is assumed to represent these reflected waves. In radial artery waveforms the second peak may be a pressure bump late in systole, or may occur early and even surpass the pressure of the incident wave. The ratio of this second peak pressure to the first peak pressure can be calculated as an augmentation index. A commercial device designed to calculate augmentation index uses a transfer function to recreate the presumed central arterial waveform from which the augmentation index is computed. The transfer function is used primarily as a means of calculating central arterial pressure, which may provide a better guide to systemic pressure than the usually measured arm cuff pressure. The augmentation index increases with age. and is increased in clinical situations associated with cardiovascular disease and prognosis.[23] In the Framingham study augmentation index, central pulse pressure and pulse pressure amplification were not related to cardiovascular outcomes in multivariable models.[24]

Analysis of the diastolic pulse contour allows the assessment of the vascular influence on arterial pressure independent of left ventricular ejection during systole. The analysis of the diastolic pulse contour is done using a modified Windkessel model, which calculates the large artery elasticity (LAE) and small artery elasticity (SAE).[25] LAE and SAE are derived from an algebraic decomposition of the diastolic waveform into one part that is primarily declining between aortic closure and aortic opening (decaying exponential function), and a second part that is largely flat but may be oscillating (sinusoidal function dampened by a decaying exponential function).[25] For this reason LAE has historically been referred to as "proximal, capacitive compliance" and relates to the loss of pressure during diastole, whereas SAE has historically been referred to as "distal, oscillatory, or reflective compliance." SAE has also been used as a surrogate marker for endothelial (dys) function.[26] A single-center retrospective study showed that reduced SAE was significantly associated with cardiovascular events, independent of age.[27]

There is substantial discussion about the meaning of each of the proposed measures of arterial elasticity **Fig. 1** illustrates the different parameters of arterial stiffness/elasticity and the information they provide along the arterial system. The PWV (derived from behavior of the large arteries), augmentation index (derived from the systolic waveform), and SAE (derived from the oscillatory component of the diastolic waveform) appear to impart some common information, given that they are correlated in several studies.[15,28] However, there are also differences among the measures, best illustrated in the Anglo-Cardiff Collaborative Trial, where a different age course was seen for augmentation index (increased rapidly during middle age and slowly in the elderly) than for PWV (changed slowly during middle age and rapidly in the elderly).[29] Morbidity and mortality studies comparing and contrasting these 3 and other measures would be useful.

PREDICTIVE VALUE FOR PROGRESSION TO HEART FAILURE

There have been several studies performed in asymptomatic subjects in whom different parameters estimating arterial stiffness/elasticity were studied to predict cardiovascular morbidity and mortality. In the majority of these studies new onset of heart failure was included in the total number of cardiovascular disease events or was not considered.

There is limited information in the literature regarding arterial stiffness/elasticity and the progression to heart failure. Sutton-Tyrrell and colleagues[17] measured aortic PWV at baseline in 2488 participants (age range between 70 and 79 years) from the Health, Aging and Body Composition (Health ABC) study. Vital status, cause of death, coronary heart disease, stroke, and congestive heart failure were determined from medical records. Over 4.6 years 265 deaths occurred, 111 as a result of cardiovascular cause. There were 341 coronary heart disease events, 94 stroke events, and 181 cases of congestive heart failure. Initially, outcomes analysis was run with aortic PWV as a continuous variable, and significant associations were found between higher aortic PWV and each of the outcomes evaluated: odds ratios per unit of log (PWV) were 1.6 (95% confidence interval [CI], 1.2–2.2) for total mortality, 1.8 (95% CI, 1.1–2.8) for cardiovascular mortality, 1.4 (95% CI, 1.1–1.8) for coronary heart disease, 2.0 (95% CI, 1.2–3.2) for stroke, and 1.5 (95% CI, 1.0–2.1) for congestive heart failure ($P<.05$ for all). When the variable was divided into sex-specific quartiles, aortic PWV was significantly associated with coronary heart disease ($P = .007$) and stroke ($P<.001$), but not congestive heart failure ($P = .328$).After adjustment of age, gender, race, and systolic blood pressure, aortic PWV remained significantly associated with all end

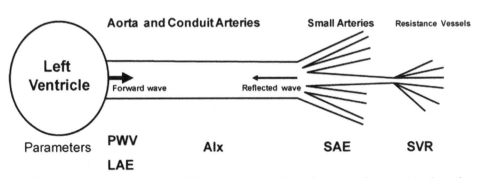

Fig. 1. The different parameters of arterial stiffness/elasticity and the information they provide along the arterial system. AIx, augmentation index; LAE, large artery elasticity; PWV, pulsewave velocity; SAE, small artery elasticity; SVR, systemic vascular resistance.

points except congestive heart failure. It is somewhat surprising that aortic PWV was not found to be associated with congestive heart failure. The increased afterload that accompanies the early reflected pressure wave in the setting of vascular stiffening results in increased left ventricular mass and eventually congestive heart failure. It could be that the blood pressure parameters are so overwhelmingly related to congestive heart failure that this masks the ability to observe a separate effect of aortic PWV.

The Multi-Ethnic Study of Atherosclerosis (MESA) found that lower small artery elasticity was the strongest predictor of incident hypertension out of several measures, including measures of large arterial stiffness and aorta distensibility.[30] At baseline of the MESA, LAE and SAE were derived from the diastolic pulse contour analysis of the noninvasive recording from the radial artery waveform using a tonometer.[31] Of the 6814 MESA participants free of overt cardiovascular disease, the procedure was performed in 6630 subjects in whom LAE and SAE were eligible for analysis. During a median of 5.8 years of follow-up, 454 adjudicated cardiovascular disease events occurred, including 256 coronary heart disease events, 93 strokes, and 126 heart failures. With 454 incident cardiovascular disease events, compared with the highest (most elastic) SAE quartile, the hazard ratio (HR) in the lowest (stiffest) SAE quartile in the fully adjusted model (model 2) was 2.28 (95% CI, 1.55–3.36) with graded risk in the intermediate quartiles. Risk for each cardiovascular entity was similarly significantly increased, generally in a graded fashion, in the presence of less elastic small arteries. For heart failure specifically, the HR for the first quartile of SAE compared with the fourth quartile was 2.47 (95% CI, 1.22–4.99; $P = .005$) after adjustment for age, race/ethnicity, gender, clinic, and height (model 1). After adjustment for all the parameters in model 1 and adding the covariates of heart rate, systolic and diastolic blood pressure, use of blood pressure–lowering medication, body mass index, ever smoking, current smoking, total cholesterol, high-density lipoprotein cholesterol, triglycerides, use of cholesterol-lowering medication, diabetes and C-reactive protein (model 2), the HR was 2.36 (95% CI, 1.12–4.94; $P = .01$). LAE was predictive for several of the cardiovascular outcome variables in model 1, but retained statistical significance in model 2 only in the prediction of heart failure ($P = .03$). Addition of SAE to model 2 for heart failure improved the P value for LAE to 0.06.

The findings in the MESA clearly demonstrated that SAE and arterial wave reflections represent important novel functional markers in the general population, which have predictive value for the development of heart failure beyond arterial blood pressure and other classic risk factors. The major question remains as to which preventive therapy and pharmacotherapy could prevent the progression toward systolic heart failure or diastolic heart failure with preserved ejection fraction.

EFFECT OF CARDIOVASCULAR THERAPY ON ARTERIAL STIFFNESS/ELASTICITY

Therapy to prevent heart failure might focus on improving SAE to reduce the contribution of wave reflections to left ventricular afterload. Attenuation of arterial stiffness/elasticity may reflect the true reduction of arterial wall damage, whereas blood pressure, blood glucose, and lipids can be normalized in a few weeks by using antihypertensive, antidiabetic, and lipid-lowering drugs, leading to a strong reduction in cardiovascular risk scores but without any improvement of atherosclerotic lesions and arterial stiffness, which requires a long-lasting correction of biochemical abnormalities.[32] A temporal dissociation is thus expected between the improvement of cardiovascular risk factors and an increased arterial stiffness.

Whether classes of antihypertensive agents vary in their efficacy to affect arterial structure and thus influence arterial stiffness/elasticity via a pressure-independent mechanism is controversial, and remains to be evaluated in large-scale trials.

Most of the published studies have included small groups of patients and are thus underpowered to conclude a lack of efficacy of one drug versus another. Moreover, several studies are short-term studies in which the effect of antihypertensives on the arterial system was studied during a period of 4 weeks or less. Long-term studies are much more important in knowing the effect of the antihypertensive agent on the vascular tree beyond blood pressure lowering.[3]

Despite these limitations, it is so far generally accepted that angiotensin-converting enzyme inhibitors, angiotensin II receptor blockers, aldosterone antagonists, calcium antagonists (especially dihydropyridines), and nitrates share a similar ability to decrease arterial stiffness.[32–38] It is also well accepted that the nonselective β-blocker propranolol and the selective β-blocker atenolol are less efficacious during long-term treatment than β-blockers with vasodilating properties.[39,40] Nitrates reduce mainly arterial stiffness of the large arteries.[41] α-Blockers appear to protect neither the vasculature nor the heart, even though they lower blood pressure. Diuretics have not been subject to as much careful study.

The effects of a given drug on arterial stiffness are complex and vary with time. The effects of a vasodilatory drug on the arterial wall may be direct, occurring by relaxation of the smooth muscle predominantly in the arterial media or by improving endothelial function. The effects may be indirect, occurring as a consequence of both a decrease in wave reflection in response to the dilation, and an increase in SAE in response to dilation of resistance vessels. Other indirect effects are structural and are due to the changes in vessel lumen or wall structure under long-term treatment. Pharmacologic trials for vascular health protection should focus not only on large arteries but also on small arteries.[42] Further studies are necessary to document whether improvements by pharmacologic interventions focused on improvement of arterial stiffness/elasticity will also be linked to improvement in cardiovascular outcome, especially in the delay of progression of heart failure. Novel therapy for heart failure should also be evaluated for its effect on arterial stiffness/elasticity.

SUMMARY

Heart failure is a major health-economic burden. Diastolic heart failure characterized by diastolic dysfunction with preserved systolic function has become a major challenge in the diagnosis of and therapy for heart failure beyond systolic heart failure. There is an urgent need for early detection of heart failure and identification of its causes. Arterial stiffness/elasticity and arterial wave reflections play an important pathophysiological role in this process. Assessment of arterial stiffness/elasticity adds further prognostic information beyond arterial blood pressure and other classic risk factors for the development of heart failure. Certain pharmacologic agents have beneficial properties on these functional characteristics, and improve the ventricular-vascular coupling. Future cardiovascular therapy should be evaluated for its effect on arterial stiffness/elasticity improvement in preventing heart failure or delaying its progression.

REFERENCES

1. Duprez DA, Cohn JN. Identifying early cardiovascular disease to target candidates for treatment. J Clin Hypertens (Greenwich) 2008;10(3):226–31.
2. Cohn JN, Duprez DA. Time to foster a rational approach to preventing cardiovascular morbid events. J Am Coll Cardiol 2008;52(5):327–9.
3. Duprez DA, Cohn JN. Monitoring vascular health beyond blood pressure. Curr Hypertens Rep 2006; 8(4):287–91.
4. Cohn JN, Duprez DA, Finkelstein SM. Comprehensive noninvasive arterial vascular evaluation. Future Cardiol 2009;5(6):573–9.
5. Chirinos JA, Segers P. Noninvasive evaluation of left ventricular afterload: part 1: pressure and flow measurements and basic principles of wave conduction and reflection. Hypertension 2010;56(4):555–62.
6. Chirinos JA, Segers P. Noninvasive evaluation of left ventricular afterload: part 2: arterial pressure-flow and pressure-volume relations in humans. Hypertension 2010;56(4):563–70.
7. Kobayashi S, Yano M, Kohno M, et al. Influence of aortic impedance on the development of pressure-overload left ventricular hypertrophy in rats. Circulation 1996;94(12):3362–8.
8. Hashimoto J, Westerhof BE, Westerhof N, et al. Different role of wave reflection magnitude and timing on left ventricular mass reduction during antihypertensive treatment. J Hypertens 2008;26(5):1017–24.
9. Borlaug BA, Melenovsky V, Redfield MM, et al. Impact of arterial load and loading sequence on left ventricular tissue velocities in humans. J Am Coll Cardiol 2007;50(16):1570–7.
10. Kass DA. Ventricular arterial stiffening: integrating the pathophysiology. Hypertension 2005;46(1):185–93.
11. Westerhof N, et al. Forward and backward waves in the arterial system. Cardiovasc Res 1972;6(6):648–56.
12. Laskey WK, Kussmaul WG. Arterial wave reflection in heart failure. Circulation 1987;75(4):711–22.
13. Pepine CJ, Nichols WW, Curry RC Jr, et al. Aortic input impedance during nitroprusside infusion. A reconsideration of afterload reduction and beneficial action. J Clin Invest 1979;64(2):643–54.
14. Chirinos JA, Segers P, Gupta AK, et al. Time-varying myocardial stress and systolic pressure-stress relationship: role in myocardial-arterial coupling in hypertension. Circulation 2009;119(21):2798–807.
15. Duprez DA, et al. Determinants of radial artery pulse wave analysis in asymptomatic individuals. Am J Hypertens 2004;17(8):647–53.
16. Duprez DA, Kaiser DR, Whitwam W, et al. Arterial stiffness as a risk factor for coronary atherosclerosis. Curr Atheroscler Rep 2007;9(2):139–44.
17. Sutton-Tyrrell K, Najjar SS, Boudreau RM, et al. Elevated aortic pulse wave velocity, a marker of arterial stiffness, predicts cardiovascular events in well-functioning older adults. Circulation 2005;111(25):3384–90.
18. Willum-Hansen T, Staessen JA, Torp-Pedersen C, et al. Prognostic value of aortic pulse wave velocity as index of arterial stiffness in the general population. Circulation 2006;113(5):664–70.
19. Mattace-Raso FU, van der Cammen TJ, Hofman A, et al. Arterial stiffness and risk of coronary heart disease and stroke: the Rotterdam Study. Circulation 2006;113(5):657–63.

20. Meaume S, Benetos A, Henry OF, et al. Aortic pulse wave velocity predicts cardiovascular mortality in subjects >70 years of age. Arterioscler Thromb Vasc Biol 2001;21(12):2046–50.

21. Shokawa T, Imazu M, Yamamoto H, et al. Pulse wave velocity predicts cardiovascular mortality: findings from the Hawaii-Los Angeles-Hiroshima study. Circ J 2005;69(3):259–64.

22. Kelly R, Hayward C, Avolio A, et al. Noninvasive determination of age-related changes in the human arterial pulse. Circulation 1989;80(6):1652–9.

23. Vlachopoulos C, Aznaouridis K, O'Rourke MF, et al. Prediction of cardiovascular events and all-cause mortality with central haemodynamics: a systematic review and meta-analysis. Eur Heart J 2010;31(15):1865–71.

24. Mitchell GF, Hwang SJ, Vasan RS, et al. Arterial stiffness and cardiovascular events: the Framingham Heart Study. Circulation 2010;121(4):505–11.

25. Finkelstein SM, Collins VR, Cohn JN. Arterial vascular compliance response to vasodilators by Fourier and pulse contour analysis. Hypertension 1988;12(4):380–7.

26. Gilani M, Kaiser DR, Bratteli CW, et al. Role of nitric oxide deficiency and its detection as a risk factor in pre-hypertension. J Am Soc Hypertens 2007;1(1):45–55.

27. Grey E, Bratteli C, Glasser SP, et al. Reduced small artery but not large artery elasticity is an independent risk marker for cardiovascular events. Am J Hypertens 2003;16(4):265–9.

28. Protogerou AD, Safar ME. Dissociation between central augmentation index and carotid-femoral pulse-wave velocity: when and why? Am J Hypertens 2007;20(6):648–9.

29. McEniery CM, Yasmin, Hall IR, et al. Normal vascular aging: differential effects on wave reflection and aortic pulse wave velocity: the Anglo-Cardiff Collaborative Trial (ACCT). J Am Coll Cardiol 2005;46(9):1753–60.

30. Peralta CA, Adeney KL, Shilpak MG, et al. Structural and functional vascular alterations and incident hypertension in normotensive adults: the Multi-Ethnic Study of Atherosclerosis. Am J Epidemiol 2010;171(1):63–71.

31. Duprez DA, Jacobs DR Jr, Lutsey PL, et al. Association of small artery elasticity with incident cardiovascular disease in older adults: the multi-ethnic study of atherosclerosis. Am J Epidemiol 2011;174(5):528–36.

32. Duprez DA. Is vascular stiffness a target for therapy? Cardiovasc Drugs Ther 2010;24(4):305–10.

33. Duprez D, De Buyzere M, Brusselmans F, et al. Comparison of lisinopril and nitrendipine on the pulsatility index in mild essential arterial hypertension. Cardiovasc Drugs Ther 1992;6(4):399–402.

34. Duprez DA, Florea ND, Jones K, et al. Beneficial effects of valsartan in asymptomatic individuals with vascular or cardiac abnormalities: the DETECTIV Pilot Study. J Am Coll Cardiol 2007;50(9):835–9.

35. White WB, Duprez D, St Hillaire R, et al. Effects of the selective aldosterone blocker eplerenone versus the calcium antagonist amlodipine in systolic hypertension. Hypertension 2003;41(5):1021–6.

36. Resnick LM, Lester MH. Differential effects of antihypertensive drug therapy on arterial compliance. Am J Hypertens 2002;15(12):1096–100.

37. Safar ME. Can antihypertensive treatment reverse large-artery stiffening? Curr Hypertens Rep 2010;12(1):47–51.

38. Safar ME, Jankowski P. Antihypertensive therapy and de-stiffening of the arteries. Expert Opin Pharmacother 2010;11(16):2625–34.

39. Schiffrin EL. Circulatory therapeutics: use of antihypertensive agents and their effects on the vasculature. J Cell Mol Med 2010;14(5):1018–29.

40. Rehman A, Schiffrin EL. Vascular effects of antihypertensive drug therapy. Curr Hypertens Rep 2010;12(4):226–32.

41. Smulyan H. Nitrates, arterial function, wave reflections and coronary heart disease. Adv Cardiol 2007;44:302–14.

42. Rizzoni D, Muiesan ML, Porteri E, et al. Vascular remodeling, macro- and microvessels: therapeutic implications. Blood Press 2009;18(5):242–6.

Aging-Associated Cardiovascular Changes and Their Relationship to Heart Failure

James B. Strait, MD, PhD[a],*, Edward G. Lakatta, MD[b]

KEYWORDS

- Heart failure • Cardiovascular aging • Cardiac function
- Cardiac reserve

Although aging does not itself cause heart failure (HF), it does lower the threshold for manifestation of the disease. As the populations of most developed countries continue to become older, on average, the importance of aging as a risk factor for all cardiovascular disease (CVD) increases in kind (**Fig. 1**). In the United States alone, it is estimated that there will be 70 million people older than 65 by 2030, representing almost 25% of the population.[1] In many respects, HF can be thought of as the quintessential final cardiovascular aging pathway, representing the convergence of age-associated changes in cardiovascular structure and function, aging changes in other organ systems, and the progressive increase in cardiovascular diseases in the elderly.

With the success of treatment options for ischemic and valvular diseases, there is an increasing number of older individuals with some degree of cardiac damage, type B heart failure at a minimum, who are increasingly imperiled by the diminished cardiac reserve associated with normal aging. Half of all HF cases are found within the 6% of the US population that is older than 75[2] (reviewed by Najjar and colleagues[3]). These individuals often go on to develop more severe cardiac dysfunction with time. In contrast to other cardiovascular disorders, the prevalence of chronic heart failure (CHF) is increasing, with approximately 5.7 million Americans with CHF.[4] The incidence of HF doubles with each decade of life and the prevalence rises to almost 10% of those older than 80 years. CHF is a highly lethal condition, with significant mortality, morbidity, and associated costs in the older population. More than 90% of CHF deaths occur in adults older than 65 years. CHF is also the leading cause of hospitalization in Medicare beneficiaries, with those older than 65 accounting for 75% of the 1.1 million HF discharge diagnoses.[4]

This article focuses on what is known about normal cardiovascular aging and the role that aging-associated changes play in reducing cardiac reserve to make the heart more susceptible to failure. There are a number of factors that link aging to HF[5] and gradually reduce the amount of cardiac reserve until finally the heart is "more likely to fail" (**Fig. 2**).

1. Structural changes: There is significant structural change in the heart and vasculature (eg, vascular stiffening, increased left ventricular [LV] wall thickness [within normal limits], and fibrosis) with aging, leading to diastolic

[a] Human Cardiovascular Studies, Laboratory of Cardiovascular Science, Intramural Research Program, Clinical Research Branch, National Institute on Aging, National Institutes of Health, Harbor Hospital, NM-500, 3001 South Hanover Street, Baltimore, MD 21225, USA
[b] Laboratory of Cardiovascular Science, Intramural Research Program, Gerontology Research Center, National Institute on Aging, National Institutes of Health, 5600 Nathan Shock Drive, Baltimore, MD 21224-6825, USA
* Corresponding author.
E-mail address: Straitj@mail.nih.gov

Heart Failure Clin 8 (2012) 143–164
doi:10.1016/j.hfc.2011.08.011
1551-7136/12/$ – see front matter Published by Elsevier Inc.

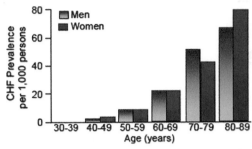

Fig. 1. Average prevalence of heart failure according to age and sex: Framingham Heart Study, 16-year follow-up. (*Data from* McKee PA, Castelli WP, McNamara PM, et al. The natural history of congestive heart failure: the Framingham study. N Engl J Med 1971;285:7796.)

dysfunction, increased afterload, and HF with preserved ejection fraction (HFpEF).[6,7] These are described individually in the *Cardiac structural* and *Central Arterial structural* sections later in this article.

2. Functional changes: There are functional changes and compensatory responses that the aged heart undergoes that diminish its ability to respond to increased workload and decrease its reserve capacity (eg, changes in maximal heart rate, end-systolic volume [ESV], end-diastolic volume [EDV], contractility, prolonged systolic contraction, prolonged diastolic

relaxation, and sympathetic signaling). These are described individually in the *Cardiac functional,* *Vascular functional,* and *Arterial-ventricular interaction* sections later in this article.

3. Cardioprotection and repair processes: The cardiac mechanisms responsible for protection from injury and injury repair become increasingly defective with age, leading to accentuated adverse remodeling and increased dysfunction.

4. Increased CVD incidence and prevalence: There is a progressive increase in the prevalence of CVD (eg, coronary artery disease [CAD], hypertension, and diabetes), leading to the development of ischemic, hypertensive, or diabetic cardiomyopathy. The reader is referred to any number of epidemiologic studies for evidence of this fact.

5. Systemic disease/Other organ systems: Aging-associated changes in other organ systems may affect cardiac structure-function and thereby contribute to HF development. This facet, however, is beyond the scope of the current review.

CARDIOVASCULAR CHANGES WITH AGING
Cardiac Changes at Rest and with Exercise

Cardiac structural changes
As described in **Table 1** and **Fig. 3**, there are structural and functional changes in the heart with

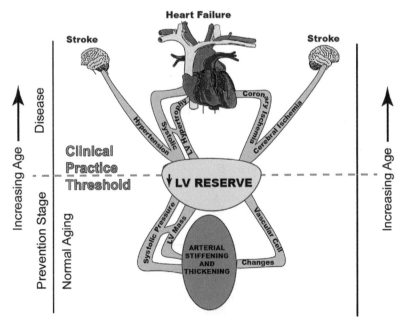

Fig. 2. Pathways linking aging to heart failure. (*Modified from* Lakatta EG. Age-associated cardiovascular changes in health: impact on cardiovascular disease in older persons. Heart Failure Rev 2002;7(1):1480; with permission.)

Table 1
Relationship of cardiovascular human aging in health to cardiovascular disease

Age-Associated Changes	Plausible Mechanisms	Possible Relation to Human Disease
Cardiovascular structural remodeling		
↑Vascular intimal thickness	↑Migration of and ↑matrix production by VSMC Possible derivation of intimal cells from other sources	Early stages of atherosclerosis
↑Vascular stiffness	Elastin fragmentation ↑Elastase activity ↑Collagen production by VSMC and ↑ cross-linking of collagen Altered growth factor regulation/tissue repair mechanisms	Systolic hypertension LV wall thickening Stroke Atherosclerosis
↑LV wall thickness	↑LV myocyte size with altered Ca^{2+} handling ↓Myocyte number (necrotic and apoptotic death) Altered growth factor regulation Focal matrix collagen deposition	Retarded early diastolic cardiac filling ↑Cardiac filling pressure Lower threshold for dyspnea ↑Likelihood of heart failure with relatively normal systolic function
↑Left atrial size	↑Left atrial pressure/volume	↑Prevalence of lone atrial fibrillation and other atrial arrhythmias
Cardiovascular functional changes		
Altered regulation of vascular tone	↓NO production/effects	Vascular stiffening; hypertension Early atherosclerosis
Reduced threshold for cell Ca^{2+} overload	Changes in gene expression of proteins that regulate Ca^{2+} handling; increased ω6ω3 PUFA ration in cardiac membranes	Lower threshold for atrial and ventricular arrhythmia Increases myocyte death Increased fibrosis
↑Cardiovascular reserve		Lower threshold for, and increased severity of heart failure
Reduced physical activity	Learned lifestyle	Exaggerated age changes in some aspects of cardiovascular structure and function. Negative impact on atherosclerotic vascular disease, hypertension, and heart failure

Abbreviations: LV, Left ventricular; PUFA, polyunsaturated fatty acids.

aging, and each of these can have significant implications for CVD. Structurally, there is a significant increase in myocardial thickness[8] as a result of increased cardiomyocyte size.[9] In addition, the heart changes its overall shape from elliptical to spheroid, with an asymmetric increase in the interventricular septum more than the free wall.[10] These changes in thickness and shape have important implications for cardiac wall stress and overall contractile efficiency.

The understanding of the changes in LV mass with aging has developed over time as researchers have made improvements in exclusion criteria, statistical correction, and technological approach. The history of this development provides a useful insight into the difficulties in conducting aging research. Initially, autopsy-based studies provided data that suggested cardiac mass increased significantly with aging.[11] Initial echocardiographic studies that calculated LV mass by wall thickness

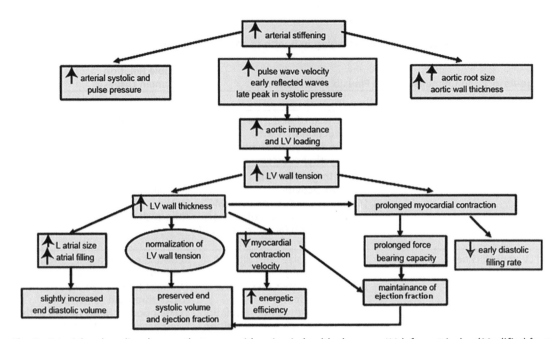

Fig. 3. Arterial and cardiac changes that occur with aging in healthy humans. LV, left ventricular. (*Modified from* Lakatta EG. Cardiovascular regulatory mechanisms in advanced age. Physiol Rev 1993;73:413–65; with permission.)

measurements corroborated these findings; however, measurements made from autopsies on subjects free from hypertension and CAD then corrected for body surface area, suggested that there is actually no change in the cardiac mass of men with aging.[7] Similarly, autopsies of hospitalized patients free of CVD did not show an increase in cardiac mass with aging. In fact, they found a decrease in the cardiac mass of men and no change in cardiac mass for women. This finding has received support from a magnetic resonance imaging–based study of healthy participants in the Baltimore Longitudinal Study of Aging (BLSA),[10] as well as multiple echocardiographic studies.[12,13] Based on these and other studies, it now appears that there is no change in LV mass in women and an actual decrease in LV mass in men with aging. The increased wall thickness represents an asymmetric increase in the interventricular septum more than the free wall redistributing cardiac muscle, but not increasing total cardiac mass.

Cardiac Functional Changes

Despite the aging-associated changes that may limit a person's functional capacity and promote vascular stiffening with consequent increased afterload, the overall resting systolic function of cardiac muscle does not change (see **Fig. 3**) with healthy aging. Examination of echocardiographic LV shortening fraction[14] and radionuclide ejection fraction (EF) in normotensive subjects

and healthy persons of different ages[15] has repeatedly confirmed the stability of cardiac EF at rest (normal average EF >65%). This is not to say that there is no change in components of cardiac systole. In fact, multiple changes occur in the mean shortening velocity and the heart's interactions with the vasculature. The combined effects of these individual changes, however, balance each other and leave the net systolic function unaltered at rest.

It is with exercise that the effects of aging are most evident (**Table 2**). An overall decrease in exercise tolerance is evident in the progressive decline in VO$_2$max, starting at age 20 to 30 and falling by approximately 10% per decade (**Fig. 4**A, B).[16] Additionally, the rate of this decline progressively increases with age. The meaning of these changes and insight into the underlying factors can be clarified through a review of the Fick equation:

$$VO_2max = CO \times (A - V)O_2$$

where CO = cardiac output, AO$_2$ = arterial O$_2$ content, and VO$_2$ = venous O$_2$ content.

Cross-sectional data reveal that the VO$_2$max falls an average of 50% from age 20 to 80 overall, which must then be a result of either/both CO and (A − V)O$_2$. CO is known to fall 25% with aging, which by definition must be because of changes in stroke volume (SV) or heart rate (HR).[17] Because SV is thought to be maintained throughout life (our

Table 2
Exhaustive upright exercise: changes in aerobic capacity and cardiac regulation between the ages of 20 and 80 years in healthy men and women

Oxygen consumption	↓(50%)
(A-V)O$_2$	↓(25%)
Cardiac index	↓(25%)
Heart rate	↓(25%)
Stroke volume	No Δ
Preload	
EDV	↑(30%) (men > women)
Afterload	
Vascular (PVR)	↑(30%)
Cardiac (ESV)	↑(275%)
LC contractility	↓(60%)
Ejection fraction	↓(15%)
Plasma catecholamines	↑
Cardiac and vascular responses to β-adrenergic stimulation	↓

Abbreviations: (A-V)O$_2$, arterial-venous oxygen concentration; EDV, end diastolic volume; ESV, end systolic volume; LV, left ventricular; PVT, peripheral vascular resistance.

laboratory is currently completing studies to test this directly), the bulk of the CO decline is likely because of impaired heart-rate acceleration (or maximal heart rate). Although the LV-EDV increases modestly with exercise, this results in an overall maintenance of SV (although our laboratory has ongoing studies to assess this assertion directly). The remaining 25% change in VO$_2$max is a result of a change in the (A – V)O$_2$ term, reflecting changes in oxygen extraction efficiency and balance (determinants include muscle mass, mitochondrial efficiency, the ability to redistribute blood flow to working muscles, and so forth[18,19]) and suggests the importance of muscle mass, mitochondrial efficiency, and so forth. Put another way, the decline in VO$_2$max is largely a result of changes in the *oxygen pulse,* which is the product of SV and the difference between peak VO$_2$ and arterial oxygen concentration or peak VO$_2$/maximal HR. Overall, this reduction in cardiac reserve is a result of multiple factors, including increased vascular afterload, arterial-ventricular load mismatching, reduced intrinsic myocardial contractility, impaired autonomic regulation, and physical deconditioning.

Cardiac Diastolic Function
Despite maintenance of systolic function at rest, there are a number of changes in the diastolic phase of the cardiac cycle that occur with aging.

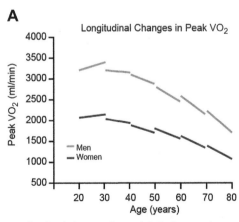
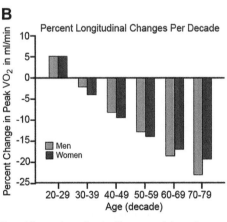

Fig. 4. Longitudinal changes in peak VO$_2$ by gender, predicted from the mixed-effects model, and separated by gender in panel *A* with the percent change by decade represented in panel *B*. (*A*) Peak VO$_2$ declines progressively more steeply with advancing age, with similar declines in men and women. Note that peak VO$_2$ is only slightly higher in men than women at younger ages, converging by old age. (*B*) Per-decade longitudinal changes in peak VO$_2$ by gender and age decade, derived from the mixed-effects model. Note that longitudinal declines in peak VO$_2$ steepen with age and that men decompensate at an accelerated, although similar rate after age 60. (*Modified by Ferrucci L from* Fleg JL, Morrell CH, Bos AG, et al. Accelerated longitudinal decline of aerobic capacity in healthy older adults. Circulation 2005;112:674–82; with permission).

Normal diastolic filling can be divided into 2 phases: passive (represented by the "E wave" on echocardiographic study of transmitral flow) and active (represented by an A wave and produced by atrial contraction) (**Fig. 5**A). The heart fills with blood more slowly in older versus younger healthy individuals, resulting in a lower proportion of total diastolic filling occurring during this passive, early diastolic phase,[8,20,21] mainly because of an increase in the isovolumic relaxation time. As the bulk of ventricular filling shifts to later in diastole and there is significant atrial enlargement with aging, the atrium contributes a greater portion of the total EDV and a decrease in the E/A ratio (see **Fig. 5**B).

Normal exercise induces an increase in SV and heart rate to increase overall cardiac output (see **Table 2**). This increased heart rate also increases the rate of isovolumic relaxation and produces a "suction" effect, which helps fill the ventricle. These responses are diminished with aging, however, as a result of slowed relaxation, reduced β-adrenergic responsiveness, and alterations in the pattern of relaxation.[10,22,23] Surprisingly, although the rate of filling declines and is shifted to later in diastole, the EDV actually remains unchanged or increases somewhat with rest and low-level exercise, largely as a result of the slower[24] heart rate, which permits longer filling time (see **Fig. 3, Table 2**) and increase in the ESV. Taken together, these reductions in early diastolic filling are partially compensated for by changes in adrenergic signaling that lower the maximal heart rate; however, these compensations are not sufficient to maintain cardiac functional reserve when a subject is exposed to maximal exercise, as shown in **Fig. 5**C. In fact, a significant deficit is uncovered in the older population when the peak-filling rate at maximal exercise is compared in young versus older individuals.

Changes in cardiac conduction system and electrocardiogram

Aging is associated with a generalized increase in elastic and collagenous tissue. Fat accumulates around the sinoatrial node, sometimes creating

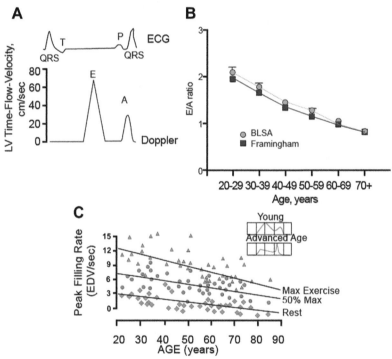

Fig. 5. Diastolic function at rest and with exercise. (*A*) The Doppler diastolic time-flow-velocity profile, showing the E and A waves from which the indexes of diastolic filling performance are derived. Time is represented on the horizontal axis. A simultaneous ECG is shown as a timing reference to indicate atrial and ventricular activation. LV indicates left ventricular. (*B*) The ratio of early left ventricular diastolic filling rate (E) to the atrial filling component (A) declines with aging, and the extent of this E/A decline with aging in healthy BLSA volunteers is identical to that in participants of the Framingham Study. (*C*) Maximum LV filling rate at rest and during vigorous cycle exercise assessed via equilibrium gated blood-pool scans in healthy volunteers from the BLSA. EDV, end-diastolic volume. ([*B, C*] *From* Strait JS, Lakatta EG. Cardiac aging: aging from human to molecules. Chapter 44. Muscle 2011; with permission.)

a partial or complete separation of the node from the atrial tissue. A pronounced decline in the number of pacemaker cells occurs after age 60; by age 75, fewer than 10% of the number seen in young adults remain. A variable degree of calcification on the left side of the cardiac skeleton also occurs. This can affect the atrioventricular node, atrioventricular bifurcation, and proximal left and right bundle branches leading to significant risk for atrioventricular conduction block.

Although there is generally no change in the resting heart rate with aging, a number of changes do occur in the cardiac conduction system that affect its electrical properties (**Table 3**). A review by Fleg and Lakatta[14] provides greater detail of this area. Likely because of a decrease in parasympathetic activity, there is a reduction in the level of phasic variation in R-R interval with respiration,[25] as well as the occurrence of sinus bradycardia. There can be an increase in pathologic sinus bradycardia owing to sick sinus syndrome and conduction pathway, although the heart rate is stable in the healthy aged heart. The P-R interval, representing atrioventricular conduction, increases from 159 ms at ages 20 to 35, to 172 ms beyond age 60.[26] The QRS axis shifts leftward, possibly because of increases in LV wall thickness, with 20% of healthy subjects having a left axis deviation by age 100.[27] Interestingly, despite increased LV thickness, there is a decline in the R-wave and S-wave amplitudes with aging evident by age 40.[28] There is an increase in nonspecific ST-T changes with aging, although the relation of these to clinical heart disease remains in question.[29]

In addition, there are increases in atrial arrhythmias, atrial fibrillation, paroxysmal supraventricular tachycardia, and ventricular arrhythmias with aging.[14] The prevalence of these arrhythmias, as well as their association with mortality, are detailed in **Table 4**. Atrial fibrillation (AF) is found in approximately 3% to 4% of subjects older than 60, a rate 10-fold higher than the general adult population. Short bursts of paroxysmal supraventricular tachycardia (PSVT) on a resting electrocardiogram (ECG) are found in 1% to 2% of healthy individuals older than 65. Twenty-four-hour ambulatory monitoring studies have demonstrated short runs of PSVT (usually 3 to 5 beats) in 13% to 50% of clinically healthy older persons.[30,31] The incidence increases with exercise, from 0% in the 20s to approximately 10% in the 80s. Ventricular ectopic beats (VEBs) undergo an exponential increase in prevalence with advancing age. Pooled data from nearly 2500 ECGs from hospitalized patients older than 70 revealed VEBs in 8%.[32]

The available data in older adults without apparent heart disease support a marked age-related increase in the prevalence and complexity of exercise-related VEBs, at least in men; however, the prognosis conferred by frequent or repetitive VEBs induced by exercise in such individuals is unclear.

In summary, aging is associated with multiple ECG changes in persons without evidence of CVD. Such changes include a blunted respiratory

---

Table 3
Normal age-associated changes in resting electrocardiogram measurements

Measurement	Change with Age	Effect on Mortality
R-R interval	No change	
P-wave duration	Minor increase	None
P-R interval	Increase	None
QRS duration	No change	
QRS axis	Leftward shift	None
QRS voltage	Decrease	None
Q-T interval	Minor increase	Probable increase
T-wave voltage	Decrease	None

Modified from Lakatta EG, Sollott SJ, Pepe S. The old heart: operating on the edge. Novartis Found Symp 2001;235:172–96 [discussion: 196–201, 217–20]; with permission.

Table 4
Relationship of arrhythmias to age and mortality[a]

Arrhythmia	Effect of Age on Prevalence	Effect on Mortality
Supraventricular ectopic beats	Increased	None
Paroxysmal supraventricular tachycardia	Increased	Probably none
Atrial fibrillation (chronic)	Increased	Increased
Ventricular ectopic beats	Increased	Probably none
Ventricular tachycardia (short runs)	Increased	Probably none

[a] In healthy elderly.
Modified from Lakatta EG, Sollott SJ, Pepe S. The old heart: operating on the edge. Novartis Found Symp 2001;235:172–96 [discussion: 196–201, 217–20]; with permission.

sinus arrhythmia; a mild P–R interval prolongation; a leftward shift of the QRS axis; and increased prevalence, density, and complexity of ectopic beats, both atrial and ventricular. Although these findings generally do not affect prognosis in clinically healthy older adults, other findings that become more prevalent with age, such as increased QRS voltage, Q waves, QT interval prolongation, and ST–T-wave abnormalities, are generally associated with increased cardiovascular risk. Abnormalities, such as left bundle branch block or AF, are strongly predictive of future cardiac morbidity and mortality among older adults, even if asymptomatic.

Changes in cellular Ca²¹ handling

Arrhythmias are a by-product of aberrant Ca^{2+} handling. Maintenance of the calcium-electrochemical gradient is an intricate process for the individual cardiomyocyte, as depicted in **Fig. 6** and **Table 1**. With aging, several changes occur (**Table 5**) that slow the cellular reactions controlling the beat of the heart as a whole (more details can be found in Lakatta and Sollott[33] and Janczewski and colleagues[34]). The action potential, transient increase in cytosolic Ca^{2+}, and rate of contraction are all prolonged, which consequently prolong systole and diastole of the heart,[33,35] consistent with the lower maximal heart rate seen in older individuals during exercise. This is because of changes in several ion currents, as well as a reduced rate of Ca^{2+} reuptake through downregulation of SERCA2 protein levels, decreased phospholamban phosphorylation, and an approximately 50% increase in levels of the

Na+/Ca^{2+} exchanger. Studies in rodents that have used gene therapy or exercise conditioning to increase the level of SERCA2 have demonstrated that impaired relaxation and Ca^{2+} sequestration that occur with aging can be reduced by these interventions. Finally, there is a compensatory increase in L-type Ca^{2+} currents with an increase in the apparent number and activity of individual L-type calcium channels that prolongs the action potential, a slower inactivation of the L-type channel, and a reduction in outwardly directed K+ currents, all of which serve to prolong the action potential.

Ca^{2+} regulation is significantly affected by reactive oxygen species (ROS) and is therefore involved in complex pathways (see **Fig. 6**) involving membrane polyunsaturated fatty acids (PUFAs). PUFAs are an important family of dietary fats (including the ω-3 and ω-6 PUFAs) that undergo lipid peroxidation to produce aldehydes, akenals, and hydroxyalkenals, such as 4-hydroxy-2-nonenal (HNE). HNE reacts with protein sulfhydryl groups to induce altered protein conformations and inflict damage on the cell.[33] With advancing age, a number of changes occur in the lipid content of the cell membrane that reduce its capacity to tolerate and adapt to stress (eg, ischemia-reperfusion) (see **Fig. 7**).

Notable among these changes are a relative decrease in the ω-3:ω-6 PUFA content ratio in cellular membranes, enhanced cellular production of ROS, and alterations in proteins governing Ca^{2+} mobilization, especially the decreased expression or function of SERCA2 and Na+-Ca^{2+} exchange protein.[33,36] These changes lead to disturbances

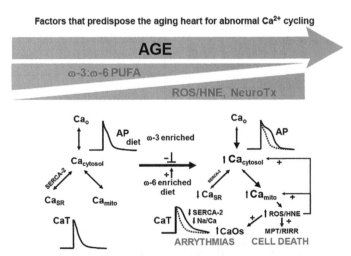

Fig. 6. An overview of change in the aging heart that predisposes to a reduced threshold for abnormal Ca^{2+} handling during acute stress. See text for details. (*Adapted from* Lakatta EG, Sollott SJ, Pepe S. The old heart: operating on the edge Novartis Found Symp 2001;235:172–96 [discussion: 196–201, 217–20]; with permission.)

Table 5
Myocardial changes with adult aging in rodents

Functional Changes	Ionic, Biophysical/Biochemical Mechanisms	Molecular Mechanisms
Prolonged contraction	Prolonged cytosolic Ca^{2+} transient	
	↓SR Ca^{2+} pumping rate	↓SR Ca^{2+} pump mRNA (no Δ calsequestrin mRNA)
	↓Pump site density	
Prolonged action potential	↓I_{ca} Inactivation	↑Na/Ca exchanger mRNA
	↓I_{To} density	
Diminished contraction velocity	↓αMHC protein	↓αMHC mRNA
	↑βMHC protein	↑β MHC mRNA (no Δ actin mRNA)
	↓Myosin ATPase activity	↓RxRβ1 and Y mRNA
	↓RxRβ1 and Y mRNA	
	↓RxRβ1 and Y protein	
	↓Thyroid receptor protein	
Diminished β-adrenergic contractile response	↓Coupling BAR-ACyclase (no Δ G_i activation, no Δ BARK activity)	↓B_iAR mRNA (no Δ BARK mRNA)
	↓TNI phospholamban phosphorylation	
	↓I_{ca} augmentation	
	↓Ca_i transient augmentation	
	↑Enkephalin peptides	
	↑Proenkephalin peptides	
Myocardial stiffness	↑Hydroxyline proline content	↑Collagen mRNA
	↑Activity of myocardia RAS	↑Fibronectin mRNA
		↑AT_1R mRNA
	↑Atrial naturetic peptide	↑Atrial naturetic peptide mRNA
Growth response		↓Induction of immediate early genes
	↓Cardiomyocyte proliferation	Δ in CyclinD1, D2, D3, pRb, p130, CDK-2
	↓Cardiomyocyte survival	Δ in TERT, IGF-1, caspases, AIF, survivin
Heart shock response		↓Activation of HSF

Abbreviations: AIF, Apoptosis Inducing Factor; BARK, Beta Adrenergic Receptor Kinase; CDK, Cyclin Dependent Kinase; HSF, Heat Shock Factor; IGF-1, insulinlike growth factor 1; RAS, renin-angiotensin system; TERT, telomerase reverse transcriptase; TNI, Troponin I.

in excitation-contraction coupling and in intracellular Ca^{2+} compartmentalization, leading in turn to spontaneous Ca^{2+} oscillations and arrhythmias (see **Fig. 6**). In addition, mitochondrial dysfunction can ensue, which impairs energy metabolism (decreased ATP production) and increases ROS production. Overproduction of ROS and the inability to scavenge excess ROS lead to damaging lipid peroxidation and relatively more diffusible but still potent, reactive intermediates, such as HNE, which affect widespread protein targets and amplify Ca^{2+} dysregulation and mitochondrial abnormalities. Finally, the abnormal Ca^{2+} handling and ROS buildup can induce

mitochondrial permeability transition, which involves the release of mitochondrial contents and activation of a sequence of events that lead to cell death. Recent research has demonstrated that these effects of aging are exacerbated by poor nutritional habits, but can be ameliorated by diets substituting ω-3 PUFAs for ω-6 PUFAs.

Cardiac adrenergic responsiveness

Adrenergic signaling is an important component of aging-associated cardiovascular change. Acute exercise and other stressors stimulate sympathetic modulation of the cardiovascular system, which increases heart rate, augments myocardial

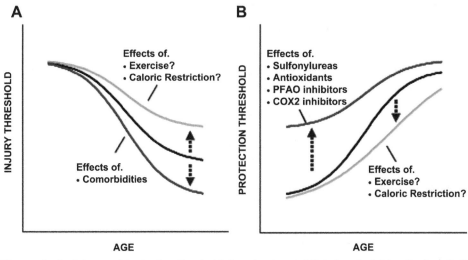

Fig. 7. Changes in the injury and protection thresholds in aging heart. (*A*) Aging diminishes the heart's threshold to sustain injury (eg, from ischemia/reperfusion). Lifestyle modifications, including exercise and possibly caloric restriction, may partially diminish the aging effect. Comorbidities (such as diabetes) have negative influence. (*B*) Aging increases the heart's threshold to activate protection-signaling mechanisms. Various pharmacologic agents (eg, sulfonylureas, antioxidants, partial fatty acid oxidation inhibitors, and cyclooxygenase-2 inhibitors) that can interfere with cardioprotective signaling pathways can exacerbate this trend and further increase the protection threshold. Exercise and caloric restriction might attenuate the age-dependent trends. (*Modified from* Juhaszova M, Rabuel C, Zorov DB, et al. Protection in the aged heart: preventing the heart-break of old age? Cardiovasc Res 2005;66:233–44; with permission.)

contractility and relaxation, reduces LV afterload, and redistributes blood to working muscles and skin to dissipate heat. With aging, however, there is a diminishment of the autonomic modulation of heart rate, LV contractility, and arterial afterload,[37] related to a decline in the efficiency of postsynaptic β-adrenergic signaling. There is a decrease in cardiovascular responses to β-adrenergic antagonist infusion at rest with aging (**Fig. 8**A) and a similarity in the hemodynamic profile of younger β-blocked subjects to older unblocked individuals (see **Fig. 8**B, C) that is consistent with this mechanistic explanation. Some smaller studies[37] provide further evidence for this effect. For example, significant β-blockade–induced LV dilation occurs only in younger subjects, the heart rate is reduced to a greater degree by acute β-adrenergic blockade in younger versus older subjects, and the age-associated deficits in LV early diastolic filling rate, both at rest and during exercise, can be mimicked by β-adrenergic blockade.

The mechanism behind these changes is not entirely clear, although several alterations in the adrenergic system have been observed. It is noteworthy that the apparent deficits in sympathetic modulation of cardiac and arterial functions with aging occur in the presence of elevated sympathetic neurotransmitter levels: during any perturbation from the supine basal state, plasma levels of norepinephrine (NE) and epinephrine increase to a greater extent in older than in younger healthy individuals.[37,38] This increase in plasma catecholamines appears to be a compensatory response to the reduced cardiac muscarinic β-receptor density and functional decline with advancing age. The amount of circulating NE rises, in part because of increased spillover from tissues (including the heart[37–39]) as a result of deficient NE reuptake at nerve endings during acute exercise, as well as reduced plasma clearance. With prolonged exercise, this diminished neurotransmitter reuptake can result in depletion of stores and reduced release and spillover in the body, thereby contributing further to the blunted cardio-acceleration and LV systolic performance seen with age during such exercise.

Renin-angiotensin system in cardiac tissue

The mechanism behind age-related cardiac remodeling is not completely understood, although a number of clues have been found[6,33]: (1) there is a strong body of evidence for the central role for the renin-angiotensin system (RAS); (2) increased oxidative stress has been implicated in age-related remodeling; (3) aging has been associated with increased production of ROS in several studies; (4) RAS activation itself may stimulate

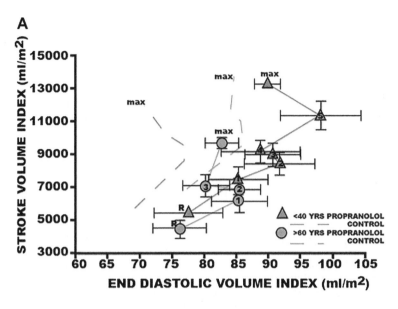

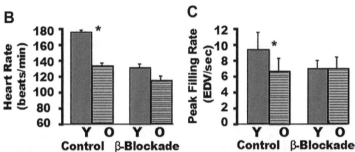

Fig. 8. (*A*) Stroke volume index (SVI) as a function of end-diastolic volume index (EDVI) at rest (R) and during graded cycle workloads in the upright-seated position in healthy Baltimore Longitudinal Study of Aging (BLSA) men in the presence and absence (*dashed lines*) of β-adrenergic blockade. R, seated rest; 1–4 or 5, graded submaximal workloads on cycle ergometer; max, maximum effort. Stroke volume versus end-diastolic functions with symbols are those measured in the presence of propranolol; dashed line functions without symbols are the stroke volume as versus end-diastolic functions measured in the absence of propranolol. Note that in the absence of propranolol, the SVI versus EDVI relation in older persons (*dashed lines*) is shifted rightward from that in younger persons (*dashed lines with points*). This indicates that the left ventricle (LV) of older persons in the sitting position compared with that of younger persons operates from a greater preload both at rest and during submaximal and maximal exercise. Propranolol markedly shifts the SV-EDVI relationship in younger persons (*triangle without points*) rightward, but does not markedly offset the curve in older persons (*circle*). Thus, with respect to this assessment of ventricular function curve, β-adrenergic blockade with propranolol makes younger men appear like older men. The abolition of the age-associated differences in the LV function curve after propranolol are accompanied by a reduction in heart rate, which at maximum, is shown in (*B*). (*B*) Peak exercise heart rate in the same subjects as in (*A*) in the presence and absence of acute β-adrenergic blockade by propranolol. (*C*) The age-associated reduction in peak LV diastolic filling rate at maximal exercise in healthy BLSA subjects is abolished during exercise in the presence of β-adrenergic blockade with propranolol. Y, <40 years; O, >60 years. * Represents $P < .0001$ (*From* Strait JS, Lakatta EG. Cardiac aging: aging from human to molecules. Chapter 44. Muscle 2011; with permission.)

ROS production; and (5) nicotinamide adenine dinucleotide phosphate (NADPH) oxidases appear to be important in linking these processes.

One important stimulus for RAS signaling is thought to be the stretch of cardiac myocytes and fibroblasts owing to the increased load imposed by the aging vasculature[40] and overall decrease in cardiomyocyte number. This initiates growth factor signaling (eg, angiotensin II [ANGII]/transforming growth factor beta [TGF-β]), which has been shown in vitro to promote cell growth and matrix production, as well as increasing apoptosis.[41] This ANGII does not likely come from circulating stores but is instead released from fibroblasts and cardiomyocytes in an autocrine/paracrine manner in response to stretch.[42] ANGII binds to both angiotensin I (AT1) and angiotensin II (AT2) receptors to activate a complex signal transduction cascade that affects a number of transcriptionally important factors.[43] Either directly or through AT1, ANGII can activate the NADPH oxidase complex to generate ROS. Understanding of the relative importance of these numerous pathways will be an important component of cardiac aging research and will provide an important link to similar signaling changes in the arterial wall.

Central Arterial Changes with Aging

In studying the effects of aging on the cardiovascular system, it is important to recall its anatomic and functional position in series with the vascular system. In fact, many researchers now believe that the greatest risk factor for development of CVD is "unsuccessful" age-associated arterial aging. Rather than acting as simple conduits for blood

flow, blood vessels are dynamic structures that adapt, repair, remodel, and govern their structural and function properties using complex signaling pathways in response to load, stress, and age.

Central arterial structural changes

Macroscopic structural changes A number of age-associated structural changes occur in the arterial system, including thickening and dilation of large arteries (see **Fig. 3**, **Table 1**).[44] Echocardiographic studies show that the aortic root dilates modestly with age, approximating 6% between the fourth and eighth decades (**Fig. 9**A). Similarly, serial chest x-rays over 17 years have demonstrated that the aortic knob diameter increases from 3.4 to 3.8 cm, although there are data to suggest that in hypertensive individuals (when aortic diameter is corrected for covariates), it may represent a relative decrease in effective diameter that may contribute to increased load on the heart.[45] In normal aging, however, such aortic root dilation provides an additional stimulus for LV hypertrophy because the larger volume of blood in the proximal

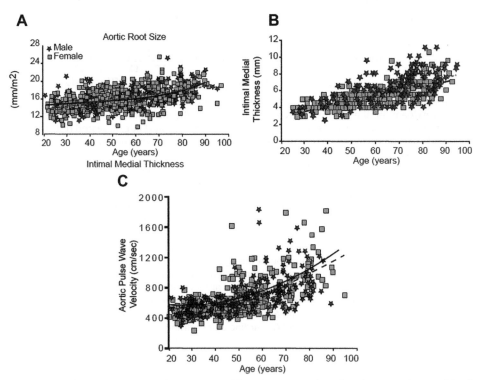

Fig. 9. Age-associated changes in arterial structure and function in men (*stars*) and women (*squares*) in the BLSA. Best-fit regression lines (*quadratic or linear*) are shown for men (*solid lines*) and women (*dotted lines*). (A) Aortic root size (measured by M-mode echocardiography) indexed to body surface area. (B) Common carotid-intima-medial thickness (measured by B-mode ultrasonography). (C) Carotid-femoral pulse wave velocity (an index of central arterial stiffness). (*From* Najjar SS, Lakatta EG, Gerstenblith G. Cardiovascular aging: the next frontier in cardiovascular prevention. In: Blumenthal R, Foody J, Wong NA, editors. Prevention of cardiovascular disease: companion to Braunwald's heart disease. Philadelphia: Saunders; 2011. p. 415–32; with permission.)

aorta leads to a greater inertial load against which the senescent heart must pump.

Autopsy reports published as early as 1910 described age-associated aortic thickening. Cross-sectional studies using ultrasound imaging have demonstrated the intimal-medial layer thickens nearly threefold (see **Fig. 9**B) between the ages of 20 and 90 years in apparently healthy individuals.[46] Both the average and range of intimal-medial thickness measurements is greater at higher ages, suggesting a variable response to chronologic age that merits further study to identify the components of "successful aging."

Microscopic Structural and Biochemical Changes

Aging is associated with structural and functional changes of the arterial wall media (hypertrophy, extracellular matrix accumulation, calcium deposits) and the vascular endothelium (decrease in the release of vasodilators and increased synthesis of vasoconstrictors) that are associated with increased vascular stiffness (see **Table 1**).[47,48] Collagen and elastin provide the strength and elasticity, respectively, of the arterial wall and are normally stabilized by enzymatic cross-linking. With aging, an increase in collagen content, nonenzymatic collagen cross-linking, and fraying of elastin fibrils occur in the medial layer,[49] all of which reduce arterial distensibility and increase stiffness. The occurrence of irreversible nonenzymatic glycation-based cross-linking of collagen to form advanced glycation end products increases with age and is associated with increased arterial stiffness in elderly people.[50] Furthermore, receptors for advanced glycation end products are stimulated to produce inflammatory and stress responses.

Through its secretion of nitric oxide (NO) and endothelin, the endothelium is a powerful regulator of arterial tone. Endothelial dysfunction has been identified in several cardiovascular disorders, including hypertension, hypercholesterolemia, and coronary and peripheral atherosclerosis.[51] Human and animal studies have revealed that aging is associated with a reduction in endothelial-dependent vasodilatation, thought secondary to reduced NO bioavailability.[49] A number of animal studies have found that NO production and NO levels[52] decline with aging, likely as a result of a decline in the level of endothelial nitric oxide synthase (eNOS).[53]

In addition to the structural alterations (described previously), arterial function is governed by age-associated changes in several signaling cascades, most prominently the RAS. The classic RAS is composed of angiotensinogen, renin, angiotensin (ANG) I and II, angiotensin-converting enzyme (ACE), chymase, angiotensin, and ANGII receptor (AT1). All of these components have been found to increase within the aged arterial wall in various species.[54,55] The local ANGII concentration is more than 1000-fold that of circulating ANGII, is independently regulated, and plays an important role in vascular pathophysiology with aging. ANGII protein abundance increases in the aged aortic wall in rats. Studies of nonhuman primates also show that ANGII, ACE, and chymase, elements of the classic RAS, are all upregulated in the aged arterial wall.[55,56] The marked increase of ANGII in the aged arterial wall appears to offset the effect of reduced plasma levels of ANGII in the elderly. In addition, the molecules linked to the ANGII signaling cascade, including calpain-1, matrix metalloproteinase types 2 and 9 (MMP-2 and MMP-9), monocyte chemotactic protein-1 (MCP-1), and transforming growth factor-beta 1 (TGF-b1) are upregulated within the aged arterial wall (see **Tables 1** and **3**).[54,57,58] A number of studies support the concept that ANGII signaling is a central pathway that mediates the cellular and molecular mechanisms that underlie arterial aging.[55]

Central arterial function

Blood pressure Arterial pressure is determined by the interplay of peripheral vascular resistance (PVR) and arterial stiffness. Stiffness, as used here, refers to time-varying cardiac elastance throughout the cardiac cycle as a result of combined effects of active contractile and "passive" structural properties, as well as the interaction of the two. Systolic blood pressure (SBP), which is influenced by arterial stiffness, PVR, and cardiac function, rises with age even in normotensive cohorts. In contrast, diastolic blood pressure (DBP), rises with increased PVR but is lowered by arterial stiffness, resulting in an increase in diastolic pressure until age 50, a leveling off between 50 and 60, then a decline after age 60.[59] Thus, hypertension in the elderly is often characterized by isolated or predominant SBP elevation. Pulse pressure, the difference between SBP and DBP, is a useful clinical index of arterial stiffness and the pulsatile load on the arterial tree and typically increases with aging. Some studies have suggested that pulse pressure is a more powerful predictor of future cardiovascular events than either SBP or DBP in older adults.[60]

Pulse wave velocity and reflected pulse waves Central arterial stiffening occurs with aging even in the absence of clinical hypertension,[61] as measured by pulse wave velocity (PWV). The Augmentation Index (AI) illustrates an important site of cardiac-vascular interaction. When the forward pulse wave reaches an area of impedance mismatch (vessel bifurcation or movement to a higher resistance vessel), a reflected wave that travels back up the arterial tree toward the central aorta is generated. This reflected wave is identified as a small notch, inflection point, in the carotid and radial pulse waveforms, measured by arterial applanation tonometry. The situation with AI is a bit more complicated (not shown). It increases until about age 50,[62] even in clinically healthy volunteers. The clinical significance of these AI changes with age is that in young subjects, the reflected wave typically arrives back at the proximal aorta in diastole and may assist in coronary artery diastolic filling. In older individuals, the reflected waves travel faster, thus arriving at the proximal aorta during late systole, thereby creating an increased load for the ventricle, a failure to augment DBP, and a potential compromise of coronary blood flow. Several studies in cohorts with CVD have observed that higher AI is associated with adverse clinical outcomes.[63] A second method of arterial stiffness assessment, PWV, is a Doppler-based method that measures the speed with which an arterial pressure wave travels along the arterial tree, typically from the carotid region to the femoral artery. Multiple studies have shown that aortofemoral PWV increases with age, typically twofold to threefold across the adult lifespan (see **Fig. 9C**).[64] Furthermore, PWV has been shown, both in clinically healthy cohorts and those with CV disease, to be a predictor of future cardiovascular events, independent of blood pressure.[65]

Arterial-Ventricular Coupling

Arterial ventricular coupling background
The concept of coupling between effective arterial elastance (E_A) and ventricular elastance measures (E_{LV}) is exceedingly important to the study of cardiovascular aging, and so merits further discussion (**Fig. 10**).[66] Oftentimes, a by-product of the need to reduce the cardiovascular system to a manageable model system is an excessive focus on individual components rather than consideration of their function and interaction with the entire system. The ratio of effective E_A/E_{LV} is an index of arterial ventricular coupling, related to the inverse of EF, and provides a more accurate measure of the complex cardiovascular system.

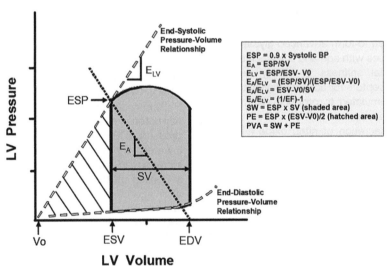

$$ESP = 0.9 \times Systolic\ BP$$
$$E_A = ESP/SV$$
$$E_{LV} = ESP/ESV\text{-}V0$$
$$E_A/E_{LV} = (ESP/SV)/(ESP/ESV\text{-}V0)$$
$$E_A/E_{LV} = ESV\text{-}V0/SV$$
$$E_A/E_{LV} = (1/EF)\text{-}1$$
$$SW = ESP \times SV\ (shaded\ area)$$
$$PE = ESP \times (ESV\text{-}V0)/2\ (hatched\ area)$$
$$PVA = SW + PE$$

LV Volume

Fig. 10. Ventricular pressure-volume diagram from which effective arterial elastance (E_A) and LV end-systolic elastance (E_{LV}) are derived. E_A represents the negative slope of the line joining the end-diastolic volume (EDV) and the end-systolic pressure (ESP) points. ELV represents the slope of the end-systolic pressure-volume relationship passing through the volume intercept (VO). The shaded area represents the cardiac stroke work (SW), and the hatched area represents the potential energy (PE). LV ESP is the LV pressure at the end of systole. EDV is the LV volume at the end of diastole. End-systolic volume (ESV) is the LV volume at the end of systole. Stroke volume (SV) is the volume of blood ejected by the LV with each beat and is obtained from subtracting ESV from EDV. BP, blood pressure; EF, ejection fraction; PVA, pressure-volume area. (*From* Chantler PD, Lakatta EG, Najjar SS. Arterial-ventricular coupling: mechanistic insights into cardiovascular performance at rest and during exercise. J Appl Physiol 2008;105:1342–51; with permission; and Sunagawa K, Maughan WL, Burkhoff D, et al. Left ventricular interaction with arterial load studied in isolated canine ventricle. Am J Physiol 1983;245(5 Pt 1):H773–80; with permission.)

The effective E_A is a steady-state arterial parameter that characterizes the functional properties of the arterial system by incorporating peripheral vascular resistance, total lumped vascular compliance, characteristic impedance, and systolic and diastolic time intervals (characterized by the relationship of end systolic pressure and stroke volume). The E_{LV} (left ventricular end-systolic elastance) represents myocardial performance and is defined by the relationship of end-systolic pressure to end systolic volume.

Arterial-ventricular coupling at rest

As detailed previously, most of the components of E_A change with age (eg, SBP, pulse pressure), so the fact that the E_A/E_{LV} ratio is maintained at rest (**Fig. 11**A–C), despite the known changes in the vascular system and consequent increases in afterload, suggests important adaptive changes in the cardiac muscle itself.[66] These strategies (in part) appear to involve LV wall thickening and increased end-systolic pressure[8] (moderates LV wall tension), increased end-systolic volume,

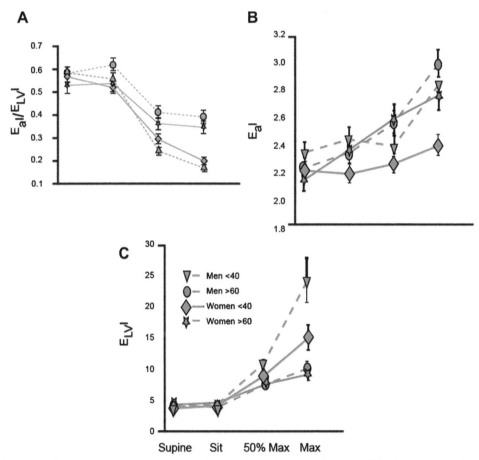

Fig. 11. (A) Arterial ventricular coupling indexed for body surface area ($E_A I/E_{LV}I$), (B) Effective arterial elastance indexed to body surface area ($E_A I$). (C) Effective LV elastance indexed to body surface area ($E_{LV}I$) in men (*dashed lines*) younger than 40 years (*triangle*) and older than 60 years (*circle*), as well as women (*solid lines*) younger than 40 years (*diamond*) and older than 60 years (*star*) in the supine and seated positions, at 50% of maximal workload, and at peak exercise. $E_A I/E_{LV}I$ decreases during exercise in both young and older men and women ($P<.0001$); however, older men and women have a blunted decline in $E_A I/E_{LV}I$ ($P<.001$). $E_A I$ increases during exercise in both young and older men and women ($P<.0001$). At maximal exercise, $E_A I$ is greater in older versus younger women ($P<.002$). In contrast, $E_A I$ does not differ between young and older men. $E_{LV}I$ increases during exercise in both young and older men and women ($P<.0001$). At maximal exercise, $E_{LV}I$ is greater in younger versus older men ($P<.001$) and tended to be greater in younger than older women ($P<.07$). (*From* Strait JS, Lakatta EG. Cardiac aging: aging from human to molecules. Chapter 44. Muscle 2011; with permission; and *Modified from* Najjar SS, Schulman SP, Fleg JL, et al. Relationship of age and sex on ventricular-vascular coupling at rest and exercise. Circulation 2000;102(Suppl); II–602; with permission.)

prolongation of systolic contraction time[67] (maintains normal ejection time in the presence of late augmentation of aortic impedance), cardiac shape,[68] and aspects of the diastolic phase.

In HF, these relationships change. In systolic HF, patients have a downward and rightward shift of the end-systolic P-V relationship and thus a reduced $E_{LV}l$ (left ventricular end-systolic elastance index) (range 0.6–2.6 mm Hg/mL^{-1}/m^2).[69] Patients with systolic HF have an augmented E_Al (range 1.7–3.7 mm Hg/mL^{-1}/m^{-2}) owing to a decrease in stroke volume index (SVI) and to increases in HR and PVR.[69] The increase in E_Al and decrease in $E_{LV}l$ result in marked, up to threefold to fourfold, increases in E_A/E_{LV} (range 1.3–4.3). This suboptimal coupling reflects diminished cardiovascular performance and efficiency of the failing heart. In contrast, patients who have HF with preserved ejection fraction (HFpEF) have an 18% and 20% higher resting E_A and E_{LV}, respectively, compared with healthy controls.[70] Studies suggest a matched increase in E_A and E_{LV} and therefore no difference in their E_A/E_{LV} when compared with normotensive controls or hypertensive patients without HF.

Arterial-ventricular coupling with exercise

Arterial-ventricular coupling with exercise has significant implications for an individual's exercise capacity with aging, however.[66] Otherwise normal arteries dilate and stiffen with age, imposing increased load in the form of inertance, reflected pulse waves, artery compliance, and resistance (reviewed by Lakatta[71]). This increased load has a significant impact on the relationship of the heart to the vascular system, as represented by the E_A/E_{LV} ratio and described previously. Furthermore, it increases tremendously when the body exercises (see Fig. 11). Although the resting E_A/E_{LV} ratio is preserved by the parallel increase in both variables (described previously), exercise requires an increase in EF that the aged heart may have difficulty providing. To increase EF, the E_{LV} must increase to a greater extent than the E_A. With increasing age, however, E_{LV} fails to increase in proportion to the increased E_A in men and there is a deficit in LVEF reserve when older subjects are exposed to acutely increased workloads (ie, exercise). Interestingly, reduction of the afterload by an acute infusion of sodium nitroprusside in healthy, older BLSA volunteers augments LVEF at rest and with exercise and provides further evidence of the importance of vascular properties.[72]

The baseline alterations in E_A/E_{LV} and its components in patients with systolic HF are also evident during exercise.[73] Indeed, E_A, E_{LV}, and E_A/E_{LV} do not appreciably change during exercise in patients with systolic HF, whereas they markedly change in healthy subjects.[73] Thus, the limited capacity of patients with systolic HF to augment their cardiovascular function during times of stress (such as exercise) involve marked deficits in both LV and arterial elastance reserves.

To date, there are no studies that have examined the change in E_A/E_{LV} or E_A during exercise in HFpEF. Researchers have examined the change in E_{LV} and EF in HFpEF during upright bicycle exercise.[74] Compared with hypertensive controls with LV hypertrophy, patients with HFpEF had a threefold smaller increase in E_{LV} and a reduced ability to lower their PVR and increase their HR during exercise. They also had a 50% smaller increase in EF during exercise. As EF is inversely related to E_A/E_{LV}, this suggests that the change in E_A/E_{LV} during exercise in HFpEF may also be severely blunted. Because female sex and systolic hypertension are risk factors for HFpEF, and because the pathophysiology of HFpEF involves a limited cardiovascular reserve,[75] the diminished E_A/E_{LV} reserve observed in systolic hypertensive women suggests that they may be exhibiting signs of subclinical (Stage B) HF. This raises the possibility that they may be on a trajectory to progressive exercise intolerance and perhaps functional limitations.

Cardioprotective and Repair Processes

Because of the many factors discussed previously, the aged heart is placed under increasing levels of stress owing to its diminished functional reserve. Furthermore, increasing age results in the increased occurrence of numerous disease processes (eg, diabetes, hypertension). Although the heart has protective systems in place to deal with such insult (see Fig. 2), these decline with age (see Fig. 7A), resulting in a lower injury threshold. It is not yet clear if there are interventions (eg, physical conditioning) that can be instituted in the elderly to delay or reverse these processes, but there are a number of promising candidates.

Physical conditioning

There is much evidence that aerobic exercise programs can provide improvements in peak oxygen consumption and its components, as well as increases in ventilatory threshold and submaximal endurance for older persons with HF.[76] A longitudinal study in older men studied in the upright position indicates that an enhanced physical conditioning status increases O_2 consumption and work capacity, in part by increases in the maximum CO by increasing the maximum SV, and in part by increasing the estimated total body (A-V)O_2 use.[15] The augmentation of maximum SVI is a result of an augmented reduction of LVESV[15] and, thus, a concomitant increase in LVEF, as the effect of conditioning status to increase Left Ventricular End Diastolic Volume Index (ml/m^2) (LVEDVI) exercise is minimal (recall that LVEDVI during acute vigorous exercise is already appreciably increased in older, sedentary, preconditioned men[77]). This minor effect of physical conditioning on maximum exercise LVEDVI in older persons is in contrast to the effect of physical conditioning in younger persons, which substantially increases LVEDVI and SVI during vigorous exercise on the basis of the Frank Starling mechanism, as well as via an enhanced LVEF. In contrast to the improved LV ejection, the maximum heart rate of older persons does not vary with physical conditioning status and exercise does not appear to offset the age-associated deficiency in sympathetic modulation. It is noteworthy that the increased pulse wave velocity, carotid augmentation index, or pulse pressure that occurs with aging is less in older persons who are physically conditioned than in sedentary persons.[59] An effect of physical conditioning to reduce these components of vascular afterload appears to be involved in the effect of conditioning to improve LV ejection.[61]

Stem cells and the promise of cardiac regeneration

It had traditionally been thought that cardiomyocytes terminally differentiate and withdraw from the cell cycle early in their development; however, carbon dating methods have established that cardiomyocytes continue to be synthesized and a low level of turnover in the heart persists throughout life.[78] New cells can arise from endothelial precursor cells (EPCs) that exist in the bone marrow or precursor cells (PCs) from other locations, including adipose tissue and the heart itself. There has been great interest in using resident EPCs as a source of myocardial regeneration after injury or other degradatory processes and many studies of cardiac cell turnover.

The field remains contentious. Some researchers contend that the rate of cardiomyocyte turnover gradually decreases with aging from 1% per year for a 25-year-old to 0.45% per year for a 75-year-old.[78] Alternatively, Anversa and colleagues[79] found that cardiomyocyte regeneration from predominantly cardiac resident stem cells actually increases with aging and remains important in the heart throughout life. These newly generated cells appear to quickly degrade in older individuals, however, to resemble those they have replaced. Necrotic cellular destruction progresses with aging until the heart is unable to keep pace with the level of required stem cell replacement, leading to a decline in cell numbers.

The cause of this "aging memory" may be reduced telomerase activity, ROS, or loss of telomere-related proteins.[79,80] The telomeres of newly generated cells in senescent human hearts quickly shorten to lengths similar to the aged cardiomyocytes they are replacing. Telomeres normally serve as protective caps for chromosomal ends, protecting them from DNA damage repair systems and activation of the p16[INK4a] pathway, with eventual senescence or apoptosis.[81] However, telomeres lose 30 to 150 base pairs during each cell division owing to the inability of DNA polymerase to fully replicate the 3' end of the DNA strand. When the telomere becomes "too short," the cell can no longer divide, and it becomes senescent and eventually dies. Telomeres can be extended by telomerase, which is composed of 2 main components, the telomerase RNA component (TERC) and telomerase reverse transcriptase (TERT), with a third component (dyskerin) working to stabilize the complex. Agonism of telomerase activity through these components may have some benefit in stabilizing cellular DNA.

If the promise of EPC mobilization in the aged heart is to be realized, the problems of telomere shortening and cellular "memory" will have to be dealt with, as well as methods to control the "internal clock" that resides in DNA-telomeres.[5] Insulinlike growth factor (IGF-1) also holds promise as a regulator of cardiac senescence. Activation of the IGF-1/IGF-1R pathway preserves telomere length and promotes cardiac progenitor cell growth and survival.[82] Injection of IGF-1 in damaged myocardium promotes the migration and homing of cardiac stem cells and facilitates neovascularization.[83]

Ischemic preconditioning

Ischemic preconditioning (IPC) is the heart's endogenous capacity to resist ischemic damage and its effects, including suppression of ventricular arrhythmias and enhanced recovery of contractile function.[84] The process is dependent on an initial, brief ischemic event usually lasting fewer than 5 minutes. It appears to have both an early protective function lasting about 1 hour after preconditioning, and also a late-delayed action that returns approximately 24 to 96 hours later. Unfortunately, aging results in decreased effectiveness of this and other protective pathways,[84] which leads to adecreased injury threshold in the aged heart (see **Fig. 7**A, B). This is but one example of a system that could be manipulated to enhance the cardiac protective systems in the aging heart (see **Fig. 7**B).

CLINICAL APPROACH TO HEART FAILURE IN AGED PERSONS
Clinical Assessment

Evaluation of the older patient presenting with failure symptoms should include a noninvasive study to determine whether the primary problem is impaired systolic function. Although systolic dysfunction is present in at least half of CHF cases, the presence of a normal, or elevated, EF is more common in older than younger patients with HF, particularly women and those with atrial fibrillation and hypertension. The number of patients with heart failure and preserved systolic function is increasing, and is likely to continue to increase with the aging of the general population.

It is often helpful to investigate whether any reversible precipitants are present in older individuals who present with new-onset or worsening HF symptoms, including anemia, infection, thyroid disease, atrial fibrillation, and dietary or medication noncompliance. Investigation for common co-morbidities is also useful, as they are frequent and associated with increased hospitalizations and adverse clinical outcomes.[85] Hypertension is almost invariably present, as well as increased central vascular stiffness and therefore impaired ventricular-vascular coupling. It should be noted that evidence of long-standing volume overload and an S3 gallop is less likely in patients with preserved systolic function and that in the general older population with HF, exertional symptoms are less common, and those related to fatigue and mental status changes more common. The diagnosis of HF with preserved systolic function is primarily one of exclusion in patients with objective evidence of pulmonary vascular congestion without findings of an ischemic, hypertensive, or valvular etiology. Amyloid should also be considered in older patients presenting with HF symptoms in the absence of other identifiable causes.

Considerations with Pharmacologic Interventions

Diuretics are particularly useful in older patients with increased vascular stiffness presenting with acute congestive symptoms, as significant reductions in pressure occur with relatively small changes in intravascular volume. HF with primary systolic dysfunction and with preserved systolic function are both associated with increased sympathetic and renin-angiotensin-aldosterone activation. In those with primary systolic dysfunction, β-blockers improve survival and other important cardiovascular outcomes in the older subsets of large randomized trials.[86] It is unfortunate that many older individuals with HF and systolic dysfunction are not receiving any β-blocker therapy, or are underdosed. In contrast to the many successful trials in those with systolic dysfunction, there are no reported randomized studies limited to the effects of β-blockers in older

individuals with HF and preserved systolic function.

ACE inhibitors are a cornerstone of therapy in patients with systolic dysfunction and their benefit extends to the elderly. Their benefit in patients with preserved systolic function, however, is less certain.[87] There is an ongoing trial of spironolactone in patients with HF with preserved systolic function, but first outcomes are not expected before 2011. There are no clear explanations for the lack of survival benefit for any medical intervention in older patients with HF with preserved systolic function. The diagnosis is more difficult and thus patients without heart disease, for whom these therapies would not be expected to be of any benefit, may be included in some of the studies. The pathophysiology may differ, with myocardial fibrosis and impaired ventricular-vascular coupling more important responsible mechanisms, and these may not respond to the tested therapies. Treatment might, therefore, be focused on blood pressure control in those with hypertension, rate control in those with atrial fibrillation, and judicious use of diuretics in the setting of volume overload. It should be noted, however, that the steep volume/pressure relationship associated with increased vascular stiffness in the older individual, might result in symptomatic hypotension when diuretics result in intravascular volume depletion.

Devices (eg, implantable cardiac defibrillators, biventricular pacing devices, left ventricular assist devices) may also significantly improve outcomes in patients with persistent failure despite medical therapy. There has been significant development on this front that has made their benefits accessible to patients throughout the spectrum of disease; however, as with any treatment, there is no guarantee of benefit and it is often just as helpful to first assess more socially relevant factors. This is especially relevant in the elderly, who have a diminished cardiac reserve to begin with and may see significantly different treatment benefits when compared with the typically younger study population on which many therapeutic recommendations are based. The importance of the individual patient's role as a partner in his or her care and of individualizing treatment and monitoring plans cannot be overemphasized.

Although patients may carry the same HF diagnosis, they differ markedly in terms of disease severity and complexity, associated comorbidities, social support, education, ingrained habits, access to medical personnel and knowledge, and understanding of health care information and directions. Noncompliance with medications or diet is often cited as a major factor contributing to hospitalization in patients with HF. In the older patient, however, noncompliance is more likely because of social isolation, financial difficulties, limited travel and meal options, decreased tolerability for some medicines, comorbidities, and difficult-to-follow complex medical regimens. In many of these patients, a multidisciplinary team approach, including simplification of the medical regimen, close monitoring, and intensive patient education, can decrease hospital admission and improve quality of life.

SUMMARY

Aging results in an increase in CVD and a decrease in cardiac reserve at the same time that the repair processes designed to deal with these problems become less active/effective. These factors combine to set the stage for heart failure: (1) structurally, the heart thickens and stiffens with age, resulting in the increased imposition of a number of functional demands; (2) functionally, changes that assist the resting heart to deal with the effects of aging cause significant functional deficits with exercise or stress, thereby lowering the cardiac reserve that the younger heart can call on to deal with disease or insult; and (3) finally, although the increased incidence of disease, less structurally efficient heart, and decreased cardiac reserve associated with aging would be well served by an effective repair system, this too declines with age. It is hoped that improved understanding of the aged heart will enable the development of therapies that prevent the genesis of HF or at a minimum help clinicians to treat the unique properties of the failing, senescent heart.

REFERENCES

1. Writing Group Members, Lloyd-Jones D, Adams RJ, et al. Heart disease and stroke statistics—2010 update: a report from the American Heart Association. Circulation 2010;121(7):e46–215.
2. Thomas S, Rich M. Epidemiology, pathophysiology, and prognosis of heart failure in the elderly. Heart Fail Clin 2007;3(4):381–7.
3. Najjar SS, Gerstenblith G, Lakatta EG. Aging and the Cardiovascular System. Cardiovascular Medicine. In: Willerson JT, Wellens HJ, Cohn JN, et al, editors. London: Springer London; 2007. p. 2439–51.
4. Jessup M, Abraham WT, Casey DE, et al. 2009 focused update: ACCF/AHA Guidelines for the Diagnosis and Management of Heart Failure in Adults: a report of the American College of Cardiology Foundation/American Heart Association Task Force on Practice Guidelines: developed in collaboration with the International Society for Heart and Lung Transplantation. Circulation 2009;119(14): 1977–2016.
5. Chen W, Frangogiannis NG. The role of inflammatory and fibrogenic pathways in heart failure associated with aging. Heart Fail Rev 2010;15(5): 415–22, 1–8.
6. Lakatta EG, Levy D. Arterial and cardiac aging: major shareholders in cardiovascular disease enterprises: part II: the aging heart in health: links to heart disease. Circulation 2003;107(2):346–54.
7. Scholz DG, Kitzman DW, Hagen PT, et al. Age-related changes in normal human hearts during the first 10 decades of life. Part I (Growth): a quantitative anatomic study of 200 specimens from subjects from birth to 19 years old. Mayo Clin Proc 1988;63(2):126–36.
8. Gerstenblith G, Frederiksen J, Yin F, et al. Echocardiographic assessment of a normal adult aging population. Circulation 1977;56(2):273–8.
9. Olivetti G, Melissari M, Capasso JM, et al. Cardiomyopathy of the aging human heart. Myocyte loss and reactive cellular hypertrophy. Circ Res 1991;68(6): 1560–8.
10. Hees PS, Fleg JL, Lakatta EG, et al. Left ventricular remodeling with age in normal men versus women: novel insights using three-dimensional magnetic resonance imaging. Am J Cardiol 2002;90(11):1231–6.
11. Linzbach AJ, Akuamoa-Boateng E. [Changes in the aging human heart. I. Heart weight in the aged]. Klin Wochenschr 1973;51(4):156–63 [in German].
12. Khouri MG, Maurer MS, El-Khoury Rumbarger L. Assessment of age-related changes in left ventricular structure and function by freehand three-dimensional echocardiography. Am J Geriatr Cardiol 2005;14(3):118–25.
13. Dannenberg AL, Levy D, Garrison RJ. Impact of age on echocardiographic left ventricular mass in a healthy population (the Framingham Study). Am J Cardiol 1989;64(16):1066–8.
14. Fleg JL, Lakatta EG. Normal Aging of the Cardiovascular System. Chapter in Cardiovascular Disease in the Elderly. 4th edition. In: Aronow W, Rich MW, Fleg JL, editors. Boca Raton (FL): CRC Press; 2008. p. 1–43.
15. Schulman SP, Lakatta EG, Fleg JL, et al. Age-related decline in left ventricular filling at rest and exercise. Am J Physiol 1992;263(6 Pt 2):H1932–8.
16. Fleg JL, Lakatta EG. Role of muscle loss in the age-associated reduction in VO2 max. J Appl Physiol 1988;65(3):1147–51.
17. Fleg JL, Morrell CH, Bos AG, et al. Accelerated longitudinal decline of aerobic capacity in healthy older adults. Circulation 2005;112(5):674–82.
18. Le Blanc PR, Rakusan K. Effects of age and isoproterenol on the cardiac output and regional blood flow in the rat. Can J Cardiol 1987;3(5): 246–50.

19. Rakusan K, Blahitka J. Cardiac output distribution in rats measured by injection of radioactive microspheres via cardiac puncture. Can J Physiol Pharmacol 1974; 52(2):230–5.

20. Miyatake K, Okamoto M, Kinoshita N, et al. Augmentation of atrial contribution to left ventricular inflow with aging as assessed by intracardiac Doppler flowmetry. Am J Cardiol 1984;53(4):586–9.

21. Bryg RJ, Williams GA, Labovitz AJ. Effect of aging on left ventricular diastolic filling in normal subjects. Am J Cardiol 1987;59(9):971–4.

22. Spina RJ, Turner MJ, Ehsani AA. Beta-adrenergic-mediated improvement in left ventricular function by exercise training in older men. Am J Physiol 1998;274(2 Pt 2):H397–404.

23. Tan Y, Wenzelburger F, Lee E, et al. The pathophysiology of heart failure with normal ejection fraction: exercise echocardiography reveals complex abnormalities of both systolic and diastolic ventricular function involving torsion, untwist, and longitudinal motion. J Am Coll Cardiol 2009;54(1):36.

24. Tarasov KV, Sanna S, Scuteri A, et al. COL4A1 is associated with arterial stiffness by genome-wide association scan. Circ Cardiovasc Genet 2009; 2(2):151–8.

25. Hiss RG, Lamb LE. Electrocardiographic findings in 122,043 individuals. Circulation 1962;25:947–61.

26. Fleg JL, Das DN, Wright J, et al. Age-associated changes in the components of atrioventricular conduction in apparently healthy volunteers. J Gerontol 1990;45(3):M95–100.

27. Golden GS, Golden LH. The "Nona" electrocardiogram: findings in 100 patients of the 90 plus age group. J Am Geriatr Soc 1974;22(7):329–32.

28. Harlan WR, Graybiel A, Mitchell RE, et al. Serial electrocardiograms: their reliability and prognostic validity during a 24-yr. period. J Chronic Dis 1967;20(11): 853–67.

29. Mihalick MJ, Fisch C. Electrocardiographic findings in the aged. Am Heart J 1974;87(1):117–28.

30. Manolio TA, Furberg CD, Rautaharju PM, et al. Cardiac arrhythmias on 24-h ambulatory electrocardiography in older women and men: the Cardiovascular Health Study. J Am Coll Cardiol 1994;23(4):916–25.

31. Fleg JL, Kennedy HL. Cardiac arrhythmias in a healthy elderly population: detection by 24-hour ambulatory electrocardiography. Chest 1982;81(3): 302–7.

32. Fisch C. Introduction: chronic ventricular arrhythmias—a major unresolved health problem. Heart Lung 1981;10(3):451–4.

33. Lakatta EG, Sollott SJ. Perspectives on mammalian cardiovascular aging: humans to molecules. Comp Biochem Physiol A Mol Integr Physiol 2002;132(4): 699–721.

34. Janczewski AM, Spurgeon HA, Lakatta EG. Action potential prolongation in cardiac myocytes of old rats is an adaptation to sustain youthful intracellular Ca2+ regulation. J Mol Cell Cardiol 2002;34(6): 641–8.

35. Lakatta E. Age-associated cardiovascular changes in health: impact on cardiovascular disease in older persons. Heart Fail Rev 2002;7(1):29–49.

36. Lakatta EG, Sollott SJ, Pepe S. The old heart: operating on the edge. Novartis FoundSymp 2001;235: 172–96 [discussion: 196–201, 217–20].

37. Lakatta EG. Cardiovascular regulatory mechanisms in advanced age. Physiol Rev 1993;73(2):413–67.

38. Lakatta EG. Deficient neuroendocrine regulation of the cardiovascular system with advancing age in healthy humans. Circulation 1993;87(2):631–6.

39. Esler MD, Turner AG, Kaye DM, et al. Aging effects on human sympathetic neuronal function. Am J Physiol 1995;268(1 Pt 2):R278–85.

40. Lakatta E. Cardiovascular aging research: the next horizons. J Am Geriatr Soc 1999;47(5):613–25.

41. Cigola E, Kajstura J, Li B, et al. Angiotensin II activates programmed myocyte cell death in vitro. Exp Cell Res 1997;231(2):363–71.

42. Sadoshima J, Xu Y, Slayter HS, et al. Autocrine release of angiotensin II mediates stretch-induced hypertrophy of cardiac myocytes in vitro. Cell 1993;75(5):977–84.

43. Cave AC, Brewer AC, Narayanapanicker A, et al. NADPH oxidases in cardiovascular health and disease. Antioxid Redox Signal 2006;8(5–6):691–728.

44. Lakatta EG, Wang M, Najjar SS. Arterial aging and subclinical arterial disease are fundamentally intertwined at macroscopic and molecular levels. Med Clin North Am 2009;93(3):583–604, Table of Contents.

45. Farasat SM, Morrell CH, Scuteri A, et al. Pulse pressure is inversely related to aortic root diameter implications for the pathogenesis of systolic hypertension. Hypertension 2008;51(2):196–202.

46. Nagai Y, Metter E, Earley C, et al. Increased carotid artery intimal-medial thickness in asymptomatic older subjects with exercise-induced myocardial ischemia. Circulation 1998;98(15):1504–9.

47. Ungvari Z, Kaley G, de Cabo R, et al. Mechanisms of vascular aging: new perspectives. J Gerontol A Biol Sci Med Sci 2010;65(10):1028–41.

48. Zieman SJ, Melenovsky V, Kass DA. Mechanisms, pathophysiology, and therapy of arterial stiffness. Arterioscler Thromb Vasc Biol 2005;25(5):932–43.

49. Lakatta EG, Levy D. Arterial and cardiac aging: major shareholders in cardiovascular disease enterprises: part I: aging arteries: a "set up" for vascular disease. Circulation 2003;107(1):139–46.

50. Semba RD, Najjar SS, Sun K, et al. Serum carboxymethyl-lysine, an advanced glycation end product, is associated with increased aortic pulse wave velocity in adults. Am J Hypertens 2009; 22(1):74–9.

51. Csiszar A, Wang M, Lakatta EG, et al. Inflammation and endothelial dysfunction during aging: role of NF-kappaB. J Appl Physiol 2008;105(4):1333–41.

52. Tschudi MR, Barton M, Bersinger NA, et al. Effect of age on kinetics of nitric oxide release in rat aorta and pulmonary artery. J Clin Invest 1996;98(4):899–905.

53. Cernadas MR, Sánchez de Miguel L, García-Durán M, et al. Expression of constitutive and inducible nitric oxide synthases in the vascular wall of young and aging rats. Circ Res 1998;83(3):279–86.

54. Wang M, Takagi G, Asai K, et al. Aging increases aortic MMP-2 activity and angiotensin II in nonhuman primates. Hypertension 2003;41(6):1308–16.

55. Wang M, Monticone RE, Lakatta EG. Arterial aging: a journey into subclinical arterial disease. Curr Opin Nephrol Hypertens 2010;19(2):201–7.

56. Jiang L, Wang M, Zhang J, et al. Increased aortic calpain-1 activity mediates age-associated angiotensin II signaling of vascular smooth muscle cells. PLoS One 2008;3(5):e2231.

57. Wang M, Zhao D, Spinetti G, et al. Matrix metalloproteinase 2 activation of transforming growth factor-beta1 (TGF-beta1) and TGF-beta1-type II receptor signaling within the aged arterial wall. Arterioscler Thromb Vasc Biol 2006;26(7):1503–9.

58. Wang M, Zhang J, Walker SJ, et al. Involvement of NADPH oxidase in age-associated cardiac remodeling. J Mol Cell Cardiol 2010;48(4):765–72.

59. Tanaka H, Dinenno FA, Monahan KD, et al. Aging, habitual exercise, and dynamic arterial compliance. Circulation 2000;102(11):1270–5.

60. Roman MJ, Devereux RB, Kizer JR, et al. High central pulse pressure is independently associated with adverse cardiovascular outcome the strong heart study. J Am Coll Cardiol 2009; 54(18):1730–4.

61. Vaitkevicius PV, Fleg JL, Engel JH, et al. Effects of age and aerobic capacity on arterial stiffness in healthy adults. Circulation 1993;88(4 Pt 1):1456–62.

62. Mitchell GF, Parise H, Benjamin EJ, et al. Changes in arterial stiffness and wave reflection with advancing age in healthy men and women: the Framingham Heart Study. Hypertension 2004;43(6):1239–45.

63. Williams B, Lacy PS. Central haemodynamics and clinical outcomes: going beyond brachial blood pressure? Eur Heart J 2010;31(15):1819–22.

64. Pearson T, Mensah G, Alexander R. Markers of inflammation and cardiovascular disease application to clinical and public health practice: a statement for healthcare professionals from the Centers for Disease Control and Prevention and the American Heart Association. Circulation 2003;107(3):499–511.

65. Najjar S, Scuteri A, Shetty V, et al. Pulse wave velocity is an independent predictor of the longitudinal increase in systolic blood pressure and of incident hypertension in the Baltimore Longitudinal Study of Aging. J Am Coll Cardiol 2008;51(14):1377.

66. Chantler PD, Lakatta EG, Najjar SS. Arterial-ventricular coupling: mechanistic insights into cardiovascular performance at rest and during exercise. J Appl Physiol 2008;105(4):1342–51.

67. Lakatta EG. Cardiac muscle changes in senescence. Annu Rev Physiol 1987;49:519–31.

68. Hees PS, Fleg JL, Mirza ZA, et al. Effects of normal aging on left ventricular lusitropic, inotropic, and chronotropic responses to dobutamine. J Am Coll Cardiol 2006;47(7):1440–7.

69. Asanoi H, Sasayama S, Kameyama T. Ventriculoarterial coupling in normal and failing heart in humans. Circ Res 1989;65(2):483–93.

70. Lam CSP, Roger VL, Rodeheffer RJ, et al. Cardiac structure and ventricular-vascular function in persons with heart failure and preserved ejection fraction from Olmsted County, Minnesota. Circulation 2007;115(15):1982–90.

71. Lakatta EG. Arterial aging is risky. J Appl Physiol 2008;105(4):1321–2.

72. Nussbacher A, Gerstenblith G, O'Connor FC, et al. Hemodynamic effects of unloading the old heart. Am J Physiol 1999;277(5 Pt 2):H1863–71.

73. Cohen-Solal A, Faraggi M, Czitrom D, et al. Left ventricular-arterial system coupling at peak exercise in dilated nonischemic cardiomyopathy. Chest 1998; 113(4):870–7.

74. Borlaug BA, Melenovsky V, Russell SD, et al. Impaired chronotropic and vasodilator reserves limit exercise capacity in patients with heart failure and a preserved ejection fraction. Circulation 2006; 114(20):2138–47.

75. Kitzman DW, Higginbotham MB, Cobb FR, et al. Exercise intolerance in patients with heart failure and preserved left ventricular systolic function: failure of the Frank-Starling mechanism. J Am Coll Cardiol 1991;17(5):1065–72.

76. Fleg JL. Can exercise conditioning be effective in older heart failure patients? Heart Fail Rev 2002; 7(1):99–103.

77. Fleg JL, O'Connor F, Gerstenblith G, et al. Impact of age on the cardiovascular response to dynamic upright exercise in healthy men and women. J Appl Physiol 1995;78(3):890–900.

78. Bergmann O, Bhardwaj RD, Bernard S, et al. Evidence for cardiomyocyte renewal in humans. Science 2009;324(5923):98–102.

79. Kajstura J, Urbanek K, Perl S, et al. Cardiomyogenesis in the adult human heart. Circ Res 2010;107(2): 305–15.

80. Urbanek K, Torella D, Sheikh F, et al. Myocardial regeneration by activation of multipotent cardiac stem cells in ischemic heart failure. Proc Natl Acad Sci U S A 2005;102(24):8692–7.

81. Wong LS, van der Harst P, de Boer RA, et al. Aging, telomeres and heart failure. Heart Fail Rev 2010; 15(5):479–86.

82. Torella D, Rota M, Nurzynska D, et al. Cardiac stem cell and myocyte aging, heart failure, and insulin-like growth factor-1 overexpression. Circ Res 2004; 94(4):514–24.

83. Gonzalez A, Rota M, Nurzynska D, et al. Activation of cardiac progenitor cells reverses the failing heart senescent phenotype and prolongs lifespan. Circ Res 2008;102(5):597–606.

84. Juhaszova M, Rabuel C, Zorov DB, et al. Protection in the aged heart: preventing the heart-break of old age? Cardiovasc Res 2005;66(2):233–44.

85. Najjar S. Evolving insights into the pathophysiology of heart failure with preserved ejection fraction. Curr Cardiovasc Risk Rep 2009;3(5):374–9.

86. Dulin BR, Haas SJ, Abraham WT, et al. Do elderly systolic heart failure patients benefit from beta blockers to the same extent as the non-elderly? Meta-analysis of >12,000 patients in large-scale clinical trials. Am J Cardiol 2005;95(7):896–8.

87. Massie BM, Carson PE, McMurray JJ, et al. Irbesartan in patients with heart failure and preserved ejection fraction. N Engl J Med 2008;359(23):2456–67.

Index

Note: Page numbers of article titles are in **boldface** type.

A

Adenovirus, cardiac involvement in, 71
Aging, and risk for heart failure, 115
American College of Cardiology and American Heart Association, classification of heart failure, 1
Aortic regurgitation, acute, 38
   as combined pressure and volume overload, 37
   therapy for, 37–38
Apoptosis, 81–82
   cardiac, molecular imaging in, 84
   role in adverse ventricular remodeling, **79–86**
Apoptosis interruptus, and remodeled myocardium, 82–83
Apoptosis-targeted interventions, in heart failure, 83–84
Arrhythmias, relationship, to age and mortality, 149
Arterial baroreflexes, 87–89
Arterial stiffness, concept of, 135–137
   contributing to progression of heart failure, **135–141**
   effect of cardiovascular therapy on, 139–140
   inflammation and, 119
   measurement of, 137–138
Arterial-ventricular coupling, 156–158
   at rest, 157–158
   with exercise, 158
Arteries, central function of, with aging, 155–156
   changes of, central, with aging, 154–158
      structural, with aging, 154–155
   physiologic role in heart failure, 135–136

B

Blood pressure, changes with aging, 155

C

Ca^{21} handling, cardiac changes with aging, 150–151, 152
Cardiomyocytes, growth regulation of, moleculat mechanisms of, 3–4
Cardiomyopathy(ies), arrhythmogenic right ventricular, definition of, 71–73
   classification of, American Heart Association 2006, 56
      diagnosis, and treatment of, **53–78**
      ESC Scientific Statement 2008, 57–59
   definition of, 53
   different forms of, systole and diastole in, 54
   dilated, changes in matrix determinants detected in plasma in, 14

      changes in matrix determinants in plasma in, 14
      changes in myocardial interstitium determinants in, 14
      definition of, 60
      familial, and genetics, 60–61, 66
      monogenetic forms of, 63–64
      myocardial remodeling with, 14
   endomyocardial biopsy in, 60
   hypertrophic, biomarkers of, 55
      causal genes for, 60
      definition of, 55
      genetics of, 55
      heart catherization and, 55–60, 62
      noninvasive imaging of, 55
   inflammatory, and postinfective, 61
      dilated, myocarditis and, 65
      treatment of, 71
Cardiovascular changes, aging-associated, heart failure and, **143–164**
Cardiovascular events, percentge of population at risk for development of, xi, xii
Cardiovascular system, inflammatory processes in, regulation of, 113
Carotid body chemoreflex, 93
Caspase 3, 81
Cytokines, circulatory proinflammatory, and risk for heart failure, 113, 114
      effect on myocardial contractility, 116
Cytomegalovirus myocarditis, 69

D

Diabetes, and dyslipidemia, 127
   and heart failure, incidence and prevalence of, 125
   and hypertension, 127
   and obesity, 127
   and risk for heart failure, **125–133**
   and vascular stiffness, 126
   autonomic neuuropathy in, 128–129
   impaired fasting glucose, and left ventricular remodeling, 126
   metabolic derangements in, 127–128
   mitochondrial dysfunction in, 128
   oxidative stress in, 128
   systolic and diastolic dysfunction in, 126
   type 2, in heart disease, 103–104
Diastolic dysfunction, inflammation in, 118–119
Dietary factors, and risk for heart failure, 115
Dyslipidemia, diabetes and, 127

Heart Failure Clin 8 (2012) 165–168
doi:10.1016/S1551-7136(11)00115-2
1551-7136/12/$ – see front matter

Moving?

Make sure your subscription moves with you!

To notify us of your new address, find your **Clinics Account Number** (located on your mailing label above your name), and contact customer service at:

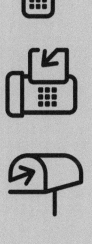

Email: journalscustomerservice-usa@elsevier.com

800-654-2452 (subscribers in the U.S. & Canada)
314-447-8871 (subscribers outside of the U.S. & Canada)

Fax number: 314-447-8029

Elsevier Health Sciences Division
Subscription Customer Service
3251 Riverport Lane
Maryland Heights, MO 63043

*To ensure uninterrupted delivery of your subscription, please notify us at least 4 weeks in advance of move.

Printed and bound by CPI Group (UK) Ltd, Croydon, CR0 4YY

03/10/2024

01040351-0012